Assistive Technology for Students Who Are Blind or Visually Impaired

A Guide to Assessment

Ike Presley and Frances Mary D'Andrea

AFB PRESS

American Foundation for the Blind

Printed in the United States of America

Library of Congress Cataloging-in-Publication Data

Presley, Ike, 1953–
  Assistive technology for students who are blind or visually impaired :
a guide to assessment / Ike Presley and Frances Mary D'Andrea.
      p. cm.
  Includes bibliographical references and index.
  ISBN 978-0-89128-890-9 (print : alk. paper) — ISBN 978-0-89128-891-6
(ascii) 1. People with visual disabilities—Education—United States.
2. Teaching—United States—Aids and devices—Evaluation. 3.
Computerized self-help devices for people with disabilities—United
States. 4. Students with disabilities—Services for—United States. I.
D'Andrea, Frances Mary, 1960- II. Title.

  HV1626.P74 2008
  681'.761—dc22

                              2008051723

Cover photograph, L. Penny Rosenblum

The American Foundation for the Blind—the organization to which Helen Keller devoted her life—is a national nonprofit devoted to expanding the possibilities for people with vision loss.

It is the policy of the American Foundation for the Blind to use in the first printing of its books acid-free paper that meets the ANSI Z39.48 Standard. The infinity symbol that appears above indicates that the paper in this printing meets that standard.

To Pat Carpenter, my mentor, who gave me the opportunity to get started with technology early in my career, and to all those who have supported me during the writing of this book.

—I.P.

To Stephen, with love and gratitude. My own personal tech guru, my best critic, and my best friend.

—F.M.D.

Contents

Foreword

Like most working professionals in the 21st century, I find that the personal computer is at the center of my day. I use my PC—which is equipped with a screen reader and text-to-speech synthesis that provide access to the information displayed on the computer monitor—to write and edit word-processing documents, send or receive e-mails, surf the Web, and perform myriad other functions. My accessible braille-enabled personal digital assistant (PDA), or notetaker, is also indispensable to my work and personal life. This small computer with speech, a one-line refreshable braille display, and a braille input keypad serves as my backup brain, containing my calendar, work-related files, and new notes. Every morning before work, I routinely visit the BookShare web site, which makes available books and other information for people with print-reading disabilities, and download my daily newspaper to get the important news and trends of the day and keep up with my sighted colleagues. I usually read the paper on an accessible digital audio player, which provides both text-to-speech access for electronic files like the newspaper or books and MP3 playback capability for music or audio files.

Was this easy access to information always available for me and for other people who are visually impaired? No, it was not. But within just a generation a dizzying array of information and communication technologies have transformed our daily lives at home, at the workplace, and in the classroom. The revolution brought about by ever-expanding computer capacity in ever-smaller packages has transformed the way we work, learn, and pursue leisure activities. Equally profound changes have taken place for people who are blind or visually impaired, as computerized technologies have broken down many information and communications barriers. The development of assistive technology—specialized software and hardware—especially over the past 25 years, has enabled children and adults who are blind or visually impaired to independently access, gather, and organize information and to communicate and share ideas. And we can do all this on terms of equality with our sighted peers.

Assistive technology does not replace the tried-and-true methods of acquiring and using information, such as hard-copy braille, Talking Books, or human readers; it expands the number of options available. We all, blind and sighted alike, now depend on information and communication technologies in ways unimaginable a generation ago. Our up-and-coming generation of students with vision loss must be as fully engaged in this world as their sighted classmates.

Despite the terrific advances made possible by these new assistive technologies, however, many teachers and other service providers in the blindness field have not had access to a comprehensive resource for helping their students fully embrace the information technology revolution. In writing *Assistive Technology for Students Who Are Blind or Visually Impaired: A Guide to Assessment*, Ike Presley and Frances Mary D'Andrea have provided a much-needed perspective, context, and, above all, clear explanations of assistive technology used by people with vision loss. The information contained in this guide will help teachers and others who work with visually impaired students not only to understand assistive technology but also to assist their students by determining their assistive technology needs and taking the necessary steps to meet them.

As readers make use of the information and strategies contained in this book with their students, they will experience over and over again the thrill of new discovery. Most of us who are blind can remember with great joy the first time we wrote and edited our own documents or did our first Web search and found and read information for ourselves. With enhanced knowledge of assistive technology and the assessment strategies gained from this book, readers can unlock the world of information and help promote independence for students with vision loss.

Even as we embrace the opportunities new technology has provided, new barriers are emerging to equal access to information. Although it is beyond the scope of this book to address these new challenges, armed with the information provided in *Assistive Technology for Students Who Are Blind or Visually Impaired*, professionals will be better prepared to help students to grapple with the changes that are coming very fast. Advances in mainstream technology far outstrip the ability of access technology developers to keep up. New operating systems, applications, interactive Web interfaces, mobile PDAs, social networking sites, text messaging systems, and many more innovations are developed at an ever-increasing rate, and it is impossible for the handful of companies that make assistive and accessible technology to keep pace. Information technology is dynamic, and our approaches to providing access for people with vision loss will need to change in the face of trends that have put the Internet and mobile computing at the center of our information world.

As you incorporate the material in this book into your instructional approaches and educational arsenal, you will be better equipped to embrace the evolution in access technology as it occurs. *Assistive Technology for Students Who Are Blind or Visually Impaired* provides the foundation you need to understand the changes that are taking place. Equally important, you will be an invaluable resource to students with visual impairments who need to successfully participate in undertaking these challenges and meeting these changes as well.

Paul Schroeder
Vice President for Public Policy
American Foundation for the Blind
Washington, DC

Acknowledgments

This book was one of those projects that seemed like it would never end, and without the help of many wonderful people, that might have been its fate. I first have to acknowledge my coauthor, Frances Mary D'Andrea. It was her vision to recognize, back in 2000, that we could take the information we were providing in a workshop called "Literacy for the Future: The Right Tool for the Job," and turn it into a book that could reach a much wider audience. FM coaxed, prodded, and supported me all along the way, from beginning to end, and I can't thank her enough.

I would also like to thank all those who participated in the workshops over the years, used earlier versions of the assessment form, and provided feedback about how it could be improved. In addition, I would like to specifically acknowledge the important contributions of Carol Farrenkopf, Kay Alicyn Ferrell, Greg Kearney, Stacy Kelly, Barbara Jackson LeMoine, Mark Richert, and Paul Schroeder, who wrote pieces for sections of this work; the substantive reviews by Peggy Bergman, Carol Farrenkopf, Pat Leader, and Cecilia Robinson; the helpful suggestions of Marie Amerson, Jim Downs, Lucia Hasty, Jay Leventhal, and Mary Ann Siller; and the wonderful photographs taken by Penny Rosenblum. I am grateful to Kim Hartsell for allowing us to use the Assistive Technology Considerations Checklist and the original assessment form on which the version in this book is based. I would also like to thank Shirley Landrum, my wonderful assistant at the National Literacy Center of the American Foundation for the Blind, who provided invaluable support by performing numerous tasks that allowed me the time to dedicate to the book, and Lisa Mauney for research assistance.

Finally, I would like to thank the editors at AFB Press, Ellen Bilofsky and Natalie Hilzen. Their ability to synthesize "techno-speak" and education terminology and ask, "What does that really mean?" shepherded me through the entire process. Their thoughtful questions and suggestions led to edits and rewrites that make this book more "user friendly" and, I hope, more beneficial to practitioners in our field.

Ike Presley

Introduction

The last decades of the 20th century were a time of great technological change and achievement, and this reality is especially evident in a visit to our public schools. Someone walking through any school today might see examples of technology in use, such as

- teachers using interactive whiteboards to post class notes that students download onto their laptops;
- teachers using online digital video clips from daily newspapers to supplement social studies and history textbooks;
- students using computer-based reading programs to improve their vocabulary, fluency, and writing skills;
- students creating multimedia projects in which they use their computers to conduct research, write the results, and print a report, as well as to create an electronic slide show to share with classmates.

By 1999, 84 percent of public school teachers in the United States reported having at least one computer in their classroom, and virtually all teachers (99 percent) reported having a computer somewhere in the school that they could use (National Center for Education Statistics [NCES], 2000). Today, desktop computers and other forms of once-revolutionary technology have become so commonplace that we take them for granted, and students going to school now do not know of a time when they did not exist.

In the past, teachers used such familiar tools as lectures and demonstrations, textbooks, worksheets, blackboards, overhead projectors, and movies to present information and concepts to students. Today, technology has become a vital and essential component of modern classrooms, and teachers have combined their traditional methods of presenting information with an ever-widening array of tools such as computers, CD-ROMs, digital video disks (DVDs), Internet access, online videos, and electronic whiteboards.

Tools used by students are also changing and increasing in complexity as they proliferate. The educational materials of the past—textbooks, periodicals, pens, and paper—are used along with a wide range of high-tech tools. Students now employ technology to reinforce instruction; support the development of skills in reading, writing, and math; and help them obtain information from both printed and electronic texts, as well as various forms of video and audio resources. The result of these changes is that both teachers and students now have a toolbox filled with a wider variety and larger number of resources that enable them to be more efficient teachers and learners.

THE NEW LITERACIES

In a broad sense, many typical educational objectives in the classroom have not changed a great deal. But in other ways, new tools have changed the nature of some tasks. Students not only write up a report on a subject, they are also asked to create multimedia presentations complete with video content, slide presentations, music, animation, and photographs or illustrations. In most schools in the United States, the technology tools to create these materials are widely available and there is now an expectation that students will complete high school adept in their use. These skills are referred to variously as "new literacies," "multiple" or "multiliteracies," or "21st century skills" (Anstey & Bull, 2006; Karchmer, Mallette, Kara-Soteriou, & Leu, 2005; Taffe & Gwinn, 2007). The National Council of Teachers of English (NCTE, 2008) has adopted a position statement related to "21st century literacies" that states that

> Twenty-first century readers and writers need to
>
> - develop proficiency with the tools of technology;
> - build relationships with others to pose and solve problems collaboratively and cross-culturally;
> - design and share information for global communities to meet a variety of purposes;
> - manage, analyze, and synthesize multiple streams of simultaneous information;
> - create, critique, analyze, and evaluate multi-media texts;
> - attend to the ethical responsibilities required by these complex environments.

Although students must still develop the literacy skills of reading and writing in order to acquire knowledge independently, teachers are also expected to prepare them to use those skills to access, process, and manipulate information from multiple sources (including electronic, audio, and visual materials); apply critical thinking skills to this information (compare, contrast, synthesize, and judge the veracity of Internet sources); and demonstrate their mastery of the information and concepts through the use of various technology tools (such as presentation software, multimedia software, and interactive web pages). So essential is the role of technology in our lives today that the International Society for Technology in Education has promoted the National Educational Technology Standards for Students, critical skills that students should develop to be prepared for the future. These standards outline "What students should know and be able to do to learn effectively and live productively in an increasingly digital world" and include creativity and innovation; communication and collaboration; research and information fluency; critical thinking, problem solving, and decision making; digital citizenship; and technology operations and concepts (International Society for Technology in Education [ISTE], 2007). For teachers, this expectation translates into new ways of teaching and of thinking about what being "literate" means. Furthermore, these expectations and high standards apply to *all* students, including those with disabilities. The literacy skills that students are now learning go beyond the familiar uses of texts and illustrations, and students today must also learn to communicate with and consider viewpoints from an increasingly global society—after all, the Internet has no physical bounds. As futurist Alvin

Toffler has said, "The illiterate of the 21st century will not be those who cannot read and write, but those who cannot learn, unlearn, and relearn" (www.alvintoffler.net/?fa=galleryquotes). To say that students in today's schools must learn to become effective problem-solvers to face the complex challenges of our rapidly changing society is, then, a mild understatement.

ACCESS AND THE NEW LITERACIES

All students may find themselves challenged in today's fast-moving and globally competitive environment, but students who are blind or visually impaired have additional challenges. They must learn the same higher levels of information-processing and manipulation skills as their classmates *and* they must have *access* to the advanced technologies such as hardware and software that make these "21st century literacies" possible. This access has been made available to individuals with disabilities through a wide range of special devices and software, referred to as *assistive technology*, which allow them to access information and the general curriculum, as well as through innovative technological tools. Visually impaired students, therefore, must develop expertise in using assistive technology, and they must develop skills in performing other complex tasks.

For educators of students with visual impairments, then, the true goal of teaching the use of assistive technology is to enable students to apply technology appropriately to complete important educational goals. The end is not in the student's learning to use the technology but in what he or she does with it.

IMPLICATIONS FOR PROGRAMMING AND ASSESSMENT

The following vignette illustrates how a particular student participates in both traditional and new literacy activities in her school.

Karen sat in her American history class, listening intently as her teacher discussed events that led to the American Civil War. She opened a new file on her accessible PDA (personal digital assistant), and took notes so she could review them later when studying for the upcoming midterm exam.

When the bell rang, Karen gathered her belongings and headed to English class. The class was reading and discussing the book To Kill a Mockingbird. *Karen had downloaded an electronic copy of this book from the National Library Service's Web-Braille service so she could read it with the refreshable braille display on her PDA. In class, she switched between the chapter in the book her class was discussing and a file that she had started, which contained her notes from the class. Another file Karen had open contained notes for a project that she and a classmate were completing about the novel. Later in the day, Karen and her partner went to the library to do more research, and while there Karen used one of the library computers to connect to the Internet. The computer had been equipped with screen-reading software that provides synthesized speech output of the text on the screen, so Karen could surf the Web to find additional resources. She printed the information that she found for her partner and also saved an electronic copy of the file on her flash drive. They decided to sift through the new information and incorporate some of it into the PowerPoint slide show that they would present to the class.*

When it was time for math, Karen headed down the hall to geometry class. An embossed copy of her braille math book was in the classroom, and she followed along with the exercises as her teacher explained theorems to the class. She also used an interactive electronic tablet with speech capacity in this class; tactile overlays depicted geometric concepts and diagrams that supplemented the class textbook, which allowed Karen to press on various parts of a diagram to hear additional information programmed into the device.

Karen is a successful high school student, keeping up with classmates, making good grades, and making plans to attend college. Because of her skills at accessing print and electronic information, she is an active learner who can gather information herself, not a student who must passively wait for material to be delivered to her in an accessible format by a teacher. In short, she is able to do what her friends and classmates are doing, and to do so in many of the same ways. Although she is blind, the use of technology has allowed her to access information, to produce materials both for others in print and for herself in braille, and to participate in activities that require her to analyze and synthesize information critically from a variety of sources.

The skills and independence displayed by this student were not learned overnight. The stage was set for Karen years ago when she was still very young. First, she received intensive instruction at the early stages of learning, when children are developing basic concepts. She also received daily reading and writing instruction in braille from a certified teacher of students with visual impairments. Equally important, Karen received periodic assessments of her educational needs and achievements. Her teachers monitored her academic progress and adjusted her program based on the results of various assessments of her reading and writing skills.

One of the important assessments Karen received was a comprehensive assistive technology assessment designed to help a student's Individualized Education Program (IEP) team determine how to enable a student to achieve his or her educational goals, particularly those a student is having difficulty achieving, by implementing specific accommodations and devices in the student's educational experience. In Karen's case, she and her educational team, including her parents, realized that some technology solutions would be needed to help her with the demanding academic tasks of a typical high school student. And, because her team recognized that the needs of students change over time, they conducted assessments several times over the years. Based on the foresight of Karen's team members in accessing her needs when she was quite young, various technology solutions were introduced early on and taught to her over time. In this way, she not only became proficient in the use of various kinds of technology well before she needed to use them for class but also developed a predisposition toward using technology in her learning process, so that when new technologies came along, she was open to trying them.

As this scenario makes clear, an assistive technology assessment is not an afterthought, but rather part of the foundation for a student's performance in school. In fact, the Individuals with Disabilities Education Act (IDEA) reauthorized in 2004 requires that the IEP team "consider whether the child needs assistive technology devices and services" (Sec. 614(d)(3)(B)(v)). It is the right of all students with disabilities to receive an assessment in the use of assistive technology.

HOW TO USE THIS BOOK

Assistive Technology for Students Who Are Blind or Visually Impaired: A Guide to Assessment is designed for teachers and other service providers who assess students with the purpose of documenting their educational needs and suggesting potential solutions through the use of assistive technology. Although the suggestions and examples provided in this book are generally aimed at K-12 students, many of the principles and issues discussed can also be applied to the assistive technology needs of college students and adults of all ages.

Since it is necessary to have knowledge of the various types of technology available to determine the devices and solutions that may meet an individual's assistive technology needs, Part 1 of this book provides an overview of a wide variety of both high-tech and low-tech assistive technology tools for students who are blind or visually impaired. These tools can be used to access print information and electronic information in different ways—visually, tactilely, and auditorily—to communicate in writing, and to produce materials in alternate formats (that is, in braille, large print, audio, and electronic formats). In general, since specific products change so rapidly, mention of particular products or brands is avoided, and categories or types of technology are discussed.

The information contained in these chapters is designed to clarify for those responsible for assessments the seemingly bewildering world of assistive technology. It will be particularly welcome for teachers of students with visual impairments, but the chapters are also important resources for members of the IEP team, administrators, program coordinators, and others who may find it difficult to keep up with the moving target that technology presents for all of us today. Service providers can use these chapters as a reference to focus on the options that will assist students with a specific type of task or to learn about the particular types of technology their students will be using at any given moment. Others may find this section useful for reviewing their knowledge of specific categories of assistive technologies or to gain information about unfamiliar technologies. Many readers may want to review the entire overview offered in this section to acquire a broad understanding of this exciting and changing field.

Part 2 describes the process of a comprehensive assistive technology assessment and provides a detailed guide that can be used by an assistive technology specialist, a teacher of students with visual impairments, and members of an educational team to capture information about how a student accomplishes essential tasks such as accessing print and electronic information and communicating through writing. These chapters also present information on how to formulate recommendations on the basis of an assessment and write up program and instructional goals. The assessment, while necessarily lengthy, provides the detail needed to make good decisions regarding what might be useful to a particular student in his or her educational environment. The process of completing the assessment includes gathering pertinent background information and considering of the student's current levels of functioning (Chapter 6); assessing the student's assistive technology needs (Chapter 7); devising recommendations based on the evaluation data and writing the final report and recommendations (Chapter 8); and implementing the team's recommendations (Chapter 9). Chapter 7 provides an assessment form that can be used to guide the evaluator, and Chapter 8 provides a simple checklist that can assist in organizing the recommendations for the student. (These forms are also reproduced in full in an appendix to this book.)

As they begin an assessment, practitioners will find it useful to read at a minimum the introductory material in each of these chapters to obtain an overview of the assistive technology assessment process, and then to focus on the detailed guidance offered in each chapter as they reach the corresponding step in the assessment. However, those who have relatively little experience in the area of assistive technology will benefit from reading the entire book before attempting to conduct an assessment for the first time. Others who are knowledgeable in this area may find the book a comprehensive resource whose descriptions ensure that participants in the assessment process do not unintentionally overlook potentially beneficial technologies for students who are blind or visually impaired.

Professionals who are working with braille users may wish to concentrate on the information about tactile and auditory tools and the sections related to assessing the individual's potential for using these tools. However, those working with students with low vision may find that having a better understanding of all types of access tools will be most helpful in determining the "right tools for the job" for these students.

The key concept that all readers should take away from this book is that no single device will fit the needs of any given student. Different students will benefit from using different technologies; the same student may use different technologies for different tasks and at different times in his or her life. Regardless of whether a student is blind or visually impaired, or has some other physical disabilities, or no disabilities at all, it takes a toolbox full of tools for students to achieve their educational and employment objectives. Technology can be the tool that can help students like Karen who are blind or visually impaired become independent and successful learners. But to enable students to use technology efficiently and to the best effect, assessment teams must apply careful thought and planning. By carefully assessing a student's needs, the means of access to information and developing skills for independence are at hand.

REFERENCES

Anstey, M., & Bull, G. (2006). *Teaching and learning multiliteracies: Changing times, changing literacies*. Newark, DE: International Reading Association.

Hatlen, P. (1996). The core curriculum for blind and visually impaired students including those with additional disabilities. *RE:view, 28*, 25–32.

International Society for Technology in Education. (2007). *National educational technology standards for students: The next generation*. Eugene, OR: International Society for Technology in Education. Retrieved from www.iste.org/Content/ NavigationMenu/NETS/ForStudents/ 2007Standards/NETS_for_Students _2007.htm

Karchmer, R. A., Mallette, M. H., Kara-Soteriou, J., & Leu, D. J. (Eds.). (2005). *Innovative approaches to literacy education: Using the Internet to support new literacies*. Newark, DE: International Reading Association.

National Center for Education Statistics. (2000, September). *Teachers' tools for the 21st century: A report on teachers' use of technology*. Statistical Analysis Report (NCES 2000–102). Washington, DC: U.S. Department of Education.

National Council of Teachers of English. (2008, February 15). *The NCTE definition of 21st-century literacies*. Position paper, adopted by NCTE Executive Committee. Urbana, IL: National Council of Teachers of English. Retrieved from www.ncte.org/announce/129117.htm

Taffe, S. W., & Gwinn, C. B. (2007). *Integrating literacy and technology*. New York: Guilford Press.

Overview of Assistive Technology for People Who Are Blind or Visually Impaired

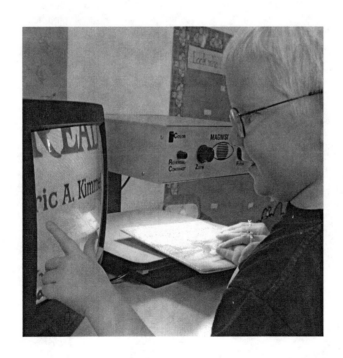

1

Technology for Learning and Literacy

Technology. Few words can rival this one in naming a force that has the potential to transform the ways in which we conduct the basic activities of daily life. All of us have to be "technologically literate" to be citizens in today's world, but this is especially true for individuals who are blind or visually impaired.

Students who are in school today have never lived in a world without computers, cell phones, or satellite transmission of news almost instantaneously around the world; they have never known a low tech world. For this reason, today's children have been called "digital natives": they are completely at home in a digital environment, using computers, playing video games, and surfing the Web (Prensky, 2001).

Like everyone else their age, students with visual impairments must also be "natives" in the digital world. They need to learn to use technology to engage in the same practices as their friends and classmates and have the same comfort level with the "new literacies" described in the Introduction to this book. Although many teachers currently in the classroom may be "digital immigrants" (Prensky, 2001) who were not born into a digital world but have adopted it over time, with varying levels of

3

comfort, teachers of students with visual impairments in general need to enable and support their students to feel at home in our complex high-tech world. The chapters that follow have been designed as an essential aid in that process, each focusing on a different aspect of assistive technology and the assessment process.

THE IMPACT OF VISUAL IMPAIRMENT

Children with visual impairments are as unique and as varied as any other group of children, but in many ways are an especially heterogeneous group, with a wide variety of characteristics and needs. Some children have a great deal of usable vision; others do not. Some have additional physical or cognitive disabilities; others do not. Because of the differences among them, it is very difficult to talk in generalities about students with visual impairments. Despite their variability, though, one overall statement can be made about most children who are visually impaired: Depending on their individual circumstances, visually impaired children may not be able to rely on the sense of sight to obtain information, observe their surroundings, and learn about the world.

What does this mean for a child? Consider how much information is derived visually from the environment. When we think about how much information those who are sighted derive just by looking around, we realize that the implications of not being able to use vision, or of being able to use it only in a limited way, can affect every aspect of life and learning. A child who may not be able to rely on his or her sight to the extent that typically sighted children do needs to learn to obtain informa-tion and access the world in other ways. Using his or her other senses to the fullest degree possible is one way. Having direct, hands-on exposure to as much of the environment as possible is another. Receiving repeated, lengthy, and in-depth explanations of objects and processes is still another. And technology, in the form of assistive technology, is yet another.

It is impossible to underestimate the importance of technology to people with visual impairments. In effect, technological devices used by someone who is visually impaired become extensions of that person and channels that support the flow of fundamental information that he or she cannot derive easily by sight.

THE CRITICAL ROLE OF TECHNOLOGY— AND ASSESSMENT

Being adept at using technology is therefore essential—in fact critical—for visually impaired students. First, in order to access the environment around them, learn about the world, and function in their daily lives, these students need to learn to use devices that help them gain that access. As the introduction to this book explains, "assistive technology" is the term that refers to the special devices—including both high-tech and low-tech tools—and software that people with disabilities can use to access both the environment *and* technology. Second, just as it has revolutionized the way we live and work, technology has revolutionized the way in which our children learn and participate in school. Visually impaired students, like all students, need to be "power users" of technology who can function at the higher levels of information manipulation that today's society demands.

But not all technological devices are effective and appropriate for all visually impaired students. Some students have more vision than others, which may allow them to read print, while others cannot. Some students are blind and read by using their tactile sense, by obtaining information auditorily, or by using both modes of input. Perhaps the most general statement that can be made about visually impaired students is that each student will have some difficulty accessing the visual environment of the classroom and will need different kinds and levels of support and instruction from a certified teacher of students with visual impairments. How a student functions best in the classroom will vary from child to child, depending on the nature of each child's visual impairment. Indeed, even children with the same eye condition will not always function the same way in the classroom. For that matter, an individual child's visual abilities and performance will vary as well, depending on environmental conditions, fatigue, the requirements of a particular task, and a number of other factors.

ESSENTIAL ASSESSMENTS FOR STUDENTS WHO ARE VISUALLY IMPAIRED

Because the needs of visually impaired students are so variable, several assessments are a critical part of their education: a clinical low vision evaluation, a functional vision assessment, a learning media assessment, and an assistive technology assessment. (For a more detailed description of these assessments, see *Looking to Learn* [D'Andrea &

Farrenkopf, 2000], *Foundations of Education* [Koenig & Holbrook, 2000], and *Foundations of Low Vision* [Corn & Koenig, 1997; Corn & Erin, in press]. The common theme of all of these assessments is to determine the extent to which a student can use his or her vision and how he or she does so. They also address the related, equally essential question of which sense the student can most effectively utilize to obtain information from the environment, thereby contributing to his or her ability to learn.

A *clinical low vision evaluation* is an assessment of an individual's vision and the way in which he or she visually functions, performed at a specialized, low vision clinic. The evaluation helps determine a student's visual abilities concerning tasks such as reading and writing and also provides the student an opportunity to try various optical and nonoptical devices, such as monocular telescopes, magnifiers, and video magnifiers (Simons & Lapolice, 2000), which may be helpful in those and other tasks (see Chapter 2 for more information). The evaluation is conducted by a trained low vision specialist whose expertise relates to the functional aspects of vision, such as the comfort and ease with which the student can do certain visual tasks. The clinical low vision evaluation is also where specific optical devices can be prescribed as appropriate for the individual needs of the student.

Another important assessment is a *functional vision assessment*. This evaluation is typically conducted by the teacher of students with visual impairments formally and informally in the settings where the student spends the most time: his or her classroom and school and in the home. This assessment should complement the clinical evaluation and document the student's visual functioning (Anthony, 2000), including how well the student uses prescribed optical devices for near and distance tasks in real-life situations.

A *learning media assessment* (Koenig & Holbrook, 1995) must also be performed. This assessment gathers information about how the student best learns: tactilely, visually, auditorily, or with some combination of these methods. In addition to determining which sensory channel (vision, touch, or hearing) is the primary and which is the secondary learning channel for the student—that is, which sense is the one the student uses most effectively to read and to learn, the assessment explores which literacy materials the student most efficiently uses in class (such as books) and in the classroom environment, as well (such as bulletin boards).

Once these assessments have been completed, a clearer picture emerges of how the student learns best, what strengths and needs he or she has, and what adaptations may be needed in the environment and in the use of educational materials. Since students' needs change over time, it is important that these assessments are done periodically as the child grows. These evaluations provide the student's Individualized Education Program (IEP) team with the information they need to make good decisions about the kinds of materials and accommodations that are useful for the student. The classroom, like the world around us, is a very "visual" place, requiring the use of vision in order to obtain full knowledge of it. Beyond the usual bulletin boards and chalkboards or whiteboards, new educational tools such as computer-based reading programs require the user to interact with them visually. How do students with visual impairments fit into a present and a future that includes the enhanced use of technology for school and work?

ASSISTIVE TECHNOLOGY: SOME BASIC CONCEPTS

As mentioned in the introduction to this book, before students can apply the 21st century skills that are expected of students in schools, they must first be able to access information independently and efficiently. Educators who wish their students to use technology for assignments or who wish to teach the use of various technology devices to students with visual impairments face an obvious problem: How do you teach someone who cannot see or has very limited vision to use a device, such as a computer, that conveys information visually and requires vision to operate it? In many cases, the answer is by modifying the device and the output (such as text in print or on a screen) that it produces. Many advances in technology have already helped develop adaptive tools that interact with devices, such as computers, and convert their output to an auditory, tactile, or enlarged visual format for individuals with visual impairments and other disabilities. These adaptive tools and devices fall into two broad categories: stand-alone devices, and hardware and software that allow the user to access computers.

Stand-alone devices refer to items that can be used independently and do not need to be connected to a computer (although many of them can be). This category includes such equipment as electronic braillewriters, advanced optical devices, electronic video magnifiers, talking calculators, talking dictionaries, modified audio recorders and players, and portable note-taking devices (personal digital assistants, or PDAs) with speech or braille output. The chapters that follow provide detailed information about these devices.

Once they have learned to use assistive technology to access electronic information, students with visual impairments can participate more equally with their sighted classmates.

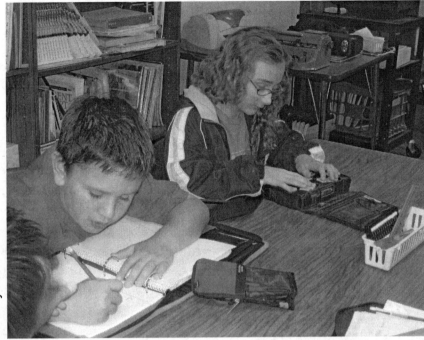

L. Penny Rosenblum

The other major category of assistive technology includes hardware and software that allow people with visual impairments to access computers and electronic information easily. Most blind or visually impaired students are able to interact with computers through the use of a standard keyboard and keyboard commands (as opposed to a mouse or other pointing device), but reading the computer monitor's typical display may present some problems. Now, however, the output of the computer that is displayed visually on a monitor can be enlarged, "read" or announced by synthetic speech, or provided in a tactile form in a refreshable braille display. In addition, many of these tools provide students with effective and efficient means of producing written communication. Once they have learned to use this equipment, students with visual impairments are on a more level playing field with their sighted classmates, able to accomplish the same tasks and participate in the general curriculum with greater ease and independence.

USING TECHNOLOGY TO ENHANCE LITERACY

Accessing Print and Electronic Text

Producing Written Communication

Producing Materials in Accessible Formats

In its central role of supporting learning and providing essential access to the curriculum and materials for students who are visually impaired, technology can support literacy in various specific ways. For example, it can be used to provide instruction in and reinforcement of early literacy skills. Numerous computer software programs have been developed to teach students such basic skills as visual tracking, letter recognition, phonemic awareness, and sound-symbol relationships.

Overall, however, there are three major ways in which technology supports literacy for students who are blind or visually impaired:

- It enables students to access print and electronic text.
- It enables students to produce written communication.
- It enables students and the professionals who work with them to produce materials in accessible formats.

Chapters 2, 3, 4, and 5 provide detailed information on each of these areas.

ACCESSING PRINT AND ELECTRONIC TEXT

The world around us is full of text in print form: books, magazines, newspapers, signs, menus, blank forms, flyers, and advertisements. Books are not the only print materials used in schools; far from it. Once students who are blind or visually impaired develop literacy skills in the early grades, it is important that a wide variety of reading material and other text-based materials are available to them so that they can practice and expand their capabilities. In addition, the print resources in the classroom that convey information—signs, bulletin board displays, notes on the chalk- or whiteboard—also need to be available. Moreover, text exists in many electronic forms as well, from the words on a computer screen, to text messages on a cell phone to PDA, or chapters in an e-book.

Both low- and high-tech tools exist that can meet students' needs to have access to the information these texts contain. As the following chapters explain, individual students need to use a combination of these tools to accomplish literacy tasks, and they will need to be comfortable using these and other tools throughout their lives. Texts produced in large print, braille, or audio recordings offer a low-tech solution to students' needs, while text displayed in a large font on a computer screen, spoken through synthesized speech, or rendered through an electronic braille display provide high-tech solutions (see Table 1.1).

Both low-tech and high-tech assistive technology tools can meet students' needs for access to information.

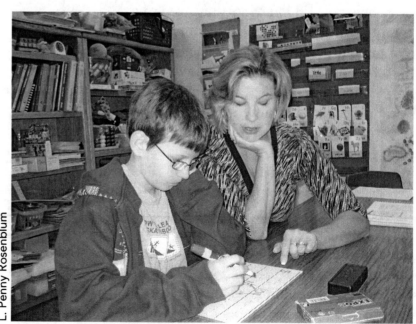

L. Penny Rosenblum

Table 1.1 Types of Assistive Technology for Students Who Are Blind or Visually Impaired

Types of Technology	Access Method		
	Visual Access	**Tactile Access**	**Auditory Access**

Technology for accessing print	Nonoptical devices
	    Large print
	    Reading stands
	    Acetate overlays
	    Lighting
	Optical devices
	    Handheld and stand magnifiers
	    Telescopes
	Video magnification systems
	Scanning and OCR systems
	Electronic whiteboards
		Braille reading
		Tactile graphics
		    Tactile math tools
			Readers
			Audio recording
			    Digital Talking Books
			    Other audio formats
			Specialized scanning systems
			    Stand-alone electronic reading machines
			    Computer-based reading machines
			E-book readers
			Talking calculators
			Talking dictionaries

Technology for accessing electronic information	Computers
	    Screen-enlarging hardware
	        Large monitors
	        Adjustable monitor arms
	    Software options
	        Operating system display property adjustments
	        Computer accessibility features
	        Cursor-enlarging software
	    Screen magnification software
	Specialized scanning systems
	Accessible portable word processors
	Accessible PDAs
	E-book readers
	Large-print and online calculators
	Online dictionaries and thesauri
		Refreshable braille displays
		Computers
		Accessible PDAs
		Touch tablets
			Talking word-processor programs
			Text readers
			Self-voicing applications
			Screen-reading software
			Accessible PDAs
			Specialized scanning systems
			E-book readers
			Talking dictionaries
			Talking calculators
			Digital voice recorders

(continued on next page)

Table 1.1   Types of Assistive Technology for Students Who Are Blind or Visually Impaired *(continued)*

Types of Technology	Access Method		
	Visual Access	**Tactile Access**	**Auditory Access**
Technology for producing written communications	Manual tools 　Bold- or raised-line paper 　Felt-tip pens and bold markers 　Bold-lined graph paper for math Electronic tools 　Dedicated word processors 　Accessible PDAs 　Imaging software 　Drawing software 　Talking word processor 　Computer with word-processing and screen magnification software 　Math software and spreadsheets 　Laptop or notebook computers	Manual and mechanical braille-writing devices 　Slate and stylus braillewriters Electronic braille-writing devices 　Electric and electronic braillewriters Computers with word-processing software Accessible PDAs Braille translation software Braille embosser	Accessible computers with word-processing software Accessible PDAs
Technology for producing materials in alternate formats	Scanning and OCR system Computer with word-processing software Laser printer	Scanning and OCR system Computer with word-processing software Braille translation software Graphics software Braille embosser Equipment and materials for producing tactile graphics Materials for collage Manual devices for tooling graphics Fusers and capsule paper	Digital and analog audio recording devices Scanning and OCR system

PRODUCING WRITTEN COMMUNICATION

Producing written communication such as reports, answers on worksheets, and letters is an aspect of literacy that has often been challenging for students who are blind or visually impaired. Many students with low vision who use traditional writing tools such as pencil and paper may find it difficult to render the correct shape of letters and punctuation marks. Sometimes the line width of writing paper and the contrast between the lines and the paper itself make it difficult for students to write legibly. The result may be written communication that is difficult for the students and their teachers, and anyone else, to read.

Students who use braille as their primary medium for reading and writing face an additional difficulty in producing written communication that others can understand, because most of their teachers and classmates cannot read braille. Learning to produce a legible signature is important, but, in general, handwriting, the traditional method of producing written communication, is not a practical methodology for students who are blind because they cannot read it back to themselves. Technology offers both low- and high-tech tools that students who read tactilely can use to produce written communication in braille and in print.

PRODUCING MATERIALS IN ACCESSIBLE FORMATS

In the past, producing materials in large print, braille, or audio format was both labor intensive and time consuming. Today, many print texts can be keyboarded or scanned into a computer system and then reproduced in large print, braille, or audio. Although it is important to ensure the accuracy of the materials by having them either produced or reviewed by a trained and qualified professional, the availability of print information to blind or visually impaired students has expanded dramatically because of the use of such technology.

THE IMPORTANCE OF ASSISTIVE TECHNOLOGY ASSESSMENTS

Determining the Appropriate Tools

Complying with the Law

Ensuring the Best Use of Resources

Given technology's fundamental and overarching importance to the ability of students who are visually impaired to participate fully in school, work, and daily life, the question becomes how to promote their development of technology-related skills. Educators and other professionals who work with students need to focus on these skills as being essential to these students' well-being. Given the wide variability of students' abilities and needs and the array of assistive technology tools now available, determining which of the many available tools will best meet the individual student's needs is a critical first step.

The purpose of this book is to provide a framework to assist service providers in identifying which adaptations, modifications, and technologies most effectively fit the needs of each student. Just as the clinical low vision evaluation, functional vision assessment, and learning media assessment provide necessary information for planning a student's educational program, an assessment conducted to inform the educational team about the appropriate technology tools for the student is necessary for planning a program, as well. This type of evaluation is known as an assistive technology assessment.

Why should we perform such an assessment? Doing so is critical to the ability of a student to participate fully in school, but there are three reasons in particular:

1. To determine the appropriate tools to help the student perform essential activities such as reading and writing, access all the information conveyed to his or her classmates, and accomplish his or her educational objectives, all of which can lead to independence and self-sufficiency as an adult
2. To comply with the law
3. To ensure the best use of financial resources

DETERMINING THE APPROPRIATE TOOLS

Because visual impairments vary from mild to no usable vision, the impact of visual impairment on students' ability to use technology will vary greatly as well. Students with mild vision loss may be able to work with technology by using optical devices or by using technology to display information enlarged. Students with little or no vision may require adaptations to technology devices that will allow them to work with a device's output in a tactile format. Other students may need to access the output by having it presented auditorily through synthesized speech. Still other students may need a combination of visual, auditory, and tactile access, depending on the task to be completed. Therefore, it is critical that educators determine how the student interacts with materials, tools, and information that are usually presented visually in the classroom. Completing an assistive technology assessment will help chart this interaction and thus help identify which tools the student needs.

Students who receive an assistive technology assessment can then be provided the appropriate tools to help them take full advantage of their educational program. (This process is described in more detail in Chapters 8 and 9.) Using these tools will help them develop efficient literacy skills and critical thinking skills and attain mastery over the manipulation of information. Often, students who are blind or visually impaired require additional time to complete certain tasks, especially when they are first developing skills. Determining the appropriate assistive technology and teaching the student to use it can dramatically decrease the time required.

The resulting increase in efficiency obtained by effective use of assistive technology can open up many opportunities for the student. For some, it will provide extra time to explore given subject matter in greater depth, or allow them to broaden their interest into other subjects. For others, it will free up time that can be used to complete separate challenging or time-consuming tasks, or to participate in social, physical, and recreational activities. When students have the right tools to improve their efficiency, not only do they have a better chance for additional educational opportunities, but more time becomes available to them to develop skills that will be valuable beyond school and that can be used as the student makes the transition into higher education, vocational training, and the world of work and independence.

What happens without an assistive technology assessment? Students who fail to receive an appropriate assessment may never have the chance to benefit from the far-reaching opportunities that enabling technology affords. For this reason, it is important for educators and other professionals to ensure that assessments are undertaken for all visually impaired students. Advocacy of this kind is critical even for students who are academically successful, who are often overlooked when it comes to assistive technology, because teachers and parents (and sometimes even the students themselves) may believe, based on the fact that they are doing well, that they do not need to use assistive technology. However, if a student never experiences the benefits of appropriate technology, the additional accomplishments he or she may have been able to achieve will never be known. A student who does not have access to beneficial technology devices—"the right tool for the job"—may spend many hours completing assignments using equipment or methods that make assigned tasks more onerous than necessary or may in fact be unable to complete an assignment at all. How will this student be able to participate in the complex multimedia activities now taking place in schools or develop the wide-ranging familiarity with technology that our society now demands?

The following situation, in which a student is using methods and materials that are inappropriate or inefficient for his needs, is an example that may be familiar to many students and teachers:

Eddie, a fourth-grade boy with low vision, is having difficulty reading materials handed out by his teacher, Mrs. O'Brian. He tells her that the print is too small for him to read. Mrs. O'Brian learns that the school has a photocopying machine that will enlarge the image of the text on a page, and she uses the copier to enlarge the handouts so Eddie can see them. However, to see the text with any level of detail, Eddie's eyes must be approximately 2 inches from the page. Reading at this distance for any length of time brings on both physical and visual fatigue for him; and in addition to being exhausted, he finds doing his assignments to be slow and time-consuming. Eddie has already found reading to be an unpleasant task, because it takes him longer than his classmates to complete reading assignments. As time goes on, he becomes more frustrated and less motivated to participate in activities that involve reading, and is unable to keep up in class, because he has not assimilated the content of the assigned readings. In addition, he has to wait until enlarged materials have been made and given to him, and this has begun to make him passive and uninvolved in learning.

Although Mrs. O'Brian's use of a photocopying machine to enlarge materials for Eddie may be of some help in certain circumstances, it is not the best tool to use for him and is not a sustainable and efficient long-term solution.

What difference might an assistive technology assessment have made for Eddie? A properly administered assessment of his needs and abilities would have determined that he needed other alternatives for reading and completing assignments. It would also have considered Eddie's need for a clinical low vision evaluation performed by a qualified low vision eye care specialist, which might have indicated his need to use an optical device. The scenario could have ended on a positive note:

After Eddie visits the low vision clinic and has a comprehensive assistive technology assessment, the evaluator recommends that he use an electronic video magnification system to view a wide variety of text, graphics, and objects. (Chapter 2 provides detailed information about this device and how it works.) When reading with the video magnifier, Eddie finds that he is able to sit in a more comfortable position and that doing so eliminates much of the physical and visual fatigue he experiences when trying to read materials enlarged on the photocopier. Now he can read materials presented in class, read for longer periods of time, and keep up with his classmates on most activities. He can also use this same device in science class to look closer at the biology specimens they are studying. He discovers that he loves science and now gets up in the morning excited about going to school.

COMPLYING WITH THE LAW

Federal law requires that all students be provided a free and appropriate public education. For students with a visual impairment or other disability, this mandate includes the creation of an IEP. The 1997 Amendments to the Individuals with Disabilities Education Act (PL 105-17) include provisions for assistive technology devices and services and requires the IEP team to address the student's need for assistive technology. Completing an assistive technology assessment and following its recommendations constitute the foundation for meeting this mandate. The appendix to this chapter, "Assistive Technology FAQs," answers some common questions about the legal and other aspects of assistive technology assessment. (See "It's the Law: Q&A about Assistive Technology and Special Education," Appendix A at the back of this book, for further information on relevant legislation and the legal definition of assistive technology.)

ENSURING THE BEST USE OF RESOURCES

In some instances, assistive technology devices and tools purchased for students are initially embraced with enthusiasm. However, after learning to use these devices, some students may realize that these new tools are not working for them after all; they may not offer features that are needed, may be too big and unwieldy or too small and inefficient for the tasks that need to be done, or are otherwise not appropriate for what the student needs and wants to do. Too often expensive equipment is purchased that does not meet the needs of an individual student and therefore ends up sitting in a closet gathering dust.

When this occurs, administrators, students, parents, and teachers may become skeptical about the benefits of assistive technology for people who are blind or visually impaired. Administrators may see technology purchases as the squandering of valuable and limited resources, which can make them reluctant to approve requests for purchasing assistive technology for other students in the future. Students themselves may see a device as one more thing they have to learn that does not improve their lives and that makes them "look different." Parents may see the equipment as one more instance of their son or daughter's being promised something to help that ends up not working and only leads to failure and frustration, which in turn results in less self-confidence. Finally, teachers may see the device as one more thing they have to learn about and teach that does not improve the student's ability to complete required educational objectives. Negative reactions such as these not only affect the student immediately involved, but also make acquiring and using assistive technology more difficult for other students in the school system. This outcome could be avoided if the student receives the appropriate assessments at timely intervals in his or her educational experience.

Determining the most appropriate assistive technology tools for students is essential for preventing the purchase of inappropriate assistive technology, and periodic assessments are the answer to preventing negative outcomes such as those just described. Although assistive technology assessments cannot completely eliminate the chance of purchasing equipment that fails to aid the student, they can greatly reduce the number of such instances and provide students with greater opportunities for success.

LEARNING ABOUT TECHNOLOGY: A GOAL FOR STUDENTS AND PROFESSIONALS

For many educators, members of a student's educational team, and related professionals, the first step toward undertaking an assistive technology assessment with a student is to become more familiar with the many types of devices and solutions now available for people who are visually impaired. It is difficult both to conduct an assessment and to know what to do with the results without knowing how to apply and translate what the assessment reveals into sound recommendations for specific devices. For this reason, the chapters included in the first part of this book—Chapters 2 through 5—present information about the different kinds of assistive technology that can be used for particular tasks. Chapter 2 describes the many kinds of devices that allow for visual, tactile, and auditory access to print materials, such as books and magazines. Chapter 3 extends this discussion to describe access to electronic information, which can include both textual and graphic content. Chapter 4 discusses technology options for producing written communication, such as homework assignments, research papers, and letters. Finally, Chapter 5 describes how to create material in alternate formats, such as braille, large print, and audio. Because of the special central role that technology can play in their students' lives and successes— or lack thereof—teachers and other professionals who work with students with visual impairments and other disabilities may find that keeping up with technology is an essential aspect of their work.

Since technological innovation is fast moving, and new devices, software, and ap-proaches are being developed all the time, it can be challenging to keep up with what is current. However, many resources exist for professionals who wish to stay informed about recent developments and ongoing trends. Within this book, Part 1, the section describing resources, and Chapter 9, which discusses follow-up assessment, provide extensive information about them for the reader. (The appendix to this chapter, "Assistive Technology FAQs", also addresses this issue, as well as many other questions that teachers often ask about assistive technology.)

A number of periodicals, web sites, electronic mailing lists, and the like offer up-to-date news about new assistive technology products. There are also several annual assistive technology conferences that practitioners and people who are visually impaired can attend for hands-on experiences with devices, as well as an opportunity to talk with manufacturers and other technology users. In addition, several agencies and organizations offer training through workshops and distance learning courses to the public and to teachers and students who want to learn more about the devices they have.

However, one of the better ways to learn about various assistive technology devices is simply to spend time with a device, exploring it, trying out its various features, and just "playing around" with it. Some busy teachers may feel unprepared or guilty for not knowing every single command or feature on every single device their students use. Although teachers of students with visual impairments need a working knowledge of the most common kinds of assistive technology and should be able to introduce a student to them, unless a teacher uses a device extensively it may be unrealistic to expect to develop in-depth knowledge about every feature. It is also counterproductive for teachers to feel that in order for their students to use a device, they themselves need to be expert users first. Instead, teachers should encourage their students who are blind or visually impaired to explore devices and their features on their own. Many devices have built-in "help files" that explain or describe how they work, or have accessible manuals that give tips and hints for using the equipment. Not only does this approach develop students' independence and problem-solving skills, it is also the way

that people learn to use new technology in everyday life—whether a new cell phone, portable music player, or a new microwave oven. By keeping an open mind, becoming comfortable about technology and its pervasive role in our lives, encouraging students to explore and use technology to the fullest extent possible, and promoting skills through opportunities for practice, professionals working with students who are visually impaired can help them excel in today's competitive world—and tomorrow's, as well.

REFERENCES

Anstey, M., & Bull, G. (2006). *Teaching and learning multiliteracies*: *Changing times, changing literacies*. Newark, DE: International Reading Association.

Anthony, T. (2000). Performing a functional low vision assessment. In F. M. D'Andrea & C. Farrenkopf (Eds.), *Looking to learn* (pp. 32–83). New York: AFB Press.

Corn, A. L., & Erin, J. N. (in press). *Foundations of low vision*: *Clinical and functional perspectives* (2nd ed.). New York: AFB Press.

Corn, A. L., & Koenig, A. J. (Eds.). (1997). *Foundations of low vision*: *Clinical and functional perspectives*. New York: AFB Press.

D'Andrea, F. M., & Farrenkopf, C. (Eds.). (2000). *Looking to learn*. New York: AFB Press.

Karchmer, R. A., Mallette, M. H., Kara-Soteriou, J., & Leu, D. J. (Eds.). (2005). *Innovative approaches to literacy education*: *Using the Internet to support new literacies*. Newark, DE: International Reading Association.

Koenig, A. J., & Holbrook, M. C. (1995). *Learning media assessment* (2nd ed.). Austin: Texas School for the Blind and Visually Impaired.

Koenig, A. J., & Holbrook, M. C. (Eds.). (2000). *Foundations of education* (2nd ed.). *Vol. I: History and theory of teaching children and youths with visual impairments; Vol. II: Instructional strategies for teaching children and youths with visual impairments.* New York: AFB Press.

National Council of Teachers of English. (2008, February 15). *The NCTE definition of 21st-century literacies.* Position paper, adopted by NCTE Executive Committee. Urbana, IL: National Council of Teachers of English. Retrieved from www.ncte.org/announce/129117.htm

Prensky, M. (2001). Digital natives, digital immigrants. *On the Horizon, 9*(5), 1–6.

Simons, B., & LaPolice, D. J. (2000). Working efficiently with a low vision clinic. In F. M. D'Andrea & C. Farrenkopf (Eds.), *Looking to learn.* New York: AFB Press.

Taffe, S. W., & Gwinn, C. B. (2007). *Integrating literacy and technology.* New York: Guilford Press.

Appendix 1A   Assistive Technology FAQs

1. *What falls under the definition of assistive technology?*

The legal definition in the Individuals with Disabilities Education Act (IDEA) states, "The term 'assistive technology device' means any item, piece of equipment, or product system, whether acquired commercially off the shelf, modified, or customized, that is used to increase, maintain, or improve functional capabilities of a child with a disability" (Sec. 602 (1)(A)). Under the laws that assistive technology includes all aids and devices that can be used to help a child with a disability perform educational activities or activities of daily living. Assistive technology includes high- and low-tech aids and devices that can be purchased or made, as well as mobility devices such as wheelchairs. High-tech devices include, for example, a computer system with synthesized speech output programs, scanners, and optical character recognition (OCR) software; braille embossers; video magnifiers (CCTVs); braille notetakers (accessible PDAs); hearing aids; and FM systems, to name a few. Low-tech devices include nonoptical devices (enlarged materials, enhanced lighting), optical devices (handheld and stand magnifiers, telescopes), pencil grips, thick black markers, and any other "tool" that enables a child with a disability to participate in activities of daily living with greater ease or independence. (See Appendix A for more information on the legal definition of assistive technology. See Chapters 2–4 for more examples of assistive technology.)

2. *Does assistive technology include training and other services in IDEA?*

Yes. According to the definition of assistive technology stated in IDEA, training for staff, students, and even parents is considered part of assistive technology services and is covered by the law. (See Appendix A about assistive technology and the law.)

3. *When can I request an assistive technology assessment of a student?*

A request for an assistive technology evaluation can be made at any time. For example, if a student experiences a change in vision (either increased or decreased visual functioning), an evaluation will help determine what assistive devices will meet the student's new needs. If a student has never had an assistive technology assessment, one should be requested to help teachers determine what devices would assist the student in class. Also, as a student becomes more capable in using certain devices, his or her needs change and become more advanced; further evaluation will help the educational team determine what devices and technology will meet the student's future needs. No child is too young or too "disabled" to undergo an assistive technology assessment. Like the learning media assessment, the assistive technology assessment should be ongoing. As children grow and develop, so too will their assistive technology needs. An assistive technology assessment will help guide the educational team in making informed decisions throughout a child's educational career. (See Chapter 9 for more information.)

4. Who should be included in an assistive technology assessment team?

Each assistive technology assessment will involve different people, depending on the needs of the student being evaluated. Generally, the people who make up the student's IEP team are involved in the evaluation, to various degrees. The IEP team members (typically made up of the teacher of students with visual impairments, the primary classroom teacher and/or subject-specific teachers, parents, and other professional support service providers, such as a speech and language pathologist and occupational or physical therapist) who work directly with the student are involved in the evaluation. One person is selected by the IEP team to coordinate the assistive technology assessment (see Chapter 6). In many cases, the teacher of students with visual impairments will conduct the assessment. However, some school districts have assistive technology specialists who might undertake the assessment. Communication and consultation among team members is critical to obtaining an accurate evaluation.

5. Is assistive technology replacing braille?

Assistive technology is *not* replacing braille. Technology has enabled students who are visually impaired to have more immediate access to the school curriculum, and it has afforded them greater speed and efficiency in producing written materials (see Introduction). However, students who are blind still need to learn how to read, to spell, and to put a sentence or paragraph together; they must learn the conventions of reading and writing in braille before they can apply those reading and writing skills to a computer. Technology is another "tool" that students can add to their literacy toolboxes.

6. How can a teacher of students with visual impairments, or a student, get exposure to the variety of devices that are available before recommending or purchasing equipment?

There are many ways that a teacher of students with visual impairments can become familiar with assistive devices. Sometimes, a low vision clinic or rehabilitation facility has various devices available for testing by clients, and by visiting the facility with your student, you and the student can both "test drive" or "play with" the devices on display. Visiting a local assistive technology vendor or manufacturer is another way to gain exposure to current devices on the market. One vendor typically does not carry every type of device on the market—different vendors hold contracts with different manufacturers. Visiting as many vendors as possible, asking vendors to show you how a device works, and gaining a little experience by testing the devices yourself will likely give you a broad perspective on what is currently available. If you ask, some vendors may be willing to loan you or your student a device to try out. Some vendors may also be willing to give you and your student a product demonstration at the school. (See Chapter 6 for more information.)

Visiting vendor displays at conferences can also be very informative. Typically, devices, manuals, and specification sheets are put on display for interested persons to examine. Vendor displays are excellent opportunities to gather a lot of information in a short period of time—you may even be able to make comparisons from one product to another. Yet another way to gain exposure to assistive technology is to observe others using assistive technology, whether it is a student or an adult. Connecting with colleagues in neighboring school districts or within your own district is another way to find out what is being used in schools. And, finally, you can conduct an Internet search of assistive technology and visit numerous sites (including vendor and manufacturers' sites) from around the world. Although hands-on experience is usually the most meaningful way to learn about technology, reading online information about devices can be informative as well. (For more information, see Chapter 9.)

7. How much will I, as a teacher of students with visual impairments, be expected to know about a particular device?

You will definitely not be expected to know everything. Students, parents, and school administrators will not expect you to know how every device works. You and the student can learn how to use a device together. Playing with the equipment and testing it out is a really good way to learn about the technology and how it works. Be sure to read the manual because it will help you get started. If possible, leave the training to the experts (that is, the vendor or trainer) and try to be a part of the training (often provided by the vendor) when the student gets trained. Teach students how to find and use the "help" files and how to troubleshoot a malfunctioning device (for example, what possible causes to consider first when solving problems, which ones may be next most likely, and so forth). Also, do not be afraid to ask questions or call the tech support number associated with a particular device.

8. What strategies can be used to get regular education teachers to support a student's use of assistive technology equipment in class?

Consider sharing information with regular education teachers about the value of assistive technology and how it promotes independence and ease of access to the school curriculum for students who are visually impaired. Demonstrate how easily the technology can be set up and used by the student (and support personnel, if needed) to help the regular education teacher realize that it can be integrated into the student's day without any major disruptions or difficulties. Make sure the teacher has an opportunity to see the student using the equipment successfully. Demystify the technology for the teacher by providing simple instructions or guidelines for use. Avoid focusing on the complexity of the software and peripherals, especially when first introducing the equipment into the classroom. Arrange a training session for the regular education teacher if the teacher does not have the knowledge to integrate the use of the student's assistive technology with the teacher's own technology. Remind teachers that the technology will be part of the student's success with the help of the entire educational team.

9. How can I make sure that students use the equipment when the teacher of students with visual impairments is not around?

It is critical that students who are visually impaired continue to use their assistive technology throughout the day as needed, every day, even when the teacher of students with visual impairments is not available. The general education teacher needs to understand the importance of continued, frequent use of the equipment in the absence of the teacher of students with visual impairments—it will help build the student's confidence and competence in using the equipment, and it will enable the student to have greater independent access to the curriculum. It may take several conversations with the teacher to get this message across. Encouraging the student to advocate for himself or herself will also help. Keeping a log nearby for the student (or teacher) to indicate when and how the technology was used may be helpful and may encourage greater accountability. Including an assistive technology goal on the student's IEP that states daily practice is required will also promote greater accountability. Providing the student with specific assignments that must be completed using the equipment is another good strategy to ensure that the student uses the equipment, while the teacher of students with visual impairments is absent.

10. What are my options as a teacher of students with visual impairments when equipment breaks down? What if the device is no longer under warranty?

Broken equipment means that a student's ability to access the curriculum and to produce materials is interrupted. The student then needs to rely on other methods to gain access to material and to complete assignments. The teacher of students with visual impairments is usually the first person who is contacted when equipment breaks down. If the equipment is still under warranty, a quick call to the manufacturer or vendor to fix the problem is the best place to start. Unfortunately, it takes time to repair equipment, which means even more time for the student without the equipment. Some vendors and manufacturers will, if asked, provide a similar device on loan to the student during repairs—each vendor or

manufacturer is different. If you have a good working relationship with a vendor, it never hurts to ask the vendor to provide a free loaner device while the broken device gets repaired, especially if your school district purchases a lot of equipment from that vendor. Sometimes, the teacher of students with visual impairments can arrange for a loaner device from a local agency or school for the blind. Similarly, if another student is not currently using a device, it could be loaned to the student who temporarily needs it. If a device is no longer under warranty, the repair costs will have to be billed to someone—most likely the school district. But, if the school district does not have the financial means to pay for the repair, the device may never get fixed. New equipment will need to be requested for the student or a loaner device will need to be obtained. (See also information on troubleshooting technology in Chapter 9.)

11. What if the teacher of students with visual impairments or a parent does not agree with recommendations on the assistive technology evaluation?

Parents have the right to voice their concerns regarding any evaluation conducted on their child. It is in everyone's best interest to make sure that parents are involved in the assistive technology assessment from the very beginning of the process. If parents have been briefed as to the purpose of the assessment and the method of data collection, they will be less likely to challenge the results because they know and understand what is being evaluated. If the teacher of students with visual impairments does not agree with the recommendations on the assessment, concerns should be addressed in a professional manner with the individuals who conducted the evaluation. Again, if the teacher of students with visual impairments has been involved in the evaluation from the outset, concerns should be minimal. But, if over the course of the evaluation a new teacher of students with visual impairments started working with the student, the new teacher may not feel connected to the process yet. It is important to maintain open communication between the IEP team and the assistive technology evaluators—everyone has something to contribute. Discussing the differences of opinion may lead to either a reevaluation or revised recommendations.

12. How is assistive technology used when students undergo formal testing (such as state tests)? What assistive technology is typically allowed for statewide testing?

Use of assistive technology for statewide testing varies from state to state. If the student's IEP addresses the use of assistive technology for testing, then there is a better chance that the accommodation will be allowed. Check with your school district and state assessment office for information about what accommodations are allowed by your specific state.

13. Can a student use more than one device on a regular basis in school? For example, could a student have two desktop video magnifiers on different floors of a school plus a portable video magnifier?

The answer should be yes, as long as there is enough funding to buy all of the devices the student needs and if the results of the assistive technology evaluation support the need for several devices. There is typically no single piece of technology that can meet all of a student's needs. Depending on the task, one device may be used over another. For example, a student who reads print and braille may use a desktop video magnifier to complete math worksheets and a portable braille PDA to take notes in English class. The results of an assistive technology evaluation should indicate which devices are needed to complete various tasks. If we follow best practices, school districts will support the use of more than one device by making the tools available to students.

14. Our students are going to be using equipment in the science lab. Do you know of any technology that will help the student who is visually impaired see what we are doing?

In the past, it has been difficult for students with low vision to see what is going on in a dissection or under a microscope. However, advances in technology have made access to such activities much easier. Lab animals can be dissected under a video magnifier and viewed on an overhead monitor, on a separate monitor, or even on a computer monitor. Size, contrast, and color enhancements can make the image easier for the student with low vision to see. Similarly, advances in eyeglasses and magnifiers (such as spectacle-mounted magnifiers or head loupes) provide a low-tech solution for activities that require precision. A microscope can also be connected to a computer and then the image can be enlarged or enhanced using specialized software. Using distance magnification devices (such as telescopes or distance video magnifiers), the student with low vision can now see what is being presented or demonstrated at the front of the class without having to move closer to the teacher. (See Chapter 2 for further information regarding accessing information at a distance.)

For students who are blind, hands-on experiences combined with rich verbal descriptions of what is being observed under a microscope are still the most reliable and meaningful instructional methods of acquiring information. Technology has not reached a point yet where visual experiences such as dissections or chemistry experiments can be reproduced tactilely or auditorily for students who are blind; the student will have to participate in the activity, with supplemental tactile graphics, diagrams, and detailed written descriptions on hand to enhance the experience. Specific items, such as talking thermometers, stopwatches, and scales and tactile graphics have been created to help students who are blind participate in some science-related activities. Teachers should not assume that students who are blind cannot participate or contribute in science class.

15. What is NIMAS? Why do I need to know about it?

NIMAS stands for the National Instructional Materials Accessibility Standard (http://nimas.cast.org). NIMAS is defined in the 2004 reauthorization of IDEA, which stipulates that textbooks and instructional materials must be put in accessible formats for students who are visually impaired or print disabled. Publishers must put their files into a format defined by NIMAS, and the files are then stored in a central repository called the National Instructional Materials Access Center (NIMAC) at the American Printing House for the Blind. These files still need to be converted into the required accessible formats by an authorized entity. (See Chapter 5 for more information.)

—Carol Farrenkopf
Vision Program Coordinator
Toronto, Ontario, Canada

2

Technologies for Accessing Print Information

<table>
<tr><th colspan="2">CHAPTER OVERVIEW</th></tr>
<tr>
<td valign="top">

Accessing Print Information Visually

- Nonoptical Devices
- Optical Devices
- Video Magnification Systems
- Scanning and OCR Systems

Accessing Print Information Tactilely

- Braille
- Tactile Graphics
- Other Tactile Tools

</td>
<td valign="top">

Accessing Print Information Auditorily

- Readers
- Audio Recording
- Digital Audio Formats
- Reading Machines
- Other Auditory Tools

Accessing Print Information Presented from a Distance

- Electronic Whiteboards
- Overhead Projectors
- Computer Slideshow Projection Systems
- Video Display Systems

</td>
</tr>
</table>

Technology provides many tools that can be used by people who are blind or visually impaired to access information presented in print form. Examples of such information are books, newspapers, and magazines, of course, but also a teacher's photocopied homework assignment, a handwritten note, a calendar, and mail. "Print" covers material that is not in the form of text, such as pictures or mathematical equations, as well.

This chapter will provide basic information about the tools that can be used to gain access to print information and the tasks that can be accomplished with them. Low-tech and high-tech tools are available that allow individuals to access print through vision, touch, and hearing—that is, visually, tactilely, and auditorily. Some of these tools permit students to access the information directly, as it remains in print form, while others convert the information into an electronic format that can then be accessed in the way that is most appropriate for the user. Given the range of options that exist for readers who are visually impaired, as well as the individuality of the needs and abilities of visually impaired readers, selecting the appropriate tool involves careful consideration of what works best for this particular person, for this particular task, and at this particular time.

ACCESSING PRINT INFORMATION VISUALLY

Nonoptical Devices

- Large Print
- Reading Stands
- Acetate Overlays
- Lighting

Optical Devices

- Magnifiers
- Telescopes
- Principles of Optical Devices

Video Magnification Systems

- Desktop Video Magnifiers
- Flex-Arm Camera Models
- Portable Models with Handheld Cameras
- Head-Mounted Display Models
- Electronic Pocket Magnifiers
- Digital Imaging Systems

Scanning and OCR Systems

- Imaging Software
- Optical Character Recognition (OCR) Software
- Specialized Scanning Systems

In general, the majority of individuals with low vision (that is, those who have some usable vision), are able to see or read print information by using their sense of sight.

Technologies that assist people in accessing printed information visually, by supporting their use of vision, can be grouped into several broad categories:

- Nonoptical devices
- Optical devices
- Video magnifiers
- Electronic devices

At times, these categories overlap. Video magnifiers are actually both optical *and* electronic devices. Although they could be categorized either way, they have their own unique characteristics and so are presented in a separate category in this chapter.

The key point to remember about the devices to be discussed here is that no single device will meet all of an individual's needs for accessing print. Most individuals with low vision will require a variety of tools to efficiently access the wide range of printed information available in our modern society. The fundamental question that must be answered is, *What is the right tool for the individual and for the specific tasks that the individual wishes to accomplish?* Having a working knowledge of the features and options available in the different devices described in these sections will offer an idea of where to start. Making decisions about selecting appropriate tools after assessing an individual's abilities, preferences, and needs will be discussed in Chapter 8.

NONOPTICAL DEVICES

Some people assume that high-tech devices or expensive lenses are required to improve an individual's ability to read print visually. Yet there are a number of methods that students with low vision can use to access print that do not require expensive electronic or optical devices. Text or graphics can be *visually enhanced*—that is, they can be manipulated to cast a larger or better-defined image on the retina—without magnifying the image. This can be accomplished by

- making the material larger;
- bringing it closer to the eye;
- illuminating the material;
- changing the contrast between the print and the background against which it is displayed.

Devices and equipment that do not use lenses to magnify an image or enhance an individual's ability to see are often referred to as *nonoptical devices*. Nonoptical devices are devices or equipment that do not optically change the material being viewed. They include a wide range of items and materials, such as

- enlarged print;
- reading stands;
- colored acetate overlays (to increase contrast between text and background);

- additional lighting sources;
- devices that control lighting.

Large Print

Traditionally, large print has been defined as printed text produced in a minimum of 16-point or, more commonly, in either 18-point or 24-point print. The larger two of these three sizes are most often used for large-print books, but with the use of computers, word-processing software, and printers, text can easily be produced in a variety of fonts and point sizes in order to meet the needs of individual users. Commercially produced large-print books and other materials can be expensive and are often produced in large formats that make them cumbersome to use and transport. With today's computer word-processing programs, however, as well as with other methods that will be covered later in this chapter (and in more detail in Chapter 5), teachers and students can produce large-print materials in any desired point and font size on standard 8½ × 11 inch paper.

Books in large print are one nonoptical tool for accessing print, here used along with a desk lamp and a notebook serving as an informal reading stand.

L. Penny Rosenblum

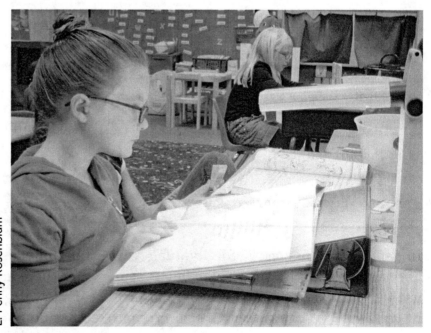

Reading Stands

Reading stands, both tabletop models and floor-standing models, allow the user to place the material to be viewed at the reader's optimum viewing angle and distance. Reading stands are useful, flexible, and low-cost tools that can bring material closer to the reader, so that he or she can maintain better posture and not become fatigued.

Acetate Overlays

Some individuals with low vision find that light-colored sheets of acetate can be helpful when placed over printed materials to increase their visibility. For example, a transparent yellow acetate sheet used in this way will increase the contrast between the print and the background against which it is displayed, making the print easier to read. Acetate sheets are sold in office supply stores for use with overhead projectors or in stores that provide theater lighting (where they are called "gels") and are available in many colors.

Lighting

Lighting is a critical factor in enhancing visibility. Some students will benefit greatly from additional lighting when performing various tasks. Others may be light sensitive and will benefit instead from adjusted lighting and efforts to reduce glare. Additional lighting—incandescent, fluorescent, halogen, or LED (light-emitting diode)—from lamps or permanent fixtures may be helpful when viewing printed materials. In addition, the ability to control the intensity and directionality of natural lighting through the use of filters, shades, and blinds is beneficial to many students who access information visually.

Helpful items such as sun visors, black felt-tipped markers, and bold-line paper are considered nonoptical devices as well. Nonoptical devices are often overlooked but can be very valuable when used alone or in combination with optical and electronic devices. (For additional information on nonoptical devices and the importance of their use, see Jose, 1983; Quillman & Goodrich, 2004; Wilkinson, 1996, 2000; and Zimmerman, 1996.)

OPTICAL DEVICES

Devices that magnify, reduce, or otherwise change the shape of the image of material

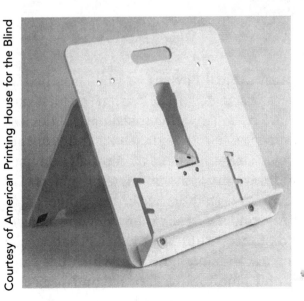

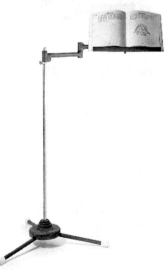

Book or reading stands, either desktop (left) or floor models (right), place reading materials in a more comfortable position for viewing.

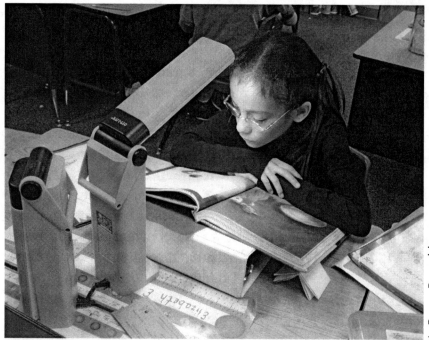

L. Penny Rosenblum

Courtesy of Independent Living Aids

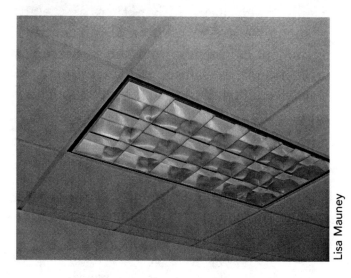

Lisa Mauney

Desk lamps, floor lamps, and overhead lighting with filters can all help students with low vision to control illumination to suit their individual needs.

being viewed through the use of lenses are referred to as *optical devices* (Zimmerman, 1996, p. 116). Optical devices, both manual and electronic (such as video magnifiers, which will be discussed in the next section), comprise a wide variety of tools designed to help people with low vision read print and view small objects. Optical devices need to be prescribed by a low vision professional based on the results of a clinical low vision evaluation.

Most optical devices can be classified as devices used for near vision or distance vision. The most widely used optical devices are spectacles (eyeglasses) and contact lenses. Other types of optical devices include *magnifiers*, for viewing objects at near range—that is, within a range of 16 inches—and *telescopes*, for viewing objects at a distance—that is, at ranges that exceed 16 inches. Video magnifiers, which use cameras and monitors to capture and project a

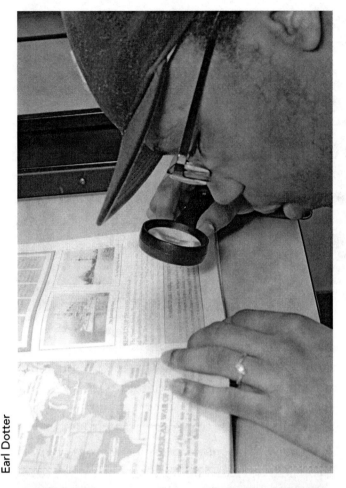

Earl Dotter

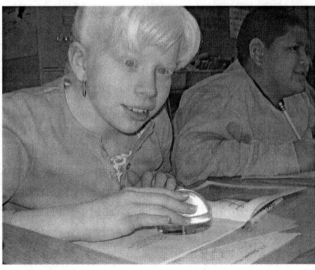

L. Penny Rosenblum

magnified image, are often classified as optical devices as well. Since they are also electronic devices, they will be described in their own section later in this chapter.

Magnifiers

Magnifiers use lenses to increase the size of the image entering the eye (Zimmerman, 1996, p. 127). They are available in various sizes, shapes, and powers of magnification and may or may not have built-in lighting. Many individuals find handheld and stand magnifiers beneficial for near-vision tasks, such as reading. *Handheld magnifiers* provide a great deal of flexibility, but require some coordination and strength to use. *Stand magnifiers* sit over the material to be viewed and do not need to be held, thus providing a fixed distance between the lens and the reading material that does not have to be maintained by the effort of the user.

Telescopes

Devices that enhance distance vision include binocular and monocular telescopes. (See "Accessing Print Information Presented from a Distance" later in this chapter for more information on options for distance vision.) These devices can be either handheld or mounted in spectacle frames. Binocular and monocular telescopes are available in various sizes and powers of magnification. Although most have a fixed power of magnification, some are able to zoom in and out, changing the level of magnification. Most telescopes can also be focused to view objects at different distances. Improvements in the

Handheld magnifiers (top) are excellent for short reading tasks, but holding them at a fixed distance from the page can be difficult for some individuals. Stand magnifiers, like this dome magnifier (bottom), can be easier to use because they are placed directly on the page, but may require additional lighting to be most effective.

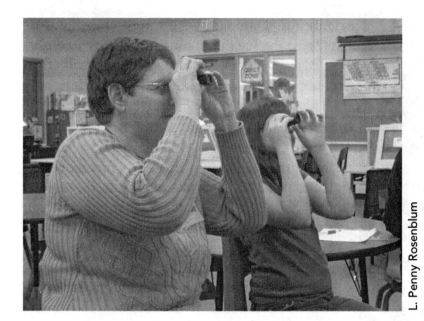

This teacher is helping her student learn to use a telescope to view posters on the other side of the classroom.

L. Penny Rosenblum

field of optics have provided many options for spectacle- and head-mounted telescopic systems—those worn either as part of spectacle frames or on separate frames worn directly by the user—that offer a wide variety of sizes, styles, and powers of magnification. Some telescopes can be fitted with *reading caps*, which are added to the end of a telescope to convert it to a *telemicroscope* and allow the user to view reading materials at an intermediate distance of 16 to 18 inches (Zimmerman, 1996, p. 170).

The electronic telescope is similar to a video camera, except that it does not record information. The device is held up to the user's eye like a manual telescope or monocular. The electronic components allow the user to zoom in or out on the object to be viewed. In addition, the unit has a brightness/contrast control that can enhance viewing in darkened environments, such as an auditorium or theater. Most of the benefits of this tool can be achieved by using an ordinary digital video camera (as discussed later in this chapter in "Accessing Print Information Presented from a Distance"). The handheld

electronic telescope is no longer in production, but there are still people using this device who find it quite helpful.

Principles of Optical Devices

Because of the many complex factors related to optical devices and because they have to be matched to an individual's visual abilities and needs, they need to be prescribed by an expert—a specialist in low vision who conducts a thorough clinical low vision examination. However, teachers who work with students who have low vision may wish to familiarize their students with various kinds of devices so they are better prepared for their visit to the low vision specialist for a low vision evaluation (Cowan & Shepler, 2000). Although most practitioners will have a limited array of optical devices on hand, it can still be beneficial for their students to be exposed to, and to experiment with, them. Students who have had some basic exposure to various types of optical devices and how they work may be better prepared to work with a low vision specialist to determine which devices will best meet their needs.

Two important properties of low vision devices that are helpful for both teachers and students to understand are *focal distance* and *working distance*.

Focal distance is the distance from the material being viewed to the lens of the optical device when the image is in focus—that is, the optimal distance from the lens to the material (Simons & LaPolice, 2000).

The focal distance of a lens determines how close the device needs to be held to the object.

Working distance is the distance from the viewer's eye to the object or reading material that is needed for the viewer to see the magnified image in focus (Dister & Greer, 2004; Greer, 2004).

Close working distances—when the individual needs to be just a few inches from the reading material—can be uncomfortable and tiring. Determining a comfortable working distance will be important and will vary from student to student depending on the focal distance of the device being used as well as such factors as the student's height and size. In general, lenses mounted in spectacles tend to have shorter focal distances than do handheld magnifiers. It is important that individuals working with a student using an optical device, particularly spectacles that have a fixed focal distance, understand that this distance must be maintained to achieve a "clear" image on the retina. Moving closer to the reading material (decreasing the working distance) will not improve the student's ability to see the information. In fact, if the proper focal distance is not maintained, the image will be less clear and become unreadable.

There are three other principles about the use of optical devices that are important to understand when selecting appropriate devices for students with low vision:

- When magnification is increased, the field of view is decreased.
- Increased magnification generally requires increased illumination.
- Training is required for the most effective use of these devices.

Field of View

The laws of physics dictate that when an image is magnified, the portion of that image that can be viewed at any one time is decreased. In other words, as the image gets bigger, the amount that can be seen gets smaller. The area that can be viewed through a magnifier at any one time is often referred to as the device's *field of view*.

Many students will at first choose near and distance optical devices that provide the highest possible levels of magnification. As they begin to use a device, however, they may become aware of the decreased field of view available and learn to select devices that provide an adequate level of magnification while offering the greatest field of view. They may also learn to select devices of different powers for different tasks. Understanding this factor can be very helpful for students and low vision specialists in determining the most appropriate optical devices for various viewing tasks.

Lighting

Viewing images or objects under increased magnification generally requires additional lighting. Lighting is a critical factor when using many stand magnifiers, some handheld magnifiers, and most distance optical devices because the available light can be blocked by the stand holding the magnifier, the user's hands, and even the user's head and body. Distance viewing devices may not work well in dimly lit environments or when viewing poorly lit targets. Providing additional lighting and controlling the available light, as explained earlier, are options that can improve the effectiveness of optical devices (Flom, 2004; Quillman & Goodrich, 2004; Watson & Berg, 1983; Wilkinson, 2000; Zimmerman, 1996).

Training

It is important to realize that effective use of optical devices requires training and practice. A teacher should not assume that because a device has been prescribed, the student will automatically know how to use it well—or at all. Parents and teachers may not understand why devices sit unused in a student's backpack or desk, when the problem is that the student is simply unable to make good use of them. Direct instruction is needed from a certified low vision therapist or a teacher of students who are visually impaired in using the device to spot, focus, scan, track, and shift gaze. Frequent opportunities for the student to practice are also needed, until the student can do these things independently and automatically. Support and understanding are important as well, because many students may feel self-conscious or uncomfortable in using prescribed devices.

VIDEO MAGNIFICATION SYSTEMS

Video magnification systems make use of electronics and video cameras to produce a magnified image. Although they contain lenses and are often classified as optical devices, they function very differently than magnifiers and telescopes. These systems provide users with a tool that enlarges reading material sufficiently for them to maintain a comfortable posture and view the materials at a comfortable distance. Although they are often referred to as closed-circuit television systems (CCTVs), this term is also used for closed-circuit televisions used in many security systems, which are used differently. To avoid any confusion, the term *video magnifier* will be used in this text.

Video magnifiers work by using a camera to capture the image of the material to be viewed and then projecting an enlarged version on a television screen or monitor. A zoom lens on the camera allows the user to vary the magnification or size of the image being displayed. There are many varieties of video magnifiers, ranging from traditional large desktop models to electronic pocket magnifiers that can be carried in a backpack or purse, but all have the camera and screen in common.

Early models of video magnifiers had few features and were relatively expensive, thus limiting their appeal. These models only offered black and white (dark on light) images that could be manipulated electronically to display a reversed or negative image (light on dark). High-resolution monitors offered brightness and contrast control of the image being displayed, but these models were relatively expensive. At first, viewing materials were simply moved around the tabletop underneath the camera. Many additional features have been developed in response to users' needs that have increased the usefulness of these systems for individuals with low vision. Features found on video magnifiers today as well as considerations for their selection and use are presented in Sidebar 2.1, "Features Commonly Found in Video Magnifiers", and discussed throughout this chapter.

FEATURES COMMONLY FOUND IN VIDEO MAGNIFIERS

Video magnifiers offer a variety of useful features beyond their basic function of displaying a magnified image. The specific features vary depending on the type of video magnifier as well as the manufacturer's offerings in a given model. Deciding which features students need on a video magnifier requires careful consideration of the tasks that they need to accomplish. Students who need to read information at a distance—for example, on chalkboards in several different classrooms—will need a video magnifier with distance viewing capabilities and portability.

Reverse polarity: Reverse polarity (positive/negative image) allows the user to select a display that features light text on a dark background instead of the typical black text on a white background. This is also known as a *negative image*. This feature can make a significant difference for some users in the ability to read efficiently. When using reverse polarity, some individuals find it necessary to readjust the brightness and contrast settings on the video magnifier. Some of the newer models make this adjustment automatically.

Color camera: Color has become such an important tool in educational materials that most students will need access to a color video magnifier. Color cameras provide more accurate renderings of information presented in a graphical format, such as photographs, diagrams, and drawings, and can increase the user's interest in viewing real objects. Black-and-white units are less expensive, but in most cases they will not be adequate. Students and individuals who need a video magnifier only for reading text may find a black-and-white model acceptable.

False color: Many readers find it easier to read when they can choose the color of the text and background. Sometimes referred to as *false color*, this feature provides the user the option to select the color of the text being viewed and the color of the background. It works in conjunction with the polarity feature of most video magnifiers. For example, one viewer might choose to read yellow text on a dark blue background, but another might prefer dark blue text on a light blue background. Because of the individuality of various visual impairments, this feature gives the user the ability to fine-tune the image being viewed to meet his or her specific visual needs.

Viewing modes: Video magnifiers may offer several viewing modes, including near, distance, self-portrait, and freeze-frame.

- *Near viewing* is the most common viewing mode.
- *Distance viewing* is available on models that allow the user to rotate the unit's camera.
- Several of the models that provide flexible camera movement also have a *self-portrait* feature. This feature allows the user to rotate the camera and point it at oneself. It can be very beneficial for activities such as grooming.

(continued on next page)

- The *freeze-frame* feature allows the user to freeze an image on the monitor as though a picture had been taken. The material being viewed can then be removed from under the camera, while the enlarged image is still visible on the monitor. This feature is especially helpful for reading directions on food packaging and other items.

Focus options: Most video magnifiers today have an *autofocus* feature. Auto-focusing is particularly useful for reading at a distance and on curved surfaces, such as a prescription bottle or the curves caused by the spine of an open book. However, there are older models still in use that require the user to focus the image to improve its clarity. For some activities, particularly handwriting, autofocus can be annoying. The unit may be focused on the page, but when the user places a pencil under the camera, it might refocus on the pencil or the user's hand. The abrupt switches in focus can be confusing to some users. Better quality models offer the option of placing the unit in a manual focusing mode for writing and similar tasks.

X-Y table: The X-Y table, which is found mainly in desktop models, provides a surface on which the material to be viewed can be placed and moved around easily underneath the camera. It usually consists of a rectangular piece of wood or plastic mounted on moveable tracks. It is placed underneath the camera on the tabletop. The X-Y table permits the reading material to be moved in a smooth and steady motion. Some models come with a motorized tray that moves automatically at a preset speed; this feature may be good for students who have physical disabilities, but it is fairly complex to set.

Line features: *Electronic blinds, masks,* and *occluders* provide users with tools to control the amount of text visible on the screen at any one time. These features allow users to block off certain areas of the display with black masks and leave viewable only the line of text that they are currently reading. This feature is beneficial to readers who have difficulty with visually tracking the same line of text from left to right. Another tracking tool found on some models is an *underline* feature. While not as dramatic as the mask, it does offer assistance for readers with milder tracking needs.

Monitor type and size: Liquid crystal display (LCD) monitors are becoming the preferred and standard choice for monitors. A larger monitor will allow more information to be displayed on the screen than a smaller monitor at any given magnification. Larger may not always be better. Shorter users may have difficulty seeing to the edges of the monitor. Monitors mounted on flexible or adjustable arms offer the best placement options for ideal viewing. Portable units offer smaller monitors that may not be adequate for users requiring higher levels of magnification.

Laptop compatibility: Several manufacturers have developed systems that connect to a laptop computer and use its monitor for the camera's magnified display. With this computer connection comes the opportunity for many additional features depending on the software added to the computer. These include a digital imaging system that eliminates the need to move the reading material under the camera, the use of optical character recognition (OCR) software to create an editable document, and the use of text-to-speech software to provide an audio reading of the text.

Computer compatibility: Computer compatibility allows a video magnifier and a computer to share a monitor. Note that these units do not magnify the computer image, only the image coming from the unit's camera. They simply allow the user to switch the view from the camera to the computer, or have a split screen displaying both images.

Twin camera system: Some systems have separate cameras for near and distance viewing, with a switch or keyboard command to allow the user to rapidly change the display from one to the other.

Other special features: Additional features offered on some models include a separate control pad for an internal clock, calendar, and calculator function.

Source: Adapted in part from F. M. D'Andrea. (2000). Activities and games for teaching children to use a CCTV. In D'Andrea and C. Farrenkopf (Eds.), *Looking to learn: Promoting literacy for students with low vision* (Sidebar 7.3, pp. 197–198). New York: AFB Press.

Video magnifiers are an extremely important tool for individuals who have low vision because they allow the user to view a variety of materials, including small objects; printed or handwritten text; and graphical materials, including photographs, drawings, diagrams, graphs, and maps. They also may help students with writing by enabling them to view their own handwriting and the paper or form they are writing on (see Chapter 4). They offer a number of advantages compared to traditional handheld or stand magnifiers, including the following:

- A higher degree and wider range of magnification than can be achieved practically with traditional magnifiers
- Reverse polarity—the ability to view light text on a dark background instead of dark text on light background—which cannot be obtained with a traditional magnifier
- The ability to function in a wider variety of lighting conditions (Most video magnifiers are equipped with a light source and do not require an external light source as do traditional magnifiers.)

Video magnifiers are particularly valuable equipment for school systems because they can be used by students with low vision of various ages and with varying visual conditions.

Most video magnifier models offer a wide range of magnification. However, some are more limited, and educators need to be careful when selecting a model to be certain that its level of magnification will be adequate for a particular student's needs. Learning more about this versatile tool will assist them in determining the best fit for each individual student.

The type and size of the system's monitor are other important considerations when matching a device to a student's needs. Although a larger monitor will allow more information to be displayed on the screen at any given magnification than a smaller monitor, larger may not always be better. Shorter students may have difficulty seeing to the edges of a large monitor. Conversely, the smaller monitors that portable units offer may not be adequate for users who require higher levels of magnification. Systems with monitors mounted on flexible or adjustable arms offer the most placement options for ideal viewing (see "Flex-Arm Camera Models" later in this chapter). In some cases, video magnifiers can be connected to a television or a laptop computer to make use of that equipment's screen.

One of the more difficult aspects of reading or viewing material with a video magnifier is shifting the camera's field of view from one part of the item to the next, since the magnified image shows only a small portion of the material at one time. With traditional desktop models, where the camera is in a fixed position, this is accomplished by moving the material so that the viewer can track a line of print from one side to the other and back again. The solution to doing this in a controlled fashion has been a moveable surface or tray, known as the *X-Y table*, on which the material to be viewed is placed. Efficient use of the X-Y table requires considerable training and practice, as explained in Sidebar 2.2, "The X-Y Table." With some of the newer, handheld models, the user moves the camera across the text rather than moving the reading material under the camera.

Numerous developments and advances in the production of video magnifiers have resulted in a variety of available models that can be divided into six broad categories:

- Desktop models
- Flex-arm camera models
- Portable models, using handheld cameras
- Head-mounted display models
- Pocket models
- Digital imaging systems

Some individual models have features from more than one category, but in general most models fit into one of the categories described in the following sections. For a quick comparison of various models, see Table 2.1 ("Advantages and Disadvantages of Different Types of Video Magnifiers"). For additional information on video magnifiers and a comparison of various models, see the *AccessWorld Guide to Assistive Technology Products*, published by AFB Press, and the Resources section at the end of this book.

Desktop Video Magnifiers

Desktop video magnifiers were the first video magnification systems to appear on the market and are still popular. These stand-alone models have a fixed or mounted camera, an X-Y table on which to place the material to be viewed, and a separate monitor. Desktop models have the widest range of magnification and features and are generally among the easiest to use, despite their size, lack of portability, and expense. Most of the controls are simple and straightforward, and most of the advanced features of video magnifiers listed in Sidebar 2.1 are found in today's desktop video magnifiers.

Placement of the monitor is a key concern when setting up a desktop video magnifier for a student. (See Sidebar 2.3, "Setting Up a Desktop Video Magnifier Workstation," for detailed information.) When the monitor is placed on the tabletop

THE X-Y TABLE

The X-Y table solves the problem of how to smoothly and efficiently move reading material under the camera of a video magnifier with a fixed camera. The X-Y table is a rectangular piece of wood or plastic mounted on moveable tracks and placed underneath the camera on the tabletop. The reading material placed on the X-Y table can then be moved in a smooth and steady motion in four directions: right, left, up, and down.

Effectively controlling the X-Y table is a key factor in the successful use of a video magnifier. Users often have difficulty keeping the table (and the reading material) from moving up and down while moving it from right to left to read text. This movement results in a wavy line of text that appears to be moving in two directions simultaneously on the screen, which can cause some users to experience nausea or seasickness. Others find it difficult to locate the beginning and end of lines of text. With material that has multiple columns, it is particularly easy to slip accidentally into the wrong column. Efficient use of the X-Y table is a motor skill that can be acquired through guided practice. Two features of X-Y tables allow the user to adjust and control its movement: the *friction brake* and *margin stops*.

Friction brake: A friction brake adjustment controls the amount of force that the user must exert to move the X-Y table in or out, thus moving the text up and down on the display screen. With practice, fine tuning the friction brake allows the user to move the reading material horizontally while maintaining a line parallel to the bottom or top of the monitor, thus easing the seasickness reported by some users. The proper adjustment prevents unwanted vertical movement as it allows easy movement up or down lines of text when needed.

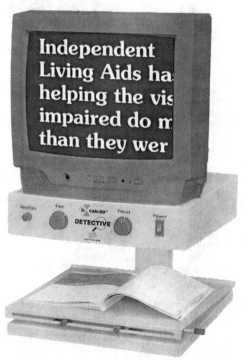

Courtesy of Independent Living Aids

The friction brake, here located on the right-hand side of the X-Y table, allows the user to control up and down movement of the text.

Margin stops: Margin stops are another feature of some X-Y tables that help when reading text with multiple columns. The margin stops control the boundaries or limits of the left and right movement of the X-Y table, so that the reader does not move from one column into another. When

(continued on next page)

SIDEBAR 2.2 (CONTINUED)

properly adjusted, the margin stops improve reading efficiency because the reader does not have to visually determine the boundaries of the column being read

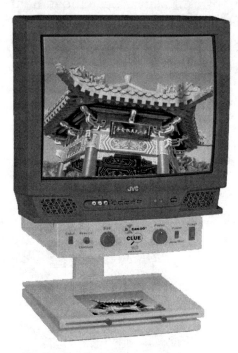

Courtesy of Independent Living Aids

The margin stops on the front of this X-Y table can be set for different column widths, improving the user's efficiency when reading.

or waste time viewing text out of order in the next or preceding columns.

Motorized X-Y tables: Students with additional disabilities may not become as efficient with the X-Y table, depending on the level of their motor skill development. However, guided practice should help them improve. Some students may do better with a motorized or automatic X-Y table, whose tray moves automatically at a preset speed. The user can set the rate at which the table moves to a comfortable reading speed and can set the margins for the left and right movement of the table. Motorized tables are expensive and not widely available, but for some users with limited motor abilities, they can make a huge difference in their ability to use a video magnifier successfully. Some models of video magnifiers no longer have the friction brake and margin stop features. Readers who do not use their video magnifier for extended continuous text reading may not miss these features, but for those who do, these two features can increase their efficiency and comfort level, which in turn can affect their willingness to use the video magnifier.

beside the camera, the user has to move the material to be viewed under the camera to one side while viewing the display straight on. The ergonomics of this arrangement (that is, the physical effects on the individual of the combination of the equipment setup and the work he or she is doing) can lead to physical fatigue in some users. Mounting the monitor over the camera, known as in-line viewing, is a better design for many users. However, in-line systems require thoughtful decisions about setup and location, so that

the monitor is at a comfortable viewing height and angle for the user. Users should be able to view the center of the monitor without having to tilt their heads back. Setting up an ergonomic in-line system for a small child can be particularly challenging, since the monitor cannot be too high for the child and therefore will need to be fairly close to the X-Y table, which can make it difficult for the child to write or turn the pages of a book under the video magnifier. This situation may require the use of an adjustable

Table 2.1   Advantages and Disadvantages of Different Types of Video Magnifiers

Type of Video Magnifier	Advantages	Disadvantages
Desktop models	Widest range of magnification levels Widest range of features Durable Easy to use	Not portable Takes up a good deal of desk space Usually the most expensive models
Flex-arm camera models	Both distance and near viewing available Fairly portable Variety of display options available	Requires time to set up and break down Need to carry monitor Need to carry X-Y table
Portable handheld camera models	Portable Less expensive Some models can connect to TV	Difficult to use handheld camera Limited range of magnification available Need to carry monitor for some models Difficult to perform handwriting tasks
Head-mounted display models	Portable Both distance and near viewing available Light amplification feature available	Unusual appearance Can be difficult to use Difficult to perform handwriting tasks Can feel awkward or heavy when worn for extended time
Electronic pocket models	Small Portable	Small range of magnification levels available Need to maneuver camera Difficult to perform handwriting tasks Some have short battery life
Digital imaging systems	Do not have to maneuver materials under camera Can view text in column, row, or single word display Many models have high-contrast color feature	Viewing graphics must be done in a "live camera" mode, in which other text viewing options are not available Difficult to perform handwriting tasks Text printed over a varying color background does not display well

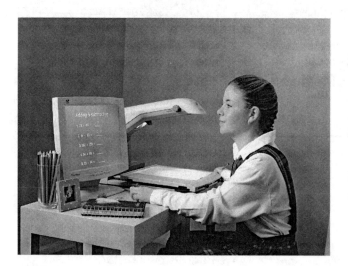
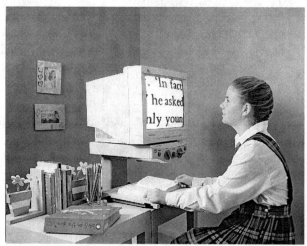

When a desktop video magnifier is set up with the monitor and camera side by side (left), it can be tiring for the student to shift her gaze from the monitor to write on the paper and back again. A desktop video magnifier with in-line viewing (right) can be a more comfortable arrangement if it is adjusted correctly.

table whose height can be varied for each individual user and for the task that the child is performing. As this illustrates, the way that physical factors and ergonomics affect the comfortable use of video magnifiers and other technology tools—and therefore the student's success in using them—cannot be overemphasized.

Many individuals who use video magnifiers also need to use a computer for school or work. The need for two separate monitors in this situation could overflow a workspace that is already crowded with other assistive technology devices. Most of the major manufacturers of video magnifiers

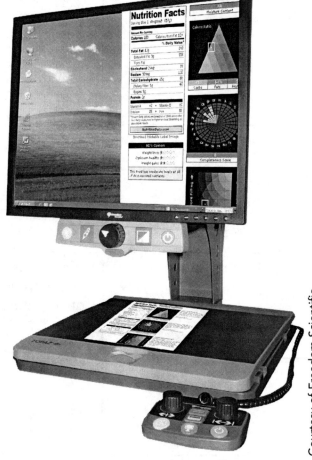

This desktop video magnifier is connected to a computer. Its monitor displays both the magnified camera image (the nutrition facts and accompanying graphics) and an unmagnified image from the computer's desktop.

SETTING UP A DESKTOP VIDEO MAGNIFIER WORKSTATION

The ideal desktop video magnifier workstation is set up so that the user can sit in a comfortable position and not become fatigued as he or she reads or writes. The monitor should be positioned so that the student's head does not tilt backward or downward while looking at it. The X-Y table should be at a height that allows the student to move the tray smoothly without straining his or her arms and also enables the student to write comfortably under the camera.

Setting Up a Fixed Unit

When setting up a workstation in which the video magnifier is a fixed unit, whose base, X-Y table, camera, and monitor cannot be adjusted, consider the following:

- Determine whether the video magnifier will be used primarily as a reading or writing tool for the student.
- If the video magnifier is to be used primarily for reading long passages of text, ensure that the student's gaze is sustained at or slightly above the middle of the monitor. A height-adjustable table and chair can be manipulated so that the monitor is positioned appropriately. However, in this position, the X-Y

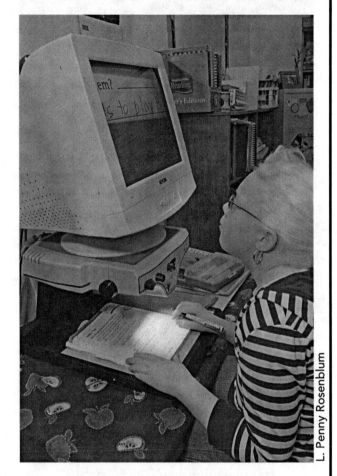

L. Penny Rosenblum

This video magnifier setup is not ergonomically appropriate for this student; her gaze is well below the middle of the monitor, so that she has to keep her neck bent backwards to look up.

table will likely be too low for the student to write on comfortably.
- If the video magnifier is to be used primarily for writing, position the adjustable table and chair so that the student's elbows are bent at about 90 degrees ("L" shaped). This will reduce strain on the arms while writing on the X-Y table. However, the monitor may then be positioned

(continued on next page)

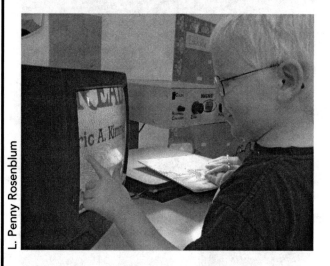

L. Penny Rosenblum

This video magnifier is adjusted properly for the viewer: the student's gaze is slightly above the middle of the monitor.

too high for the student, who will have to tilt his or her head backward to view what has been written.

Setting Up an Adjustable Unit

If the student's video magnifier is not a fixed unit and various parts of the unit can be adjusted, then consider the following when setting up a workstation:

- Adjust the monitor so that the student's gaze is centered at or slightly above the middle of the monitor.
- Adjust the X-Y table so that the student's arms will be "L" shaped when writing under the video magnifier or when moving the X-Y table. Note that the student's arms should not be completely extended or straight when writing under the unit or when moving the X-Y table.

- Use a height-adjustable table or chair as needed.
- Teach the student how to adjust the device as needed for reading or writing tasks. Since desktop video magnifiers can be quite heavy, it is best to have an adult make changes to the workstation for younger students.

For All Types of Video Magnifiers

- Make sure that the student's feet are flat on the floor. Smaller children may need a footrest if their feet do not touch the ground.
- Position the workstation so that light from overhead lamps or windows does not reflect directly on the monitor.
- Avoid placing the workstation directly in front of a large bank of windows, as the light from behind the workstation may interfere with the student's ability to focus on the monitor.
- Ensure that enough table space is available next to the video magnifier for the student's books and other materials.
- Be cognizant of the position of the monitor in relation to other students in the classroom when it comes to test taking. Students may not want their work and test responses to be easily seen by their classmates.

Carol Farrenkopf, Vision Program Coordinator
Toronto, Ontario, Canada

offer computer-compatible models that can be connected to the computer monitor, allowing the computer and the video magnifier to share the same monitor, as noted in Sidebar 2.1. The video magnifier unit has a switch to control the image going to the monitor, which can be set to display the image from the computer, the image from the video magnifier, or in some models, one of the images on the top and the other image on the bottom of a split screen. It is important to note that the image from the computer will not automatically be enlarged in this situation; the user will need to run a screen magnification program on the computer to enlarge its display. (See Chapter 3 for information on screen magnification software.)

Most computer users choose to place their monitors directly behind their keyboards, leaving the camera off to the side. If this arrangement is chosen, however, the ergonomic benefit of in-line viewing is lost. In-line viewing can be maintained by placing the monitor on top of the video magnifier and installing a pullout keyboard tray under the work surface or using a wireless keyboard that can be placed on the student's lap. This arrangement will be adequate for some users to give them access to the computer keyboard, the X-Y table, and the controls for the video magnifier. In setting up this arrangement, it is again important to make sure that the height of the equipment allows the user to have a comfortable viewing angle to decrease physical fatigue. An occupational therapist can be of great assistance in determining the best arrangement of the computer and video magnifier, a perfect example of the need for a team approach to assessing the technology needs of students, which was stressed in Chapter 1 and will be further discussed in Chapter 6.

Since it is often difficult to quickly locate the desired area for viewing when a user places something on the X-Y table, some manufacturers have provided a red light that focuses on a set spot under the camera. The red light pinpoints where to place the material so that it can be easily located and viewed.

In an effort to increase the usefulness of video magnifiers, some manufacturers have sought to combine tools that a user might like to have all together in one place. The introduction of an enlarged calculator function can assist individuals wishing to use their video magnifiers to keep banking records. The numbers and operations of the calculator are displayed on the screen and the user has control over the size of the numbers. In addition, some models have an enlarged electronic clock and a calendar that can be displayed on the screen.

Desktop models offer the widest variety of features and in most cases the greatest ease of use, which makes them ideal for elementary school classrooms where young students spend most of their day. Because video magnifiers have proved to be such valuable tools for students with low vision, many students and their teachers would like to use them in all of their classrooms. However, transporting the equipment from room to room is challenging. Teachers and students have devised numerous creative systems to provide basic mobility, but none have been an ideal solution. The usual problem is with rolling carts that become top heavy when a video magnifier is sitting on them or when the unit is not securely fastened to the cart. In such cases, the video magnifier can end up falling or sliding off—a dangerous situation at best.

This lack of portability is one of the greatest disadvantages of desktop video magnifiers, for adults as well as students, along with their inability to allow the user to perform distance viewing. The ideal device would be a video magnifier that could be carried easily from place to place, offers both near and distance viewing, and has the same variety of features as a desktop model. Many manufacturers have attempted to design this perfect tool, but to date no one has completely succeeded. As demonstrated in the following sections on other types of video magnifiers, however, many improvements have been made in the areas of portability, near viewing, and distance viewing.

Flex-Arm Camera Models

The flex-arm camera video magnifier is a variation of the desktop model in which the mounted camera can be rotated or moved around to view materials. Flex-arm camera models are more versatile than standard desktop models because they can be used for both near and distance viewing. The camera can be positioned over an X-Y table or some other flat surface for near viewing and then rotated for distance viewing—for example, to see a whiteboard or chalkboard

in a classroom. Flex-arm camera models can be configured as either desktop or portable systems. The lightweight camera and stand can be disassembled, placed in a case, and transported to other locations. However, these systems still need a separate display monitor, unlike some of the portable and pocket models that will be discussed later, which often restricts their portability.

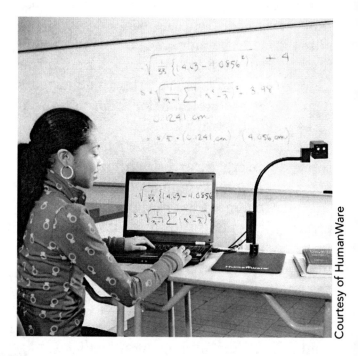

This student (top) uses a flex-arm camera video magnifier to view mathematical equations written on the whiteboard in her classroom. The same device can also be used for reading books and other materials (right).

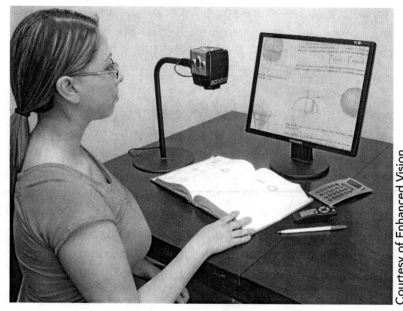

Courtesy of HumanWare

Courtesy of Enhanced Vision

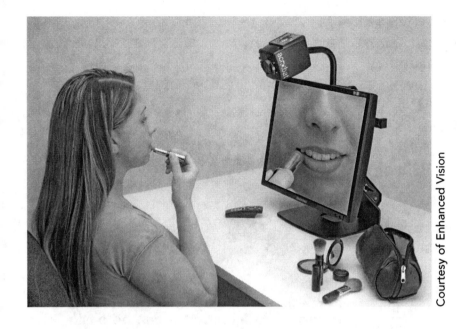

This flex-arm camera video magnifier has the camera mounted on the monitor and can be used for inter-mediate distance tasks such as applying makeup.

Courtesy of Enhanced Vision

In the early models of video magnifiers, before the advent of in-line viewing, the camera was mounted on a stand over the X-Y table. One advantage of this arrangement was that the camera could be rotated 90 degrees and pointed at a chalkboard or other display for distance viewing. However, this feature proved difficult for many users. The availability of cameras with autofocusing has made the use of video magnifiers for reading information displayed at a distance more feasible, since automatic focusing eliminates the need to spend time adjusting and focusing the camera. (See "Accessing Print Information at a Distance" later in this chapter for more information on distance viewing.) Even with autofocusing, many individuals still find it difficult to move the camera efficiently from side to side to read at a distance. However, some students are able to master the physical coordination required to read material at a

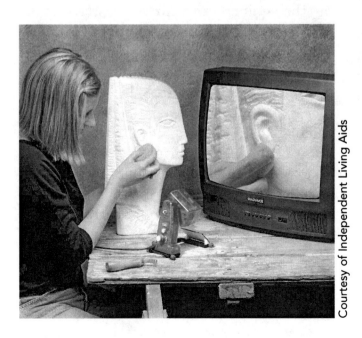

Courtesy of Independent Living Aids

This artist appreciates the flexibility of a rotating camera, which can be used for near, intermediate, or distance viewing, when working on small details of her sculpture.

distance—for example, writing on a white-board or chalkboard—and copy it onto paper while using the video magnifier. Autofocusing is also very useful for near reading on curved surfaces such as a prescription bottle or the curves caused by the spine of an open book.

Portable Models with Handheld Cameras

Portable video magnifiers rely on a handheld camera that the user rolls or slides over the material he or she wishes to have magnified, which then sends the image to a separate small monitor or another display, such as a television. These types of video magnifiers work well for spot reading or tasks of short duration but tend to be inefficient for longer assignments and continuous reading.

Models that connect to a television or external monitor include the appropriate

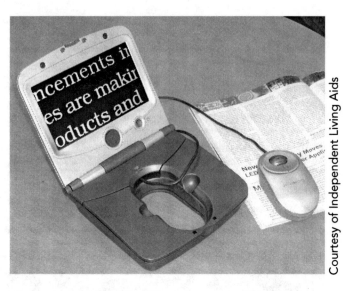

Portable video magnifier models that include a small monitor can be easily transported for use in a wide array of settings.

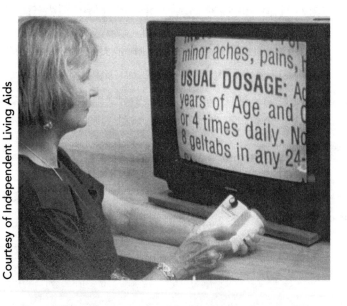

Some portable models of video magnifiers with a handheld cameras connect to a standard television, providing an inexpensive option for spot reading and short reading tasks.

cables and power supply with the camera and can be transported easily in the accompanying case. Although these devices are portable, their use relies on the availability of a monitor or television in each location where the system will be used. The logistics of connecting to a monitor or television and locating the equipment within a classroom make it a less-than-desirable solution for many students, although in some situations, it can be useful. If a television or unused computer monitor is readily available in various class-rooms, this type of video magnifier could be a useful tool for some students who need to accomplish tasks requiring only spot reading.

Some portable video magnifiers include a 9- or 10-inch monitor with a handheld camera, which fits into a carrying case about the size of a large briefcase. This type of unit is light enough to be quite portable. The downside of these systems is the small size of the display and the coordination required to manipulate the handheld camera effectively. Other models that connect to a laptop computer offer the use of a somewhat larger monitor but require the user to obtain and transport a laptop in addition to the video magnifier.

Head-Mounted Display Models

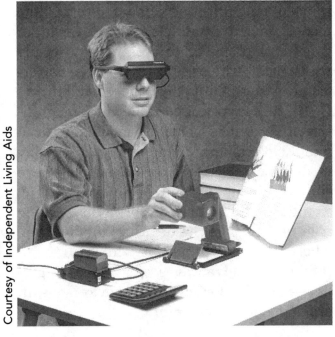

Head-mounted display video magnifiers increase portability by eliminating the need to transport a monitor.

Head-mounted display systems offer an additional option for portability. The user wears the unit like a pair of spectacles or goggles while rolling a handheld camera over the material to be viewed. A cable connected to the camera carries the signal to a control unit that is connected by an additional cable to two small displays positioned inside the goggles directly in front of each of the user's eyes. At this distance from the eyes, the image can be manipulated electronically so that it appears as large as it would on a desktop monitor. This type of system eliminates the need for an external monitor, thus providing a degree of portability. Rechargeable batteries and an adapter to plug into a wall socket allow these systems to be used in a wide variety of locations. However, the weight and appearance of the goggles detracts from the appeal of this equipment and makes it an unacceptable alternative for many students.

Some manufacturers have taken this idea one step further by mounting the camera in the goggles. A sliding lens mounted on the front of the goggles can be positioned for reading or distance viewing. Reading with this device can be somewhat difficult because users have to move their heads right and left to view the text. The system can be mounted in a specially designed stand and connected to an external monitor for extended reading tasks. The weight of the device and the head movement required

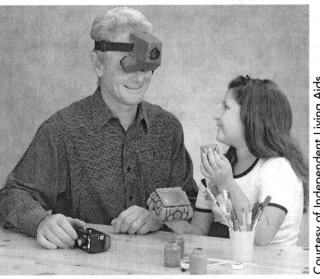

Units that mount the camera in the goggles also increase portability. They are especially good for students or adults to use in distance viewing of classroom demonstrations, sporting events, plays, concerts, and exhibits.

deter many students from using this device as a reading tool, but many find this system useful for distance viewing and for viewing information presented on chalkboards, overhead projectors, and computer projection systems, in addition to viewing plays, concerts, and live presentations.

Electronic Pocket Magnifiers

Another type of portable video magnifier, known as an electronic pocket magnifier, contains both the camera and visual display in one unit and is approximately the size of a paperback book. The device is placed directly on top of the material to be viewed, and the user moves the device around to read the information. Pocket models are similar to portable models with handheld cameras in that they require the user to have a good deal of coordination to maintain the camera perpendicular to the print for continuous text reading.

Some pocket magnifiers locate the camera directly under the viewing surface, while others place it at one end of the device. In models with the camera to one side, the user must be able to grasp the concept that what he or she is seeing is actually slightly displaced, not directly beneath the screen being looked at. Most users can quickly adjust to this situation, but it can be confusing for others.

Electronic pocket models offer a limited range of magnification compared to desktop models and a small viewing area, but in general they are quite portable and easily transported. The use of rechargeable batteries gives these units even more flexibility.

All three types of portable video magnification systems—portable models with a handheld camera, head-mounted display models, and electronic pocket models—have similar advantages and disadvantages. The significant advantage of portability—being able to transport the device to any location where a user might need it, while still maintaining the advantages of a video magnifier—is traded for several disadvantages. In order to obtain portability:

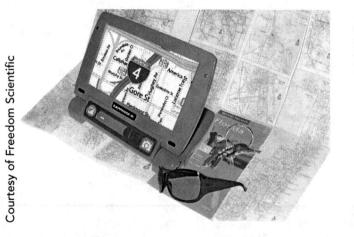

Courtesy of Freedom Scientific

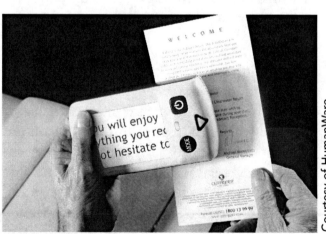

Courtesy of HumanWare

Electronic pocket model video magnifiers (left), which incorporate the camera and visual display in one unit, are excellent tools for short spot-reading tasks, such as reading a map. Some models locate the camera to one side of the unit (right), which requires users to learn to place the camera, not the screen, directly over the text to be viewed.

- the user trades a large display for a device that can be easily transported to any location. The user accepts a smaller viewing screen, which may be more difficult to see, or a head-mounted device that can cause head and neck strain with prolonged use.
- the user trades the weight of the traditional camera and X-Y table for a handheld camera with some significant disadvantages. As the user moves the handheld camera over the text to be read, it must remain perpendicular to the line of print. This is not too difficult to master for short reading

passages, but when a student needs to read for an extended period of time, the coordination required for this task can become quite tiring, and he or she can develop fatigue in the fingers, hands, arms, and shoulders from the repetitive movement of the camera.

Although these trade-offs may seem severe to some, other users find them acceptable for certain tasks, particularly short reading tasks.

Digital Imaging Systems

Because of ongoing advances in technology, various methods of accessing printed information involve converting the material into electronic formats. Once the information is in a digital or electronic form, the individual user can read or access it in the way that is most effective for his or her needs. Thus, the line between print and electronic information has been blurred, if not eliminated, by assistive technology.

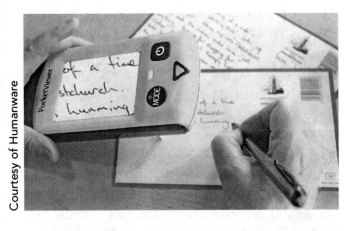

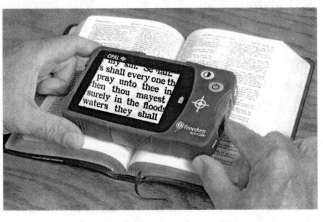

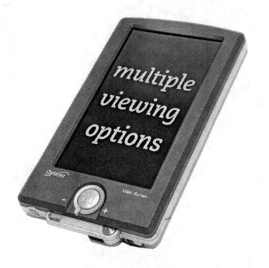

Courtesy of Humanware

Courtesy of Freedom Scientific

Courtesy of APH

There is a wide variety of models and styles of electronic pocket video magnifiers from which to choose. Some can be used for very short writing tasks, but students may find the necessary coordination difficult.

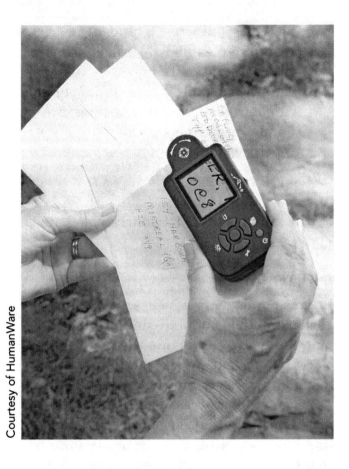

This unit is less expensive than most other electronic pocket video magnifiers, but offers a very small viewing area. Since most of these devices are used for spot reading, some users find this an acceptable trade-off.

Some video magnification systems have been merged with computer technologies to provide visual access to print information that is converted into electronic information. This new category of video magnifiers takes a distinctively different approach from the traditional desktop models and portable models by allowing the user to manipulate a digital image of printed text. Video magnification systems of this type are therefore categorized as digital imaging systems, and they offer some of the best features of several of the different categories.

These systems use a digital camera to take a picture of a page. The image is then processed by software running inside the unit or in a computer connected to the camera. The software analyzes the image and determines where the text is located on the page and where the page is blank. By sampling the contrast at various locations on the page, the system is able to determine where words begin and end. It is then able

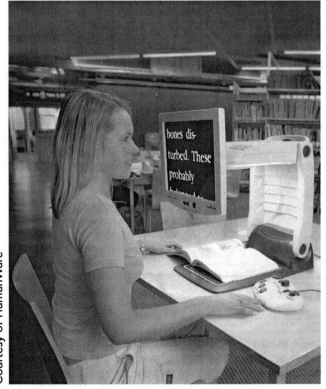

This student is using a digital imaging system video magnifier in the column mode to read a book in the library.

to display the text on a monitor in the user's desired magnification and format. If there is insufficient room on a line for the next word, the system moves the word down to the next line (similar to the "word wrap" feature found in most computer word-processing programs). Since the page is not moved in order to view it, there is no need for an X-Y table or for the user to develop the skills necessary to manipulate one.

The system can display the text in one large column the same way a teleprompter does for a newscaster or speaker. The user can set the rate at which the text scrolls up the screen or move it manually. Or, the text can be presented across the page in one continuous horizontal line in a "tickertape" fashion—again, with the user having complete control over the rate at which the text is presented. A third presentation option displays the text as single words presented individually on the screen. The user selects a desired speed or presentation rate for this option as well, but the system displays longer words for a longer period of time and short words for less time. Several such systems are currently available, but this technology is in its infancy and significant improvements will in all probability be made in the future.

Although these systems manipulate the digital images of the text produced by the camera, they are still dealing with magnified images of words that are projected onto a screen. Some video magnifiers that use digital imaging technology have gone one step further by combining visual access to text with synthetic speech that "reads" or announces it aloud. These computer-based systems use optical character recognition (OCR) software to analyze the image of the text and convert it into electronic, editable text (see the discussion of OCR systems in the next section), which is then converted into synthetic (or synthesized) speech created by text-to-speech software. As the system speaks each word, the corresponding text is highlighted on the screen for easier viewing. The combination of highlighted text and synthesized speech—in which the use of two sensory modalities, vision and hearing, reinforces comprehension—has proved to be very valuable to many users (Evans, 1997, 1998; see also the section on "Specialized Scanning Systems" and in Chapter 3). In addition, once the printed text has been converted into electronic text,

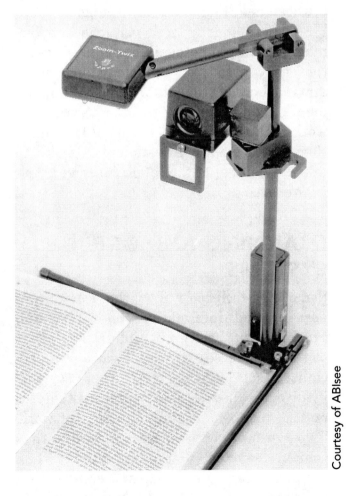

Courtesy of ABIsee

This digital imaging system offers distance viewing capabilities through the use of a second camera.

other programs running on the computer can be used to produce the information in large print, braille, or a variety of audio formats (see Chapter 5).

In addition to options for text and background color and polarity, some of these systems also offer an option for distance viewing. This is accomplished by either the use of a second camera or by rotating the main camera 90 degrees. Some systems require the user to also rotate a lens for distance viewing, while others have circuitry that compensates for the greater distance. The two-camera systems require only the use of keyboard commands and then pointing the camera at the desired target to switch easily between near and distance viewing.

As new and updated versions of video magnifiers become available, it is imperative that assistive technology specialists and teachers of students with visual impairments keep abreast of these advances and work with their students' clinical low vision therapist to ensure that students are able to take advantage of the latest improvements in this area.

SCANNING AND OCR SYSTEMS

Some high-tech tools allow the user to convert printed information, both text and graphics, into electronic information that can then be accessed with a variety of specialized tools (see Chapter 3). These systems involve the use of a computer system, an optical scanner, and appropriate software. Two types of software can be used with a computer system that is equipped with a scanner: imaging software and optical character recognition (OCR) software. It might be said that the scanner "takes a picture" of the page of text and graphics, and that imaging

software displays that picture or image on the computer screen. The user can save the image as an electronic file that can be retrieved and viewed later. OCR software, in contrast, starts out with the same image or picture taken by the scanner and then converts the image into an electronic text file, which can be manipulated or edited by other software programs on the computer.

Although the processes involved are similar, the use of OCR software results in an electronic file that can be edited or revised by the user. The use of imaging software does not offer this option. For example, the electronic text file created by an OCR program can be opened with word-processing software and displayed in various fonts and point sizes, enlarged and viewed with screen magnification software, or listened to as synthetic speech with screen-reading software. Each of these two access approaches, imaging software and OCR software, have advantages and disadvantages. Table 2.2 ("Imaging Software vs. OCR Software") provides a quick comparison of imaging software and OCR software.

Imaging Software

As its name implies, imaging software allows an optical scanner (once it is installed and configured for a computer) to scan graphical images, including images of text, into a computer and provides basic tools for manipulating the appearance of that image. Although commercial imaging programs are available, major operating system software often includes imaging software as an accessory. In addition, many scanners include imaging software as well.

Images of printed text scanned into a computer and displayed by the imaging software are seldom large enough to be readable by most students with low vision.

Table 2.2   Imaging Software vs. OCR Software

Features	Imaging Software	OCR Software
Converts printed information into electronic information	Yes	Yes
Provides visual access to text with screen magnification software	Yes	Yes
Provides auditory access to text with screen reading software	No	Yes
Retains graphics and original formatting	Yes	Yes, in some cases
Provides text that can be edited by user	No	Yes
Provides a writing tool to complete forms and worksheets	Yes	Yes, but reformats document
Can be used to complete matching activities (in which students need to draw lines between items in two columns that match)	Yes	Yes, but is much more complicated

Many of these programs do provide a zoom feature that can be used to enlarge the image being viewed, including text, which can be useful for some individuals. However, the zoom feature in this software is designed to provide a detailed view of a section of an image for editing or redrawing, not for viewing the entire image under magnification. Consequently, this feature was not designed to facilitate the process of moving or navigating over the entire image to read the text, as a visually impaired user would need to do. In general, the lack of navigation tools makes the use of this type of software tedious and inefficient for most students with low vision, although there are some students who can master it for short reading passages.

The attraction of imaging software, however, is its price: free. It is typically either "bundled" (sold together) with the optical scanner or included as part of a computer's basic operating system software, as it is with both Macintosh- and Windows-based computers. Imaging software can also be useful as a writing tool for students with low vision who wish to complete forms or worksheets. (See Chapter 4 for further explanation of this feature.)

Another way to take advantage of imaging software is to use it with screen magnification software (see Chapter 3). Most screen magnification programs have excellent navigation controls. The user can scan the image of text and graphics into the computer and then use the magnification and navigation features of the screen magnification program to read and review the image easily. With just a few keystrokes, the text and graphics can be viewed at the optimum magnification for the individual. In addition, the magnification can be easily adjusted to zoom in for details or zoom out to view the entire layout of the text or graphic.

In this way, the combination of a scanner, imaging software, and screen magnification software offers a computer-based alternative to a dedicated video magnification system. Imaging software may provide some of the same controls found on video magnifiers, such as polarity selection and options for text and background color combinations. Some even offer features similar to the occluders, masks, or blinds that allow the user to control the number of lines of text being viewed at any one time. However, many users find the navigation controls of imaging software by itself somewhat cumbersome to manipulate efficiently and prefer to use a dedicated video magnification system.

Optical Character Recognition (OCR) Software

OCR software takes the use of optical scanners and computers a giant step further as a tool to provide access to printed text on paper for individuals with low vision. OCR starts with the scanned image of a page and analyzes the shapes it contains, comparing them to stored images of text characters. As it begins to find matches between the shapes and the characters, it "recognizes" the characters as a specific text font. In this way, it reproduces text by producing an electronic file of the actual text characters printed on a page.

This text file can then be saved in a wide variety of word-processing formats. Once the text is available electronically, the user can access it in a variety of ways. (This will be discussed further in Chapter 3.) Screen magnification software can be used to open the file in the user's favorite word processor,

select the desired magnification, and allow the user to read the text using the navigation controls. Or, other types of programs can be used to access the text auditorily or tactilely, through a screen-reader or braille display. This process works very well for many users.

The major disadvantage of OCR software is that it is not 100 percent accurate and does make errors, especially in regard to the format and layout of the text and graphics. Many individuals with low vision can use an optical device to view graphics in the original document and determine the format and layout of the text, but doing this kind of checking involves an extra step. In contrast, imaging software offers accuracy. The text that the viewer sees on the computer screen is the same exact text printed on the page because it is basically just a picture of the text. The disadvantage of imaging software is the lack of good navigation tools for viewing the image when it is enlarged. But it does provide the text in a format that can be viewed with other software programs that do provide excellent navigation tools. Imaging software and OCR software can both be valuable tools for people who are blind or visually impaired, but each has advantages and disadvantages; what is needed is a program that offers the best features of both tools in a single package. A variation of the specialized scanning software, which will be discussed next, attempts to provide this option.

Specialized Scanning Systems

Attempts to overcome the disadvantages just described have led to the development of software that combines the benefits of both imaging and OCR software. Design of this software was motivated by the needs of individuals with reading difficulties who are not visually impaired. These systems display the exact image of a page on the computer screen, while OCR software, running in the background, enables the text to be read aloud without affecting the image. The OCR software "recognizes" the text, and passes it on to software that reads and speaks it using synthesized speech. At the same time, the imaging software allows the user to control visual aspects of any graphics and text displayed, such as size, polarity, and color. Additional navigation features give the user the ability to have each word highlighted with a selected color combination while it is spoken by the speech synthesizer.

Navigation is automatic; the user does not have to move the display of the text from left to right or up and down. The program knows where each word of the text is located and displays the words on the computer screen as they are spoken. Any inaccuracies produced by the OCR processing may be spoken, but since the student is viewing the visual image of the exact text, he or she can see the correct word or words and recognize them. This can be confusing to some students, but once they become familiar with the system they will know that they need to stop on such occasions and determine whether the auditory or the visual information is correct. This type of tool for accessing printed information, which combines visual and auditory access to text, has great potential for students with low vision who could benefit from auditory reinforcement as well as for other students with reading difficulties.

Other specialized scanning systems go beyond the basic OCR software. Using OCR technology, these systems convert printed information into editable text that is then displayed on the computer's monitor. These programs allow the user to choose the desired font and point size for the display. In addition, polarity and color combinations can be selected. These specialized systems also offer text reading through synthesized speech, which can be synchronized with visual highlighting of each word as it is spoken. These specialized scanning systems also exhibit errors in recognition and formatting similar to those found with the OCR programs discussed earlier. Many students find this dual modality input to be an extremely effective tool for reading large quantities of printed information. Readers using such systems are better able to comprehend the content of the information being presented. Hearing each word spoken decreases the effort required to visually identify each word being read, while seeing each word highlighted decreases the effort required to hear and understand each word spoken by the speech synthesizer, especially words that are easily mispronounced by synthetic speech. Using this combination approach can increase the student's reading rate and can result in better comprehension and less fatigue for longer reading tasks (Evans, 1997, 1998).

Students and individuals who wish to access printed information visually have a wide variety of optical, nonoptical, and electronic tools available to accomplish such tasks. Because circumstances, the demands of a given task, and an individual's sensory capabilities can vary, even from day to day, the person who is successful at accessing information visually will use a variety of tools. Thanks to technology, students can have a "toolbox" full of resources for obtaining information with flexibility and effectiveness, and for achieving their educational, career, and personal goals. But, to ensure success, students will need appropriate training in the use of these tools, experience with their use, and knowledge about which tools are best for short or spot reading tasks, lengthy continuous reading tasks, and distance viewing tasks. Selecting and using the right tool for the job will be the key. Assessing a student's needs and abilities is the critical determinant in identifying the appropriate tool.

ACCESSING PRINT INFORMATION TACTILELY

Braille

Tactile Graphics

Other Tactile Tools
- Tactile Math Tools

When a student's primary means of learning and obtaining information is through his or her sense of touch, tactile methods of reading and performing other tasks may be recommended on the basis of such assessments as a learning media assessment. As indicated in Chapter 1, however, students may use one sensory modality for certain tasks and another for other tasks, and they may change the use of those respective modalities over time. When it comes to accessing printed information through touch, braille is central.

BRAILLE

The need for braille as a tool for literacy for students who are blind or visually impaired cannot be overemphasized. For students who use their tactile sense as the primary way in which to obtain information, and for those whose visual abilities may not sustain visual reading efficiently or for extended periods without fatigue, braille provides direct, immediate, and reliable access to information. Auditory access to written text cannot replace the direct access braille provides. *Hard-copy*, or *paper*, braille provides to visually impaired readers information equivalent to that provided by print to sighted readers, and a knowledge of braille is the cornerstone of literacy, educational achievement, and successful employment for many students and adults.

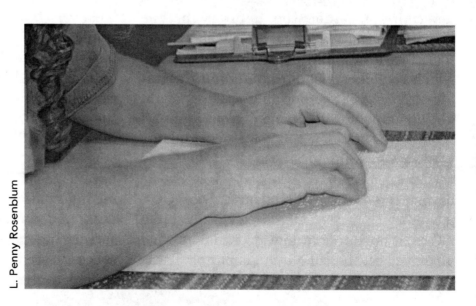

Braille, a system of raised dots that represent the written word, provides an excellent tactile tool for accessing print information.

L. Penny Rosenblum

In addition to the content of the text, braille provides information about the following:

- *Spelling of words and terms.* It is essential for learners to repeatedly see or feel the letters to correctly spell words. Having information in braille allows the user exposure to the spelling of words each time the information is read and at any time that the reader wishes to return to specific text and review it.
- *Structure and format of printed information.* Information about headings, subheadings, and paragraphs cannot be easily conveyed in an auditory format. The understanding of the relationship of these elements within written information adds significantly to the reader's comprehension of the information.

Thus, there will always be a need for braille materials, braille tools, and competent braille instruction for students to maximize their educational potential.

Some portion of the information provided in print, such as books and magazines, is available in hard-copy braille. The selection is limited, however, compared to the vast amount of information available in print, even though new methods of producing braille have shortened the time required to produce material, and braille publishers and producers continue to expand their offerings. Technology has significantly improved the options for producing braille, which is now often generated electronically. Appropriately prepared electronic files can be used to produce hard-copy braille by means of braille embossers and printers, or can be read on electronic braille displays.

Different braille codes are used to present certain types of material, such as mathematics, computers, or music. These options are covered in detail in Chapters 3 and 4.

As mentioned throughout this chapter, when printed text is converted into electronic text files—for example, by using a scanner and OCR software—tactile readers can then read the text using methods for accessing electronic text, such as refreshable braille. These methods are discussed in Chapter 3.

TACTILE GRAPHICS

Over the ages people have found that some information is best communicated via a graphical or pictorial representation such as maps, charts, and graphs. Often this type of information cannot be communicated effectively with verbal descriptions, regardless of whether they are embossed in braille or spoken aloud. When this is the case, people who are visually impaired need a tactile representation of the graphical information. A good tactile graphic is one that provides a tactile representation of the important information in the original graphic, not necessarily one that reproduces tactilely every visual element of the original.

A variety of techniques exist to produce graphical information in a tactile format. Specially trained transcribers use both low-tech manual tools and high-tech electronic tools to produce tactile graphics. Tactile graphics can be created on braille paper or on thin aluminum sheets that are used in a thermal vacuum process to produce multiple copies of the graphic. Because most of these production methods are time consuming (although less so than in the past), they do not allow for the quick communication of simple concepts. (Some additional methods

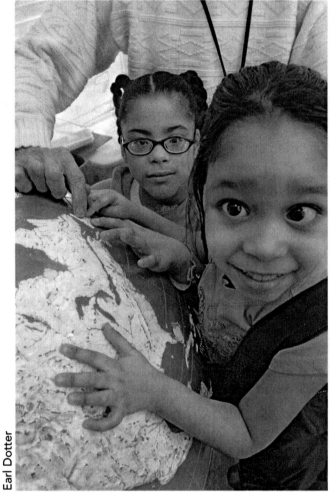

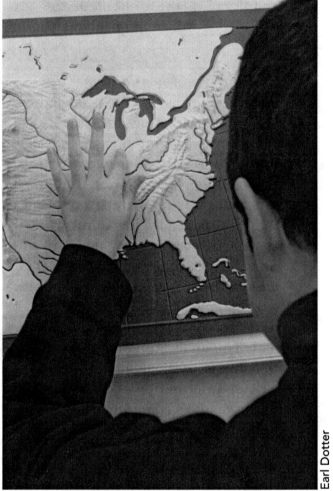

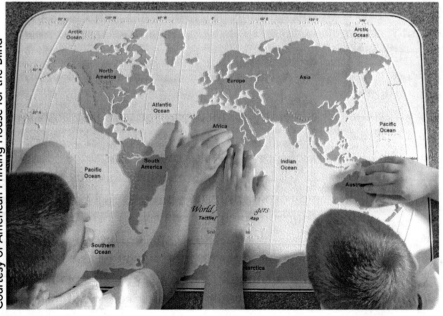

A tactile globe and commercially produced tactile maps help these young students grasp basic geography concepts.

for making instant tactile graphics in the classroom are described in Chapter 5, along with more details about the techniques mentioned here.)

The methods for producing tactile graphics include, but are not limited to,

- tooling;
- collage;
- capsule paper and fuser;
- computer-assisted tactile graphics.

Tooling is a method of producing tactile graphics that uses specially designed tools to work from the back side of braille paper or a heavy-duty foil. Textures, lines, and points are embossed, creating a raised image on the front. Copies of the tactile graphic, particularly those created on foil, are made using a vacuum form process called thermoform.

Collage is a method in which materials of different but compatible textures are selected to represent the components of the print graphic (areas, lines, and point symbols). The textures are adhered to a base surface that also contains labels, written in braille, that identify the various components of the graphic. The collage method is often used to create a master tactile graphic that is then copied using the thermoform process.

Another production technique is based on *capsule paper and a fuser*. The capsule paper is coated with microcapsules that respond to irradiation (light energy) and heat. An image is transferred to the capsule paper by drawing with a special marker, photocopying, or using a computer printer. The paper is fed through a fuser that irradiates and heats the paper. The ink interacts with the light, heat, and chemistry of the paper to swell, creating a raised line drawing of the original graphic. Also called swell graphics, puff pictures, and toaster graphics, this method is often used in schools because it offers quick production with minimal supplies. Simple diagrams can be prepared and immediately delivered to the student. Students can also create their own graphics.

Computer-assisted tactile graphics use drawing software to create an image to be produced as a tactile graphic. The image is printed on the production medium using one of the methods just described. The image can also be sent directly to a braille embosser capable of producing graphics.

These tools make production of tactile graphics less time consuming and more efficient, which increases the availability of graphical information that can be accessed tactilely. (For further information on tools and techniques for producing tactile graphics, see Edman, 1992.)

OTHER TACTILE TOOLS

In certain school subjects, students work not only with print in its traditional forms,

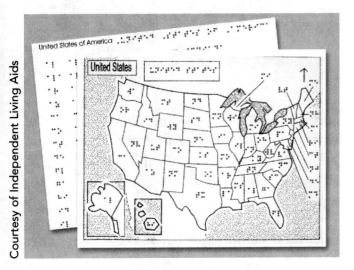

This tactile map of the United States was produced using capsule paper and a thermal fuser.

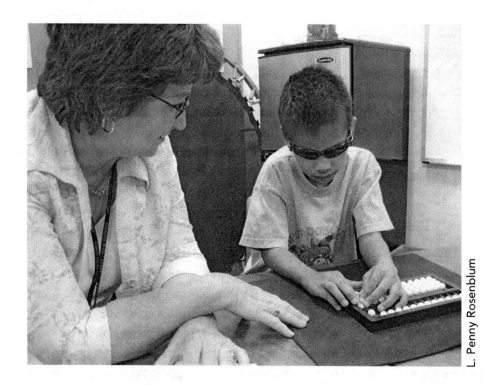

Students can execute basic math calculations using an abacus. A large abacus (below) is easy for young students to manipulate.

L. Penny Rosenblum

but also with other materials such as maps or mathematical calculations. The methods already discussed are useful for creating teacher-made maps, and ready-made maps are also available from a variety of sources (see the Resources section at the end of this book). Other solutions may also be needed to help students with little or no useful vision to access the mainstream curriculum when the class is working with a variety of materials. Several tactile tools provide such solutions. (Another product that allows tactile access to graphic information, the Touch Tablet, is described in Chapter 3.)

Tactile Math Tools

Mathematical concepts and calculations can be difficult for students who are blind or visually impaired because they cannot see the numbers that have been arranged traditionally in columns and rows. Although doable, setting up math problems on a braillewriter can be time consuming and

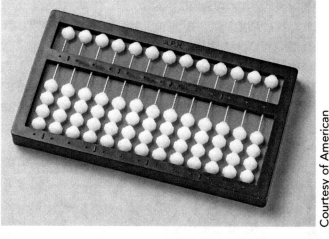

Courtesy of American

cumbersome. A number of other tools, two of which are the abacus and the Cubarithm, allow students to use their tactile sense in the comprehension and application of mathematical concepts.

The abacus is an old and valued instrument for computing calculations in many cultures. The Cranmer abacus, designed for use by people who are blind, essentially consists of beads mounted on rods. The rods are divided by a plastic bar that separates four beads on the bottom from one bead on the top of each row. The user slides the beads from the bottom up to the bar to indicate numerals 1 through 4. The bead on the top can be slid down to represent the numeral 5. By setting combinations of these beads, almost any number can be entered on the abacus. The four basic functions of addition, subtraction, multiplication, and division can be performed using this tool. It is a portable, battery-free device, that many individuals find very useful. An abacus is also available with large beads for people who might have difficulty manipulating the smaller beads.

The major benefit of the abacus over other tools such as the talking calculator (discussed in Chapter 3) is that it is helpful in the instruction of mathematical facts. Use of the abacus requires students to learn about mathematical functions and to understand basic concepts. Because of this, many states allow the use of an abacus as an accommodation when students are taking state-mandated assessments. (Teachers can check with their state department of education for guidance on allowable test accommodations.) With it, mathematical problems such as long division calculations are easier for children to compute.

The Cubarithm is another time-tested tool that can be used to teach the layout of arithmetic problems to students who are blind or visually impaired. Weighted cubes that are embossed with braille characters are placed on a workboard divided into sections. These cubes can easily be removed to allow the user to make corrections when necessary. Cubes are placed in the appropriate locations to perform arithmetic calculations. The cubes are relatively small, thus necessitating a certain level of fine motor skills for their use. (For additional information and instructions for using the Cubarithm, see Gissoni, 2005.)

Other tactile math tools include raised-line measuring tools, such as rulers, protractors, and compasses. (These and other tools are available from American Printing House for the Blind and other suppliers listed in the Resources section. For more information on tools for mathematics, see Osterhaus, 2008.)

ACCESSING PRINT INFORMATION AUDITORILY

Readers

Audio Recording

Digital Audio Formats
- Digital Talking Books
- Other Electronic Formats
- Convergence

Reading Machines
- Stand-Alone Electronic Reading Machines
- Computer-Based Reading Machines
- Multisensory Access

Other Auditory Tools

Although vision and touch are the primary senses through which many students obtain information about their environment, print information can also be accessed through the sense of hearing, which can be an important learning channel or reinforcing method for some students. Many years ago, before the advent of tactile reading systems and devices for magnification, auditory access was the only way in which people who were blind or visually impaired could gain access to print. Many methods and tools that support auditory access to print are now available, including, but not limited to the following:

- Human readers
- Tape recorders and players
- Digital recorders and players
- Digital Talking Book players
- E-book readers, including MP3 players
- Talking calculators
- Talking dictionaries
- Accessible personal digital assistants (PDAs)
- Specialized scanning systems with speech
- Talking computers
- Talking compasses
- Talking global positioning system devices

The use of these types of tools to access printed (as well as electronic) information is often referred to as *auditory access*. Auditory access can assist some students in completing lengthy reading assignments in less time than required to read the same information in print or braille alone. Literature, social studies, and some sciences can be comprehended easily by listening, although mathematics and the applied sciences can be more difficult to understand in this way.

The major disadvantage to accessing information auditorily is that doing so does not help students develop or reinforce certain literacy skills. When students are listening to material in an audio format, they do not receive information about the spelling of words, punctuation, or the structural format (for example, headings or subheadings) of the information. As a result,

they do not receive exposure or practice that helps them increase their understanding or knowledge of these basic components of literacy. Therefore, it is strongly recommended that students not rely on auditory access as their only method of acquiring information, particularly students who are learning English as a second language.

Auditory access should not be confused with the audio-assisted reading mentioned earlier. Audio-assisted reading involves reading along in print or braille with what the student is hearing read aloud. When using the combination of auditory and print or braille input, readers can obtain the literacy information just discussed while accessing the information faster than they might be able to with print or braille alone. This method of accessing information is not more efficient for all students, but many find it to be very beneficial. The technologies discussed in this section provide tools that can assist students in the process of auditory access and audio-assisted reading.

READERS

One of the methods most widely used by individuals who are blind or visually impaired to access printed information is having another person read it aloud to them. Working with readers may not usually be thought of as using technology, but assistive technology, as explained in Chapter 1, is the use of any methodology, device, or equipment in support of the performance of a task.

Like other access tools, using a live reader in real time to access information has advantages and disadvantages. Readers can be used successfully for tasks in the areas of education, employment, and activities of daily living. The keys to working successfully and efficiently with a reader are making sure that

- the reader is well trained and has some knowledge of the subject being read;
- the listener is organized, focused, and knows how to direct the reader courteously and efficiently.

Knowing how to work with a reader efficiently can be extremely important for both education and employment, especially when dealing with issues of testing, assessment, and promotional exams.

When using a reader, listeners will need to make notes at times about something that they are hearing. Note taking can be done by writing a notation in braille or print, or making an audio recording. In fact, some individuals choose to record the reader speaking the entire document for later review. At other times, readers will be asked to record themselves reading a book or magazine and later provide the recording to the person who is visually impaired. To produce an effective recording, the reader needs to know how to operate the recording equipment efficiently, how to organize his or her tasks, and how to receive direction from the visually impaired student or other individual. (For additional information on using readers, see Leibs, 1999; Whittle, 1995; Cheadle & Elliot, 1995; Castellano, 2004.)

AUDIO RECORDING

Readers who had developed effective skills in reading books and magazines aloud were instrumental in the development and implementation of audio recording, one of the first technologies used to give people who are blind or visually impaired access to printed information through the auditory sense. "Talking Books," as they became known, were first recorded on vinyl records or discs by readers. These devices were refined and improved, and they served the public well until the advent of affordable cassette tape players and recorders in the 1970s. As more books became available on cassette tape, manufacturers began to develop new features for the tape players designed to provide more information on each tape and to improve the efficiency with which listeners could use them. The primary supplier of Talking Books has been the National Library Service for the Blind and Physically Handicapped (NLS), part of the Library of Congress. Most of the titles from NLS are considered pleasure or recreational reading, but recordings of textbooks have been provided by Recording for the Blind and Dyslexic (RFB&D) (see the Resources section for more information).

Recorded books on analog cassette tape are now being replaced by other media and technologies that will be discussed later in this section, but a wide variety of materials still exists that was recorded in this format and may still be available during the transition to digital media. It is important for teachers to be aware of all the technology options for their students.

Talking Books were intended for people who are unable to read print and were typically recorded on four-track cassettes, which can contain a recording twice as long as can fit on a conventional two-track tape. They were also recorded at a slower speed to increase the capacity of the tapes. A specially adapted tape player is required to listen to four-track cassettes. These adapted players and recorders have a number of features that allow listeners who are visually impaired to use the recordings more efficiently, including

- variable speed control;
- variable pitch control;
- tactile controls;
- tone indexing.

These features are described in more detail in Sidebar 2.4, "Features of Adapted Cassette Tape Players.". Many of these features, or updated versions of them, have been included in the newer technologies that are rapidly replacing cassette tape players, such as digital Talking Books.

Even though recorded information on tape cannot substitute for information in braille or print, its use has greatly expanded the availability of information for many individuals who are blind or visually impaired. Literature and pleasure reading in particular can be enjoyed in the form of Talking Books, since they are generally read in sequence from beginning to end. However, this type of linear access is less effective for the study of information used for education, training, and research, or in other situations in which specific portions of the material need to be accessed out of order and sometimes repeatedly. Digital Talking Books offer an effective solution to this problem.

SIDEBAR 2.4

FEATURES OF ADAPTED CASSETTE TAPE PLAYERS

Although cassette tape players have been helpful and essential equipment for many visually impaired readers, newer forms of equipment and technology are replacing them. However, there are many recorder/players still available, and they can still be used to assist students with auditory and audio-assisted reading. Adapted cassette tape players incorporated a number of features that allowed listeners of Talking Books to control the way recorded information is presented. These features significantly improved the user's reading experience over previous recorded formats, and it is useful for visually impaired readers and the professionals who work with them to have a basic understanding of their value.

Variable Speed Control

Most individuals can listen to and absorb information faster than a reader can read aloud in making the recording. Variable speed control allows listeners to adjust the speed of the soundtrack to suit their individual preferences and ability to absorb information auditorily, depending on the subject matter. For example, a student can slow down the presentation rate of mathematical, scientific, or highly technical material, or speed it up when listening to literature and information in the social sciences.

Variable Pitch Control

Playing back a taped voice at a speed faster than it was recorded raises the pitch of the voice so that it sounds like the kind of voice often associated with a cartoon character. Although some people are able to listen to this high-pitched voice and absorb more information at a faster rate, many listeners find it distracting and difficult to understand. A feature of adaptive tape players known as *variable pitch control* allows listeners to adjust the pitch of the reader's voice so that they can play the tape as fast as they are able to understand the recording while still hearing it in a normally pitched voice.

Tactile Controls

The design of the tactile controls on an adaptive tape player greatly increases the efficiency with which users can operate the device. Tactile markings help users identify the Play, Pause, Fast Forward, Rewind, Record, and other buttons. Other control knobs or sliders have notches or varying resistance to mark the adjustment scales for features such as volume, balance, variable speed control, or variable pitch control.

Tone Indexing

Because analog tape is a linear medium—it only goes forward or backward—locating specific information and navigating around a taped recording can be complicated. Students frequently need to locate particular reading passages or homework assignments in a lengthy textbook recorded on multiple cassettes, each with four tracks. To help listeners navigate in situations such as this, a feature was created on adapted tape players and recorders known as *tone indexing*. When a reader makes a recording for a student using one of these players, he or she can press a tone-indexing button that embeds a low-frequency tone at desired locations on the tape. Usually, page numbers are marked with a single beep and chapters with two beeps. When the listener plays the tape normally, these tones are barely audible. However, another feature of the special cassette players, known as *cue and review*, allows the user to listen to the tape in play mode while it is fast forwarding (cue) or rewinding (review). When the tape's rapid movement raises the sound of the recording to a higher pitch, the narration will sound garbled, but the listener will hear a high-pitched tone or beep wherever the indexing tone was placed by the reader. The listener can count the number of tones to reach the desired page and then release the fast forward or rewind button to play the tape at regular speed. Although tone indexing was a big improvement over tapes with no navigational tools, some students find this system cumbersome and have difficulty identifying each indexed tone. Moreover, this system is still not capable of identifying a particular passage or word on a page.

DIGITAL AUDIO FORMATS

The advent of digital recording—recordings stored as electronic data, rather than in a physical format as in analog recording—has led to audio formats for Talking Books that are far superior to audio recording on cassette tapes in the quality of the recording and the benefits that they offer to readers. Audio recordings of books and other materials can be saved on compact discs, various memory storage devices, or simply as files stored on a computer's harddrive. Playback devices have been developed for all of these media, and each device and medium has its own set of advantages and disadvantages. (For a discussion of digital voice recorders, see Chapter 3.)

Digital Talking Books

Like the audio formats they have superseded, Talking Books are in the midst of a great revolution—the migration from tape to digital formats. Digital Talking Books (sometimes abbreviated as DTB) are based on a standard format for accessible digital recordings known as DAISY (Digital Accessible Information SYstem). "DAISY" refers to a set of guidelines and a structure for producing books in a digital format. The most useful DAISY files have both recorded audio and text, but some DAISY books are only audio or text that is read aloud with synthetic speech. The great advance that DAISY books represent for individuals who are blind or visually

Courtesy of Independent Living Aids

One of the first portable Digital Talking Book players.

impaired is that they allow markers to be inserted into the digital book file to identify the location of chapters, sections, subsections, pages, paragraphs, sentences, words, and even letters, which makes it easy to navigate within a recording and find any information of interest.

The first Digital Talking Books were recorded on compact discs (CDs) and played on adapted CD players with the ability to locate and identify the embedded markers. Early desktop players have been joined by portable players that are similar to portable music CD players, as well as by a Digital Talking Book player that consists of software running on a computer. This software program enables the user to place the Digital Talking Book CD in the appropriate computer disc drive and listen to the recording through the computer's sound card and speakers. Some DTBs are saved as files on various storage media and can be accessed with software DAISY players on computers and other devices.

As already noted, Digital Talking Book technology has greatly increased the efficiency with which a listener can navigate through recorded information using the keys on the adapted CD player, allowing a reader to access and manage the use of material with great flexibility. Digital Talking Book players have also improved the user's ability to control playback speed without affecting the pitch of the reader's voice. Finer adjustments in playback speed allow listeners to set the player to their optimum rate for comprehension and speed.

Software Digital Talking Book players offer the promise of full-text searching; the ability to have text highlighted as it is read aloud as well as displayed in the user's preferred font, point size, and color combination; and the ability for users to place their

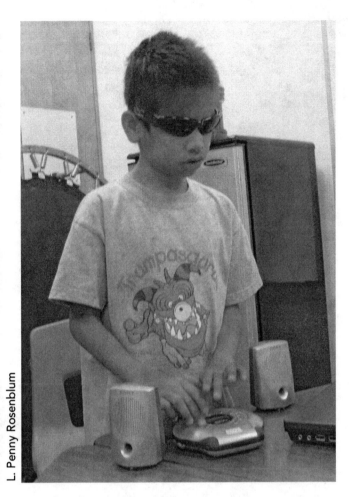

L. Penny Rosenblum

Users can easily access various parts of a book when it is recorded in the DAISY format.

drives. The playback units developed by NLS access audio recordings stored on a memory storage device housed in a plastic cartridge about the size of a cassette tape. (For additional details, see www.loc.gov/nls.) As these technologies continue to develop, users will have access to greater quantities of information on smaller and more convenient systems.

Digital Talking Books offer students significant advantages over cassette recordings. The machines and storage formats are sturdier and more portable. Students can read their school assignments or leisure reading anywhere that they find themselves. The search capabilities and improved controls can save them hours of time each week simply in finding the assignments they need to read and the passages that contain the data required to complete homework questions and reports. If they record classes, they can also bookmark important points so they can easily find them later for studying. The potential of Digital Talking Books for transforming the lives of students who read at least some material auditorily is just beginning to be realized.

own markers in a file so they can review the marked passages later or save them to a separate file. As Digital Talking Book technology improves and achieves its potential, users will continue to increase their efficiency in accessing recorded information.

Producers of recorded information continue to explore newer and more efficient storage media. As of this writing, NLS's transition from tape to digital Talking Books is in midstream. It has skipped the compact disc format altogether and started producing its recordings on devices known as memory storage cards, similar to flash

Other Electronic Formats

Mainstream audio books have become widely available in bookstores and over the Internet. These recordings are available on compact discs and in digital audio formats such as MP3 files, which can be downloaded to various electronic devices. These formats provide excellent sound quality and represent another accessible medium. However, they do not posses the navigational features of books recorded in the DAISY format.

At the same time, more and more books and other printed materials are becoming available as electronic books, or e-books. These are not audio recordings but rather

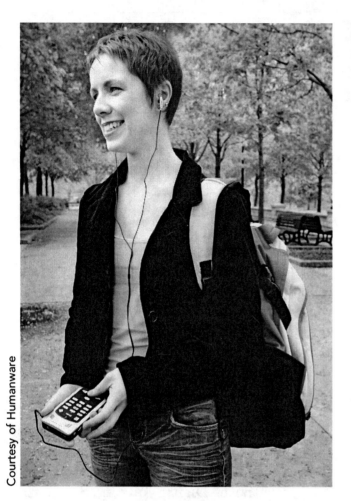

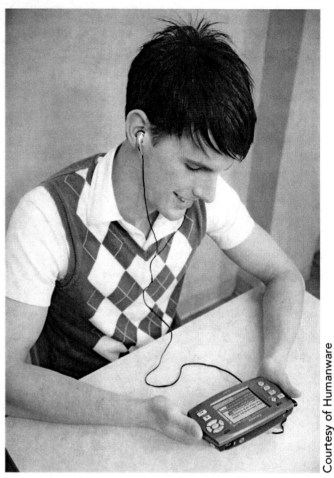

Small, lightweight players (left) allow users to access electronic files more easily. Other devices (right) that play e-books in a variety of formats, including audio, can also display the text in fonts up to 20 points and have text-to-speech capability.

electronic files, so the information in the file is electronic text that can be accessed with a wide variety of devices that produce synthesized speech. As with other files accessed with synthetic speech, the user can control the rate and other aspects of the speech and navigate by characters, words, sentences, and paragraphs (see Chapter 3). However, many e-books are created in proprietary formats and can be read only on certain players, such as iPods or the Amazon Kindle, that are not accessible. Readers need to be careful in choosing e-books to make sure that they are in fact accessible to them.

Convergence

With the development of Digital Talking Books and e-books, the line between printed information and electronic information has been further blurred. Information that was once printed is now being converted into electronic information to be made accessible for individual users. Numerous devices can access this electronic information, which will be explored in Chapter 3.

Books on tape, CD, and other storage media are excellent tools for accessing some printed information auditorily. When students need to obtain textbooks and other materials in these formats, however, the process of ordering them from a central depository or requesting production from a producer of alternate media can be time consuming. (For information about producing and obtaining materials in alternate formats, see Chapter 5.) Students often need immediate access to printed information, which is why old-fashioned, low-tech human readers continue to be useful in many situations. However, a reader is not usually needed on a continuous basis, and one may not always be available precisely when an individual has some text that he or she needs read. For many years, people who are blind or visually impaired have dreamed of a device that could simply read printed text aloud whenever they needed it. Modern technology is making progress in this area.

READING MACHINES

Stand-Alone Electronic Reading Machines

What at one time seemed like a dream is commonplace today: an individual places printed text on the scanning bed of an electronic reading machine, which converts the image into electronic text and reads it aloud.

Ray Kurzweil began developing the first reading machine toward the end of the 20th century. Early reading machines were quite large and contained many electronic circuit boards and microprocessors. They were also limited in their accuracy and were prohibitively expensive. Although today's stand-alone reading machines are much smaller, cheaper, more accurate, and easier to use, they consist of the same four main components as the early versions:

- Optical scanners that produce electronic images of text

- OCR software that converts the pictures of text into characters
- Software that converts the text into synthesized speech
- A speech synthesizer that makes the sound of the text being read aloud

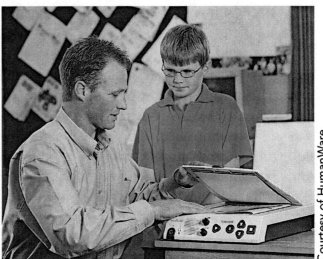

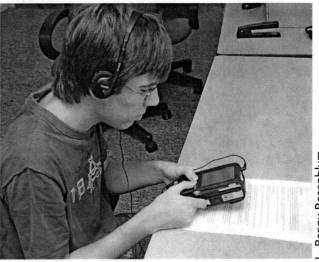

A stand-alone scanning and reading machine (top) can be used to access books and other printed information in the classroom or elsewhere. The portable specialized scanning system used by this student (above) offers additional flexibility.

These components are generally housed in a wooden or plastic box. The optical scanner part of a reading machine is a flat piece of glass, similar to that found in a photocopying machine, and a scanning mechanism that shines light onto the page.

As described earlier in this chapter in the discussion of scanners and OCR software, the scanner takes a digital picture of the page and converts the image into an electronic file that is analyzed by the OCR software and recognized as characters and words. Then this information is passed on to the speech software. (For more on synthetic speech, see Chapter 3.) The speech software determines how the text should be spoken and instructs the speech synthesizer to make the appropriate sounds. This results in the text being spoken aloud with a synthesized voice. Rudimentary control of the speech synthesizer allows the user to adjust the volume, reading rate, and tone of the synthesized speech. A few commands can be issued to navigate forward and backward through the document.

Tremendous improvements have been made in all four of the major components of reading machines in the areas of cost and accuracy. The cost of stand-alone reading machines has decreased dramatically, and the ability of OCR software to correctly recognize text is in the range of 98 percent accuracy for most fonts.

Continued miniaturization of integrated circuits and other computing components has led to the development of a portable handheld reading machine. The first of these portable systems married a digital camera and a PDA that runs OCR software and a software speech synthesizer. The second generation of this device moved the technology into a cell phone. The portability of this device makes it an attractive and flexible tool for students and others who wish to have instant access to printed information. Its price is comparable to a stand-alone reading machine. As this technology continues to grow and mature and it becomes quicker and easier to convert printed information into an electronic form, the distinction between tools for accessing print and accessing electronic information continues to diminish.

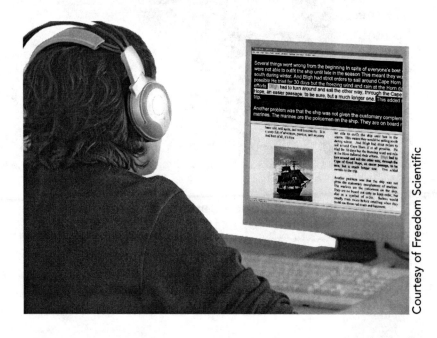

Courtesy of Freedom Scientific

This computer-based specialized scanning system allows this student to scan printed text and access it on his computer using synthesized speech, or enlarged print, or both.

Computer-Based Reading Machines

One alternative to a stand-alone electronic reading machine is a reading system built around a personal computer. Such a system requires the same four components as a stand-alone reading machine. Once an individual has a basic computer system with a high-quality sound card, all he or she has to purchase is an optical scanner and specialized scanning software that uses the computer's sound card to produce synthesized speech. If the user already has a computer, a reading system such as this is considerably less expensive than a stand-alone device. To read a document, the user places it in the scanner and executes a command to start scanning. After a document has been scanned and recognized with the OCR software, it is displayed on the computer screen. The print document has now been converted into an electronic file that can be saved for later use or read aloud with the software speech synthesizer.

Specialized reading system software is available from several manufacturers (see the Resources section at the back of this book). These programs offer many features and options that afford the user flexibility, choice, and support for individual needs and abilities. Although specialized reading system software does an acceptable job of converting printed text into electronic text, its speech and reading features are what make it such a powerful tool for visually impaired students. When a user begins to read a scanned document, he or she has the option of hearing it in its entirety or hearing it read by character, word, sentence, or paragraph. The user can also navigate forward or backward through the document in any of these units. Electronic bookmarks may be set at various points in the document for quick and easy navigation, or the user can search for specific text and jump straight to that location. The reading voice can also be modified in several ways to meet the needs and preferences of each individual user, with a variety of male or female reading voices that can be listened to at the desired speed. And if the reader encounters an unknown word, a few simple keystrokes will provide a spoken definition from the program's internal dictionary.

One very useful, but often overlooked, scanning feature that enhances the efficiency of this reading tool is the ability to do *batch scanning*. With batch scanning, the user can scan and store multiple pages before the computer begins the recognition process, rather than processing the pages one at a time. Once all of the pages are scanned—which usually takes less than 30 seconds per page—the user is able to do something else while the computer runs the OCR process. When the recognition process is complete, the user can listen to the information at his or her convenience. This flexibility allows users to employ their time more efficiently when scanning long documents.

Specialized reading system software not only can save information as an electronic file, it can also open other electronic text files stored on the user's computer and read their content aloud to the user. Large quantities of printed documents that have been converted to electronic text files can easily be accessed with this software. (For additional information on accessing e-text, see Chapter 3.) The combination of all the features available in computer-based reading systems provides the user with a tool to efficiently access printed information through audition.

Multisensory Access

Although technology that is designed for people who are blind or visually impaired can be categorized by how the user chooses to access information—visually, tactilely, or auditorily—specialized reading software crosses this divide in several ways. The software produces an electronic file containing the text of a print document, and the user can choose to access that electronic information through vision, touch, or hearing. A reader may choose to produce the information in hard-copy braille, using braille translation software and embossing it with a braille embosser (see Chapter 5). Or an electronic braille display can be connected to the computer, and the text can be read by means of refreshable braille (see Chapter 3). Those who prefer to access the information auditorily can use the speech output provided by the specialized reading system software.

Individuals who wish to access the text visually have two options available. One is to use a separate screen magnification program (see Chapter 3) to enlarge the text as it is displayed on the computer screen. Users can select point size and font style of the text displayed, in addition to the color of both the text and the background. With the text displayed in a font, color, and point size big enough for the user to see at a comfortable distance from the monitor, the user may choose to read the information visually.

The second option is visual reading of the text accompanied by audio-assisted reading. In this case, each word in the display is highlighted as it is spoken by the reading voice. For example, a user could choose to have the text displayed on the screen in an 18-point Verdana font with yellow characters on a black background. The colors for the highlighted text could be set to the reverse, with black text displayed on a yellow background as each word is spoken. Many readers find it easy to follow this highlighting visually as it progresses from word to word. As noted earlier, using a combination of visual and auditory displays of information can be a valuable tool for many students with low vision.

OTHER AUDITORY TOOLS

A variety of self-voicing or "talking" devices are available to assist students with various aspects of their schoolwork. In subjects where students are dealing with information or concepts represented in forms other than traditional text—such as mathematics, science, and geography—different solutions are needed for accessing the mainstream curriculum. Since many of these devices are electronic in nature—such as talking dictionaries, talking calculators, and Touch Tablets, which incorporate both tactile and audio features—they will be covered in Chapter 3.

ACCESSING PRINT INFORMATION PRESENTED AT A DISTANCE

Electronic Whiteboards

Overhead Projectors

Computer Slideshow Projection Systems

Video Display Systems

Accessing print and other information presented at a distance is a major challenge for students with visual impairments and requires solutions different from those that will work with print material that can be read up close. No single solution will provide the necessary access to print information in all circumstances. Using a combination of solutions and tools can ensure that a student receives equal access to the educational environment his or her fellow students enjoy.

Information presented at a distance in a classroom can include text or graphical information displayed on a

- chalkboard or whiteboard;
- overhead projection system;
- computer projection system;
- video display system.

In each of these instances, the basic problem is the same: information is too small to be viewed by the student with low vision from his or her seat in the classroom.

The traditional solution to the problem of accessing information presented at a distance has been to have the student sit closer to the board or display. Although some students will be able to read some of the information presented, most likely they will not be able to read all of it. Having a student with low vision sit in the front row can decrease his or her working distance to the chalkboard or whiteboard to possibly 5 feet or less. Although this may be adequate for some students to be able to read text directly in front and at eye level, it may not be sufficient for text placed higher on the board or a few feet to either the right or left of the student's seat, or for information written on a side wall of the classroom for students to read or copy. Therefore, other options must be explored. Because some of them involve converting the text into electronic information, they straddle the line between print and electronic material as well as among different other formats, offering students the

ability to access the information tactilely or auditorily as well as visually.

One simple, essentially "no-tech" solution to accessing information presented at a distance is to provide students with a copy of the information in their preferred format, be it braille, regular print, large print, or electronic file. They then have the material in a format that they can use in class at the same time that other students are reading it. The information will also be available to them at any point in the future to review or to use to study for exams. For this strategy to be successful, however, the classroom teacher must ensure that materials are provided in advance to the teacher of students with visual impairments so that there is sufficient time to produce the materials in the required alternate format. (For additional information about producing materials in alternate formats, see Chapter 5.)

Having the teacher provide the information to the student directly can work well if the instructor has it available in an electronic format and the student has an accessible device that can read it. Many instructors use computer-based word-processing software to produce handouts for their students rather than handwritten materials. In turn, students can be taught to copy electronic files onto a device that will output the information in their desired alternate format—such as large print, braille, or synthetic speech. Thus, information that is presented to the class in print can be provided as electronic information to the student who is blind or visually impaired. (For a discussion of devices designed to access electronic information, see Chapter 3.) Another solution that can be practical in some situations is to have another student, a paraeducator, or the teacher read the information to the student, who can then use one of the writing tools that will be discussed in Chapter 4 to make a personal copy of the information. This is not always a practical or long-term solution, however, as there may be times when no one is available to read the material to the student, and the student also needs strategies to access distant information independently.

As these examples illustrate, one solution will not fit all students or situations. In addition to these environmental and simple "no-tech" solutions, there are a variety of both low-tech and high-tech tools that can help students in the classroom, depending on where and how the information is presented. The use of manual and electronic optical devices, such as telescopes and some video magnifiers, to read print and view other information at a distance was discussed earlier in this chapter.

One other option for distance viewing is to use a regular digital video camera—the kind that many families use to take vacation videos. This device offers the user a wide range of magnification through the use of a zoom lens. This feature allows the user to zoom in for a good look at the details of an object under study and then zoom out to observe the object's relationship to its surroundings. The other major advantage of these systems is a feature that effectively amplifies the available light. By using this feature to increase contrast, the user can increase the perceived illumination of a distant object, such as a demonstration in a poorly lit classroom or an exhibit at a museum with low illumination. The feature allows the viewer to perceive details that he or she would not ordinarily be able to see. However, using video cameras in a classroom can make other students and teachers uncomfortable, especially if the student is recording the activities for later review.

Therefore, there needs to be some conversation about the use of this device beforehand (as discussed in Chapter 8).

Although these devices will help some students with some tasks, no single device will allow the student to efficiently access all of the information that might be presented in an educational setting. Some other options are discussed in the following sections.

ELECTRONIC WHITEBOARDS

Whiteboards have replaced chalkboards in many classrooms across the country. Whiteboards consist of a glossy surface, usually white, on which erasable markings can be made using a special type of marker. This new low-tech tool has had both a positive and negative impact on students who are visually impaired. It has eliminated the frustration of trying to see low-contrast writing in white or yellow chalk on a green or gray board, which in all likelihood contains chalk dust from multiple erasures. But it has *introduced* the problem of trying to view text and graphics displayed on a shiny, reflective surface, which produces a good deal of glare. With experimentation, some students with low vision can adjust their seating and the lighting in the room can be modified to compensate for the glare. The students can then read the board with a handheld telescope, a video magnifier, or a digital video camera connected to a monitor.

Technological solutions have also been used to make whiteboards more accessible for students with low vision. Electronic or interactive whiteboards and devices that attach to a standard whiteboard to make it electronic can eliminate the visual challenges created by whiteboards in the classroom. Electronic whiteboards are specialized, pressure-sensitive whiteboards. As the teacher draws or writes on the board, sensors register the pressure exerted and transmit signals to a computer, which in turn translates the signals indicating where the user is touching the board's surface into a display on the computer monitor. Thus, a student with low vision can view whatever the teacher writes on the electronic whiteboard on his or her computer screen. The student can then use screen magnification software (see Chapter 3), if needed, to enlarge or magnify the image to the desired size. Snapshots of the information on the whiteboard can also be saved as files on the computer for later review. This process can be an effective tool for working on math problems; as the teacher explains various steps and procedures, the student can record or save the individual screens and review them as often as desired in an enlarged format.

A similar result is produced by a device that clamps onto the corner of an existing whiteboard and works with special holders for the markers used on the board. When the teacher writes, the device tracks the motion of the marker in the holder and converts it into an image that can be transmitted wirelessly or via a cable to a computer, where it is displayed on the monitor. Again, the student sees exactly what the teacher is writing, and the information can be viewed, saved incrementally, and reviewed as often as desired.

These two solutions have proved effective for some students with low vision, but they are not effective for students who prefer tactile or audio access because the process creates images, not editable text. Handwriting recognition software exists for these systems to convert the writing into editable text that can be manipulated by the computer, and once the printed information has been converted into electronic information, it can be accessed with some of the tools discussed in Chapter 3. However, these programs require the writer to form characters in a specific way. Teachers do not always find it easy to write in this way, and this can result in numerous recognition errors by the software. Improvements in this technology over time may increase its usefulness for visually impaired students.

OVERHEAD PROJECTORS

Although use of overhead projectors is dwindling in classrooms as other technologies become more common, some instructors still choose to display information for their classes with this device. Although tools specifically designed to provide easy access to this projected information are not available, some students have been successful in using handheld telescopes and video magnifiers to access materials presented in this manner.

If the teacher has prepared the overhead transparencies in advance, he or she can provide a photocopy of the materials to a student with low vision, who can then use one of the devices or methods to read print described earlier, such as a video magnifier. Sometimes, however, instructors write on their transparencies during a presentation, particularly when explaining math problems, and then erase the information before moving on to a new topic or problem. In this case, one possible solution might be to use a digital video camera to capture the images of the information on the overhead and display them on a separate monitor. For some students, the image on the monitor would be large enough to read. An added advantage of this option is that a video recording of the presentation can be made for later review. If none of these options seem adequate for a particular student, then the instructor may need to provide his or her materials ahead of time to the teacher of students with visual impairments to prepare them for the student in an accessible format such as braille, large print, or an electronic file.

COMPUTER SLIDESHOW PROJECTION SYSTEMS

Many teachers present information using computer-based slideshow presentation software, such as PowerPoint, in conjunction with projection systems that display the information on movie screens or specialized interactive whiteboards. Students are also being required to create presentations to present to classmates about individual and group projects. Most of the options already discussed for accessing information presented at a distance can also be used to read this type of presentation.

In addition, because slideshows such as these are constructed as electronic files, it is possible for the content to be accessed in ways similar to other forms of electronic information. Most electronic slideshows can be created in such a way that their contents can be imported into a standard word-processing program. This electronic information can then be accessed with the tools discussed in Chapter 3 or used to produce large print or braille with the tools discussed in Chapter 5. (For information on how to create an accessible electronic slideshow, see Web Accessibility for All, n.d.[a], n.d.[b]).

VIDEO DISPLAY SYSTEMS

Although they are not strictly print information, films have been used in the classroom as an educational tool for many decades, and viewing them presents students who are visually impaired with many of the same challenges as viewing print. Despite the great advances in the delivery of films through video and DVD technology, until recently very little has been done to make film accessible to students who are blind or visually impaired. Several of the options discussed previously for viewing information at a distance can be used to view videos presented in the classroom with televisions, computer monitors, or computer projection systems. All have limitations, however, especially for longer presentations.

Another option to explore for students with low vision is to provide a separate monitor for viewing. Most video display systems can be configured to play on two separate displays, so that the class can view the film on one monitor and the visually impaired student can have a separate monitor, although a signal booster may be required to ensure a high-quality image on both. The size of the monitor needed will vary from student to student, but in many cases there will be older television sets within the school that can serve this purpose. The television or monitor will need to be properly located within the classroom with regard to light sources that could create glare and reflections that decrease visibility.

Another approach to providing viewers who are blind or visually impaired with access to videos, both educational and recreational, is the use of *audio description*, in which key visual elements presented in a video or multimedia product are described on a separate soundtrack that is integrated into the final presentation. This process allows individuals who are blind to be informed about content that would not be evident to them simply by listening to the audio. In audio description, narrators typically describe "actions, gestures, scene changes, and other visual information. They also describe titles, speaker names, and other text that may appear on the screen" (AccessIT, The National Center on Accessible Information Technology in Education, n.d.). Other terms used for audio description include video description or descriptive video. The development of standards for description of educational videos and other multimedia materials is under way, and the description of educational media promises to be an extremely beneficial tool for students who are blind or visually impaired.

SUMMARY

A wide selection of tools for accessing print information is available to students who are blind or visually impaired. Some are adequate for accessing small quantities of print information, or spot reading, while others are more effective for reading longer passages. Students can choose tools that will allow them to access information visually, tactilely, or auditorily. In some cases they will want to choose tools that provide access in more than one modality. When appropriate, these can be some of the most powerful learning tools available. At times, the best tool to use will be one that converts print information into electronic information, which allows students to access material in a number of different ways, as discussed in the next chapter. Having the opportunity to select tools from a well-stocked toolbox is essential in assisting students who are blind or visually impaired to access print throughout their school years.

REFERENCES

AccessIT: The National Center on Accessible Information Technology in Education. (n.d.). What is audio description? AccessIT. Retrieved from www.washington.edu/accessit/articles?1079

AccessWorld 2008 guide to assistive technology products (2008). New York: AFB Press.

Castellano, C. (2004). Using readers. *Future Reflections, 23*(3).

Cheadle, B., & Elliott, P. (1995). Of readers, drivers, and responsibility. *The Braille Monitor, 38*(3). Retrieved from www.nfb.org/Images/nfb/Publications/bm/bm95/brlm9503.htm#7

Cowan, C., & Shepler, R. (2000). Activities and games for teaching children to use monocular telescopes. In F. M. D'Andrea & C. Farrenkopf (Eds.), *Looking to learn: Promoting literacy for students with low vision* (pp. 137–166). New York: AFB Press.

Dister, R., & Greer, R. (2004). Basic optics and low vision devices. In A. H. Lueck (Ed.), *Functional vision: A practitioner's guide to evaluation and intervention* (pp. 61–88). New York: AFB Press.

Edman, P. (1992). *Tactile graphics*. New York: AFB Press.

Evans, C. (1997). *Changing channels—Audio-assisted reading: Access to curriculum for students with print disabilities*. Austin: Texas School for the Blind and Visually Impaired. Retrieved February 29, 2008, from www.tsbvi.edu/Education/audioassisted.htm

Evans, C. (1998, June). Audio-assisted reading access for students with print disabilities. *Information Technology and Disabilities Journal, 5.* Retrieved from http://people.rit.edu/easi/itd/itdv05.htm

Flom, R. (2004). Visual functions as components of functional vision. In A. H. Lueck (Ed.), *Functional vision: A practitioner's guide to evaluation and intervention* (pp. 25–60). New York: AFB Press.

Gissoni, F. (2005). *Instructions for the cubarithm slate.* Lexington, KY: American Printing House for the Blind, Fred's Head Companion. Retrieved February 29, 2008, from http://freds headcompanion.blogspot.com/2005/11/instructions-for-cubarithm-slate.html

Greer, R. (2004). Evaluation methods and functional implications: Children and adults with visual impairments. In A. H. Lueck (Ed.), *Functional vision: A practitioner's guide to evaluation and intervention* (pp. 177–256). New York: AFB Press.

Jose, R. T. (1983). Treatment options. In R. T. Jose (Ed.), *Understanding low vision* (pp. 211–250). New York: AFB Press.

Leibs, A. (1999). How to find and manage readers. *A field guide for the sight-impaired reader.* Westport, CT: Greenwood Press.

Osterhaus, S. A. (2008). Teaching math to visually impaired students. Texas School for the Blind and Visually Impaired, Austin. Retrieved February 29, 2008, from www.tsbvi.edu/math

Quillman, R. D., & Goodrich, G. (2004). Interventions for adults with visual impairments. In A. H. Lueck (Ed.), *Functional vision: A practitioner's guide to evaluation and intervention* (pp. 423–475). New York: AFB Press.

Simons, B., & LaPolice, D. (2000). Working effectively with a low vision clinic. In F. M. D'Andrea & C. Farrenkopf (Eds.), *Looking to learn: Promoting literacy for students with low vision* (pp. 84–116). New York: AFB Press.

Watson, G., & Berg, R. (1983). New training techniques. In R. T. Jose (Ed.), *Understanding low vision* (pp. 317–362). New York: AFB Press.

Web Accessibility for All. (n.d.[a]). *How to create descriptive text for graphs, charts & other diagrams.* Madison: Center on Education and Work, University of Wisconsin–Madison. Retrieved February 29, 2008, from www.cew.wisc.edu/accessibility/tutorials/description Tutorial.htm

Web Accessibility for All. (n.d. [b]). *Tutorial for creating accessible PowerPoint presentations.* Madison: Center on Education and Work, University of Wisconsin–Madison. Retrieved February 29, 2008, from www.cew.wisc.edu/accessibility/tutorials/pptmain.htm

Whittle, J. (1995). On how to use readers more effectively. *The Braille Monitor, 38*(12).

Wilkinson, M. (2000). Low vision devices: An overview. In F. M. D'Andrea & C. Farrenkopf (Eds.), *Looking to learn: Promoting literacy for students with low vision* (pp. 117–136). New York: AFB Press.

Wilkinson, M. (1996). Clinical low vision services. In A. L. Corn & A. J. Koenig (Eds.), *Foundations of low vision: Clinical and functional perspectives* (pp. 143–184). New York: AFB Press.

Zimmerman, G. J. (1996). Optics and low vision devices. In A. L. Corn & A. J. Koenig (Eds.), *Foundations of low vision: Clinical and functional perspectives* (pp. 115–142). New York: AFB Press.

3

Technologies for Accessing Electronic Information

Many of the assistive technology solutions for providing students who are blind or have low vision with access to the same information that their sighted classmates are reading involve using high-tech tools to convert print information into electronic, or digital, information, as described in Chapter 2. This chapter will explain the different ways in which students can access that information once it is in electronic form.

Much of the information generated in today's society, however, has not been converted from print but has been created and shared via electronic means. It is digital in origin. And though it is true that accessing that information does not necessarily involve different methods or technology than those used to access information that was originally in print, it is also true that an increasing number of interactions and activities today are done through computers and related technology. Therefore, visually impaired students need to be able to access the mainstream technology that makes up a rapidly growing component of education in today's schools, as discussed in Chapter 1. Technology is not just a tool in the classroom but also a subject in itself—it is part of the core curriculum that all students, including those who are blind or visually impaired, need to study. According to the International Society for Technology in Education (2007), students are expected to "demonstrate a sound understanding of technology concepts, systems, and operations" and "apply digital tools to gather, evaluate, and use information."

For the most part, accessing electronic information in an educational setting means being able to use personal computers and computer applications—running various programs such as word processing, spreadsheet, programming, and database applications; surfing the Internet to do research and use online information tools, such as library catalogs and search engines; and using e-mail. Moreover, a vast array of information that has traditionally been available only in print is now becoming available electronically. (For an introduction to what is available, see Dresner, 2004.) It may also involve using other devices, such as personal digital assistants (PDAs), that provide similar access to electronic files, software, and other information. More broadly, access to electronic information also encompasses being able to use cell phones, MP3 and other music players, and the household and commercial electronic devices that are becoming more ubiquitous every day, such as ATMs (automatic teller machines) at the bank, ticket-purchasing machines at subway stations or movie theaters, and even microwaves and programmable thermostats in the home. (The online technology magazine, *Access World: Technology and People Who Are Blind or Visually Impaired* [www. afb.org/aw] is a good source for information about access to

such mainstream technology.) Although access to electronic information in this broader sense will not be the focus of this chapter, in order to participate fully in today's world—whether going to school, conducting research, working, shopping, or socializing—visually impaired individuals need to access electronic materials and the devices used to support them. The technologies described in this chapter provide access to information in electronic forms as well as computers and other electronic or digital technologies.

ADVANTAGES OF ELECTRONIC ACCESS TOOLS

Portability

Flexibility

Efficiency

Once information is in an electronic format, there is a wide selection of tools from which students can choose to read it, and they can do so through the means that is most effective for them: visually, tactilely, or auditorily. As the descriptions of these devices and other tools throughout this chapter will demonstrate, most of these resources for accessing electronic information have certain characteristics that make them especially valuable: portability, flexibility, and efficiency.

PORTABILITY

Electronic information can be saved in files on a variety of small memory storage devices such as a compact disc (CD), thumb drive (also called a flash drive or memory stick), compact flash card (such as those found in digital cameras or similar devices), or an SD (secure digital) card, such as those found in PDAs. These storage devices are all very small compared to either print or braille books and are exceedingly portable, thus providing users with an easy way to carry information with them between home and school, or from computer to computer. For example, a student can work on a report on her computer at home, store it on her portable thumb drive, and bring it to school to finish it on a computer there.

FLEXIBILITY

Tools for accessing electronic information generally offer the user a great deal of flexibility in how the information is accessed within a particular sensory modality. For example, information accessed visually can be read in a student's preferred font, point size, and text and background color combination. Information accessed through touch can be read via hard-copy or refreshable braille using methods that allow the user to navigate quickly and efficiently through the information. Information accessed auditorily can be manipulated to meet a listener's preferences for rate, volume, and pitch, as well as for male and female voices.

EFFICIENCY

One of the great advantages of using technology to access information electronically is that readers are enabled to access the information in more than one modality at once. For example, a student can view magnified text and hear it spoken simultaneously, or access the information tactilely and

hear it spoken at the same time. It is even possible for the student to access information visually, tactilely, and auditorily all at once. It is much easier for the user to achieve this kind of multimodal access with electronic text than it is with print information. As will be discussed in more detail later in this chapter, reading with two sensory channels at the same time gives a student two kinds of clues to deciphering the text and can thus greatly improve his or her comprehension and ability to access information easily and efficiently.

ACCESSING ELECTRONIC INFORMATION VISUALLY

Computers
- Screen-Enlarging Hardware
- Software Options
- Screen Magnification Software

Other Devices That Provide Electronic Information

As already noted, electronic information is displayed visually throughout the environment in the form of computer displays, automatic teller machines (ATMs), electronic signs, information kiosks, credit and debit card readers, cell phones, PDAs, e-book readers, and so on. Most of these devices display information in a 12-point or smaller font, a size that is not easily legible for most people with low vision. Consequently, individuals with low vision need some type of adaptive hardware or software to read the information displayed on these devices. Some people will be able to use the low vision devices discussed in Chapter 2, such as handheld magnifiers, to read electronic information displayed on screens or monitors. In many cases, though, this will not be efficient or comfortable for reading for long periods of time, and other alternatives, such the ones offered here, will need to be explored.

COMPUTERS

When read or accessed visually, electronic information is typically presented through a visual display on a personal computer's monitor. People with low vision who use computers can choose from hardware or software options to enhance and enlarge the image on the screen. Both options have advantages and disadvantages.

Screen-Enlarging Hardware

Three primary types of hardware adaptations can assist individuals wishing to access a computer visually: larger monitors, screen-magnifying lenses, and adjustable monitor arms.

Larger Monitors

One of the simpler ways to enlarge the information displayed on a desktop computer is to use a larger monitor. Personal computers equipped with 14- or 15-inch monitors generally display text that is too small to be read by people with low vision. Today, 17-inch, 19-inch, 21-inch, and even larger monitors have become affordable. These larger monitors provide a larger image of the text or graphic being displayed by the computer, and for some users, a larger monitor allows a greater working distance. However, many users with low vision find only a slight improvement with the increase in image size afforded by a 21-inch monitor as opposed to a 17- or 19-inch model, but the larger image displayed by a monitor that is 25 inches or larger may be a significant improvement. Larger dedicated computer monitors can be quite expensive, but some flat-screen televisions in the range of 30 to 32 inches can be used as the display for a computer with the appropriate cable

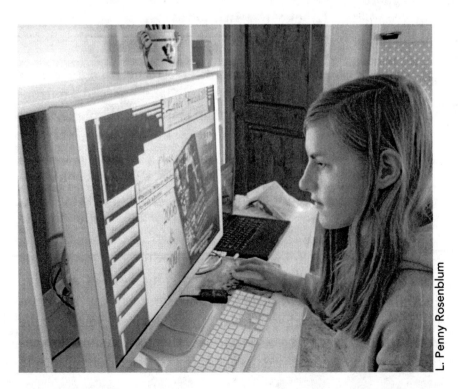

L. Penny Rosenblum

For some students a larger monitor can improve access to the computer and electronic information.

and connector, and these can be more reasonably priced.

Two types of monitors are commonly used with computers. CRT (cathode ray tube) monitors are the older style of large, heavy monitors used on early computers. LCD (liquid crystal display) monitors are generally lighter and offer a flat screen. Many LCD monitors are also available in a wide *aspect ratio*—that is, a display that is wider than it is tall. A wider screen can display even more text that has already been enlarged by one of the methods described later in this chapter. Some users feel that CRT monitors offer a better image than LCD monitors, but others prefer the reduced weight and wider aspect ratio of the LCD.

The major disadvantage of using a larger monitor (25 inches or larger) is that the distance between the user and the edges of the display is also increased, making it more difficult to read the text that is on the periphery. For some individuals, particularly younger students and shorter people, the advantage of the larger image size provided by a larger monitor is cancelled out by the increase in the distance between the user's eyes and the edges of the monitor. Users who want to try a large monitor need the opportunity to explore various sizes of displays with common software applications (such as word processors, spreadsheets, e-mail, and Internet browsers), to be sure that a larger monitor size is an efficient solution for them.

Screen-Magnifying Lenses

Another simple way of enlarging the image displayed on a computer monitor is to attach a Fresnel lens to the front of the monitor. This special type of lens, which serves as a magnifier, comes in a thin, plastic sheet and is marked in concentric sections. The

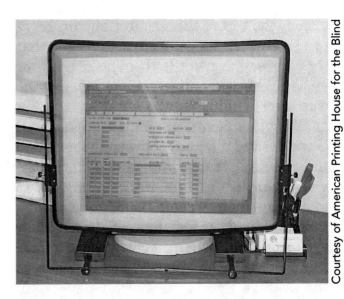

Courtesy of American Printing House for the Blind

Screen magnification hardware, such as this magnifier, can be useful for some students with low vision.

Fresnel lens can either be mounted directly on the monitor or may come with a stand that allows it to be placed in front of the monitor. These types of lenses magnify the image displayed on the monitor up to 2 times its original size. For some users this is adequate magnification, but for many it is not. Most of these magnifiers offer a filtering system that helps to reduce glare. Additional glare filters that do not magnify are also available for computer monitors.

Adjustable Monitor Arms

Sometimes the size of a computer monitor is adequate, but it is placed too low, too high, or too far from the user for the best viewing. Monitor stands or holders that allow users to place the monitor in a better viewing position are produced in various styles and are readily available from office supply dealers. When evaluating or using a monitor stand, there are two factors to consider: the height of the monitor and the working distance of the user. For people with low vision, the top of the monitor should be at eye level when they are sitting erect so that they never have to tilt their head back for viewing. Most monitor stands will provide this level of adjustment.

The other factor that must be considered is the desired distance between the user and the display. Many individuals with low vision can use a standard monitor, but to maximize their vision, their working distance—that is, the distance between their eyes and the visual display (see Chapter 2)—needs to be less than 12 inches, whereas the average working distance for individuals with typical vision is 13 to 16 inches. When individuals have a viewing distance of less than 12 inches, they tend to bend over to get closer to the monitor, which increases back fatigue and decreases the time that the individual can work on the computer before becoming uncomfortable. In addition, when the individual bends forward, the position of his or her abdomen can interfere with the hands and restrict the ability to use the keyboard efficiently.

A monitor stand mounted on a flexible arm can eliminate both of these problems.

This type of monitor stand is usually clamped onto the back edge of the desk or table. The clamp secures a two-part flexible arm that is attached to the monitor. Some arms offer only two or three fixed positions for height adjustment, but more useful models offer a continuous adjustment for monitor height. The monitor arm can also be adjusted to move the monitor forward or backward to position the monitor at the optimal viewing distance, allowing the user to sit comfortably with his or her back against the chair. If an individual with low vision can read text on a regular monitor at less than 12 inches, a flexible monitor arm can be used to place the monitor at the desired working distance and appropriate height.

When purchasing a flexible-arm monitor stand, it is essential to make sure that when it is being used, both the height and working distance can be adjusted to meet the user's needs. Also, monitor stands are rated for different monitor *weights*, not monitor *sizes*. It is therefore also essential to acquire a monitor stand that can support the weight of the monitor to be used. For some individuals with low vision, a flexible-arm monitor

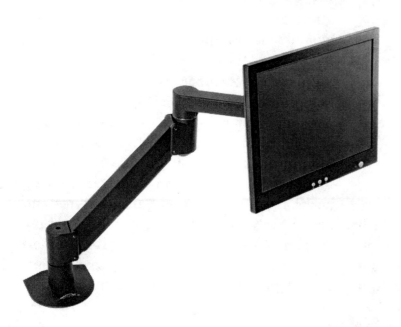

An adjustable monitor arm for a liquid crystal display monitor allows the user to place the monitor in the ideal viewing position.

stand can provide the adaptation necessary to access electronic information displayed by a computer system.

Software Options

There are several different types of programs that can help users with low vision to access the information on their computer screen. Some are built into computers' operating systems, so that individuals can set up features according to their preferences. Cursor-enlarging software is one specific type of program that may either be found in the operating system or added on. Finally, screen magnification software refers to programs that can be installed on a computer that not only allow the user to magnify text or images on the screen but also offer considerable control over the appearance and presentation of text as well as a variety of other features.

Operating System Accessibility Features

Numerous adjustments can be made to the basic operating system software of computers that can increase accessibility for some individuals with low vision. In the Microsoft Windows operating system, these adjustments can be made using the Display Properties menu in the Control Panel and the Accessibility Wizard program. In the Macintosh operating system, the adjustments are found in the System Preferences and Universal Access menus or in the Finder's View menu. Instructors and students can explore these options to determine whether they will provide adequate access to information displayed on the computer monitor or whether they need to investigate other solutions.

Display Properties. Several adjustments in the Windows Display Properties settings

may prove beneficial to users with low vision. These adjustments offer the greatest control and fine tuning of the display but they can be time consuming to explore. The first option to investigate is the setting for the screen resolution. A screen resolution at the lower end of the spectrum (800 × 600 pixels) will increase the size of text, graphics, and other screen elements (such as menus, dialog boxes, and buttons). Many users will find this adjustment helpful. However, choosing a lower screen resolution will cause some applications, particularly those with a great deal of graphics, to appear less clear or sharp, and some applications may not display the desired images at all. Also, some screen elements, particularly menus that have submenus and sub-submenus, may not be fully displayed—that is, parts of the sub-submenu may disappear off of the right edge of the monitor. This problem can be circumvented by using

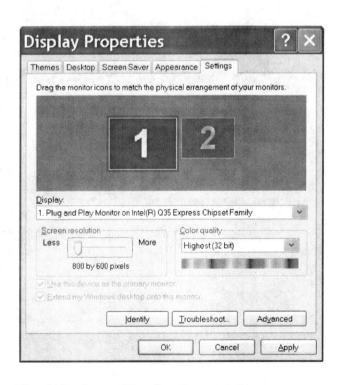

The Windows Display Properties menu.

alternative methods of choosing these menu items, such as shortcut keys or hot keys. The same caveat applies when changing the screen resolution on a Macintosh by going to Displays in the System Preferences.

An alternative to lowering the screen resolution is to adjust individual screen elements using the Appearance/Advanced options in Windows. These options allow the user to select the size of icons, the vertical and horizontal distance between icons, and the font, point size, and attributes (such as bold or italics) of the text used to label icons. The user can also select the font, point size, and attributes of text used for menus, title bars, message boxes, selected items, and tooltips (the text that appears within a box when the cursor or pointer is hovered over an item). The text and background color of many of these screen elements can also be controlled. The combination of settings and adjustments selected by the user, known as a "theme," can be saved in Display Properties; the theme can be used on the current computer

or transferred to other computers. On a Macintosh, the same can be done in the Finder by pressing the Command key with the letter "J." This opens up the View options, and users can change icon size, the size and position of text associated with icons, and other features.

Built-In Accessibility Features. A less time-consuming option than adjusting all of the options in the Display Properties menu in the Microsoft Windows operating system is to use the accessibility features. These are easily navigated by running the Accessibility Wizard program, found in the Programs menu under Accessories/Accessibility. The Wizard asks a set of questions to determine which features should be adjusted for the user. The final result can be a useful adjustment for students wishing to access the computer visually, but most users will find the Wizard itself to be inaccessible, because the vast majority of the text in the Accessibility Wizard dialog boxes is displayed in the standard point size. Students wishing to use this feature may need to

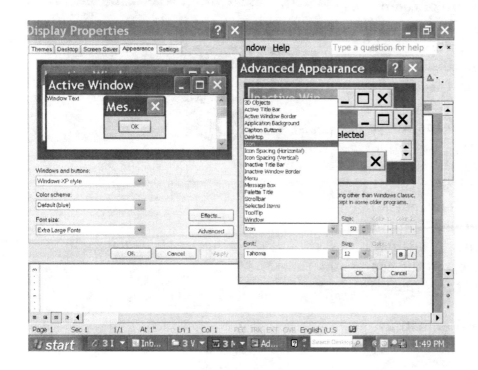

The Display Properties Appearance and Advanced Appearance menus in Microsoft Windows.

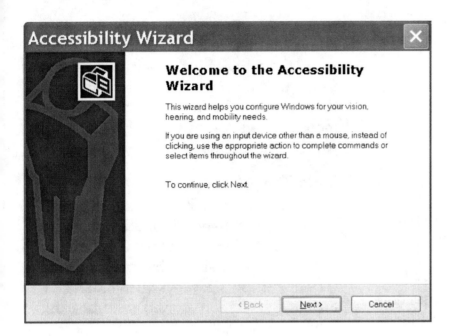

Accessibility features built into the Microsoft Windows operating system are set up by running the Accessibility Wizard program, found in the Programs menu under Accessories/Accessibility.

enlist the assistance of a friend or teacher who has some general knowledge about basic computer modifications to help them run the Accessibility Wizard.

On Macintosh computers, the options in the Universal Access area of the System Preferences are an easy way to make individual adjustments to the visual display. (See Sidebar 3.1, "Accessibility on Macintosh Computers," for more information about the Macintosh built-in accessibility features.)

Cursor-Enlarging Software

For people with low vision, one of the more frustrating aspects of using a computer can be trying to find one's place while typing or trying to select text to highlight. A simple solution that will benefit most users is software that enlarges and enhances the computer cursor (also known as the mouse pointer). Cursor- or pointer-enhancing software provides two relevant features for users with low vision. These programs allow the user to choose from a selection of larger cursors or pointers of different shapes, and they also allow the user to select the color so that the pointer provides better contrast with the background. Additional features include choices for shapes and actions, such as pointing fingers or different kinds of arrows. The shapes, or icons, representing the cursor are almost endless and can point to either the left or right. Actions associated with a cursor include flashing or blinking; color changes or movement within the pointer (for example, the standard hourglass "busy" symbol may be shown turning over, or a clock's hands may move); visual trails displayed when the pointer is moved; and concentric circles targeting the pointer when a keyboard command is used. Most of these features are available as adjustments to the computer's operating system software so that changes made apply to all programs running on the computer.

Cursor-enhancing software is available commercially, as both shareware and freeware. (See Sidebar 3.2, "Assistive Technology for Free: Freeware, Shareware, and Public

ACCESSIBILITY ON MACINTOSH COMPUTERS

In the Macintosh environment, accessibility features are a built-in part of the operating system software and not, as in Microsoft Windows, third-party programs—that is, software developed and sold by companies other than Apple (although there are some shareware and freeware access applications available). The Macintosh accessibility features are found in the System Preferences under Universal Access. Two features are available to assist people with visual impairments in accessing the computer: Zoom, for enlarging the screen for people with low vision, and VoiceOver, the screen reader. All current Macintosh computers include these two functions.

Zoom

Zoom is a screen magnifier that can enlarge the screen content from 1 to 20 times the original size. It is turned on from the Universal Access menu or by pressing the keyboard shortcut Command + Option + 8.

Once activated, the amount of magnification is controlled by using the equals sign (=) key to enlarge the image or Command + Option + Hyphen to decrease the magnification. Several other options can also be set, including showing a preview rectangle (enlarging only a portion of the screen, rather than the whole thing), smoothing the image (making sure the edges of the enlarged image are not jagged), and having the enlarged section follow the cursor around the screen as the user types on the keyboard or moves the mouse. Users can also enable zooming with a mouse scroll wheel.

VoiceOver

VoiceOver is the built-in Macintosh screen reader and is been included with every Macintosh running system 10.4 Tiger or better. It is enabled by pressing the Command + F5 keys (Command + Function + F5 on portable keyboards). When activated, it announces that it is running and then stands by for VoiceOver commands. VoiceOver is run by holding down the Control and Option keys and using the arrow keys to navigate. On Mac OS 10.5 or better, it is also possible to use the number pad on a full-sized keyboard to control VoiceOver.

With VoiceOver, unlike Windows screen readers, every action taken is visible on the screen to a sighted teacher, classmate, or co-worker. This permits collaboration between visually impaired users and their sighted associates. In addition, accessibility is achieved at the application level rather than at the screen reader level. This means that users can achieve major improvements in accessibility by updating an application (assuming that the developer has followed the accessibility guidelines), rather than needing to update the screen reader for each application.

VoiceOver provides access to on-screen controls such as application windows, menus, and icons and is compatible with most built-in Macintosh applications such as the Mail e-mail program, Safari and Opera web browsers, and TextEdit and OpenOffice Version 3 text applications. A wide range of other applications are also accessible. Apple sets guidelines for software development so that developers must make their programs accessible in VoiceOver.

VoiceOver also supports many modern USB-based braille displays and permits system navigation with them. It also allows users to save their VoiceOver preferences on a USB flash drive, permitting users to access their customized setting on any Macintosh computer. Macintosh features a high-quality text-to-speech voice (referred to as "Alex") that is still understandable even as speed increases. In short, VoiceOver is a full-fledged screen reader, similar to JAWS or WindowEyes, running on the latest version of Microsoft Windows.

Running Windows on Macintosh Computers

Since 2006, all Macintosh computers have been produced with the Intel processor, allowing them to run the Windows operating system in addition to the Macintosh operating system. One method of doing this is to dedicate a portion of the hard-drive space (referred to as "partitioning" the drive) on the Macintosh to running Windows. The user can simply restart the computer to switch to either Windows or the Macintosh environment.

However, by installing certain software (referred to as "desktop virtualization" software) the user is able to move seamlessly between the Mac desktop and Windows. This means that a student can install popular accessibility software, such as screen magnification or screen-reading software, that runs only in Windows into a Macintosh. The student can then easily switch between the two desktops (that is, between either the Macintosh or the Windows environment) to take advantage of both. It is important to note that the Windows-based software will only run in the Windows environment; even though it is installed on the Macintosh, it will not run on the Macintosh desktop. But for schools that use the Macintosh operating system on their computers, it is good to know that the option exists for students to benefit from third-party programs designed for Windows-based machines.

More information on VoiceOver and Zoom can be found at www.apple.com/accessibility or on the Curtin University Centre for Accessible Technology web site at www.cucat.org. The Curtin University Centre site also includes VoiceOver documentation in various accessible formats at www.cucat.org/books/vogs. For a product evaluation of VoiceOver, see "An Evaluation of VoiceOver, the Macintosh Screen Reader," by Jim Denham, in *AccessWorld*, 9(6), November 2008, from www.afb.org/afbpress/pub.asp?DocID=aw090603.

Greg Kearney, *programmer, Wyoming Medical Center, Casper, and trainer in Macintosh accessibility*

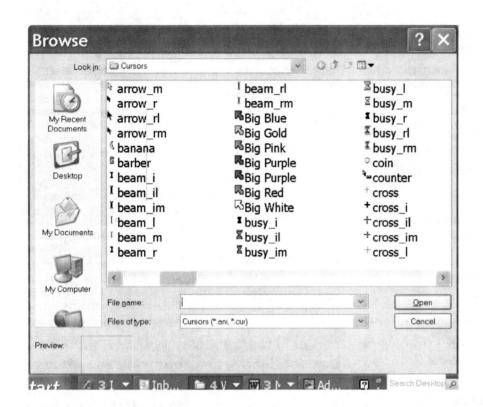

Most cursor-enhancement programs install their larger pointers in the Window/Cursors folder. The list in this screen shot contains files for the Big Blue, Gold, Pink, Purple, Red, and White cursors.

Domain Software." Windows- and Macintosh-based computers also provide some built-in options for adjusting the appearance of the cursor, but the choices for size are limited and may not be adequate for low vision users.

Combining Hardware and Software Adjustments

For some individuals with low vision, a combination of the hardware options and system software adaptations that have been discussed can provide adequate access to electronic information on a computer. For example, Stacey might choose to use a 25-inch or larger monitor mounted on a flexible-arm monitor stand, which allows the monitor to be positioned at the ideal height and working distance for her. In addition, she might change the setting on the computer by adjusting the basic operating system to lower the screen resolution to 1024 × 768 pixels. She might also increase the icon size and the size of the text used in the icon title (referred to as the "text title"), as well as expand the horizontal and vertical spacing between icons to improve visibility. Font, point size, and color combinations could be selected for menus, title bars (the line that is usually at the top of the screen and contains the title of the window), and other screen elements to make it easier for her to see these items. She might also download a free cursor-enhancement program from the Internet to make it easier to locate and work with the pointer. All of these adjustments would then be saved as the student's new theme in Display Properties.

With the combination of these adjustments and the use of the larger monitor on the flexible-monitor arm, students can now sit in a comfortable position for keyboarding and view the monitor at an adequate working distance. This, or a similar arrangement, can provide an enlarged display that will be useful to some individuals with low

SIDEBAR 3.2

ASSISTIVE TECHNOLOGY FOR FREE: FREEWARE, SHAREWARE, AND PUBLIC DOMAIN SOFTWARE

Versions of assistive technology software can sometimes be found for free on the Internet and are variously known as freeware, shareware, and public domain software. There are some slight differences among these designations:

- *Freeware* is copyrighted software given away for free by the author. Although it is available for free, the author retains the copyright, which means that you cannot do anything with it that is not expressly allowed by the author. Usually, the author allows people to use the software but not sell it.

- *Shareware* is available free of charge, but the author usually requests that you pay a small fee if you like the program and use it regularly. By sending the small fee, you become registered with the producer so that you can receive service assistance and updates. You can copy shareware and pass it along to friends and colleagues, but they too are expected to pay a fee if they use the product. Shareware is also copyrighted.

- *Public domain software* refers to any program that is not copyrighted. Public-domain software is free and can be used without restrictions.

Users should always be cautious about downloading programs from the Internet, so it is a good idea for individuals wishing to take advantage of freeware, shareware, and public domain software to enlist the assistance of a knowledgeable technology specialist.

---

vision, although in many cases it will not provide enough enlargement. Determining the most beneficial options for enlarging information on the screen will be discussed in Chapter 8.

Screen Magnification Software

Screen magnification software is a type of computer program that allows the user to magnify or enlarge the image being displayed on a computer's monitor. It is a more all-encompassing solution than the adjustments discussed previously, which only affect certain screen elements. An important point to remember about this type of software is that as the screen magnification increases, the field of view—the amount of the original screen that can be seen at any one time—is decreased. Users must adjust to this smaller field of view to use this type of software successfully.

Numerous types of screen magnification software are available, and they vary widely in price and features. People with low vision who wish to access the computer screen visually can select from freeware and shareware,

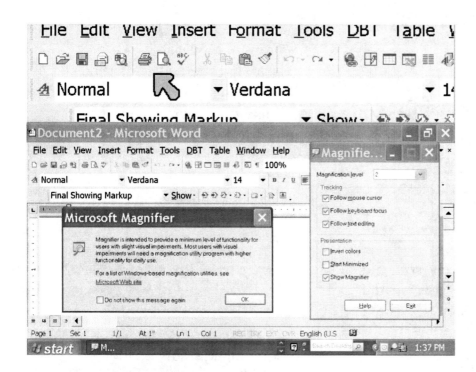

The Microsoft Magnifier program enlarges all screen elements but does not offer the more robust features found in specialized screen magnification software.

as well as from commercial programs. Although the commercial products offer a vast array of features, there are times when the less expensive alternatives may offer the features that a student or other user needs most.

Simple screen magnification software is included in most computer operating systems. Unlike the adjustments that can be made to the operating system accessibility features, discussed previously, screen magnification software provides enlargement of all screen elements (menus, icons, dialog boxes, etc.). In the Windows operating system, this feature is called Microsoft Magnifier, and it is found in the Programs/Accessories menu. In the Macintosh operating system (systems 10 and higher), the program is called Zoom and is found in the Universal Access area in the System Preferences (as already described in Sidebar 3.1). These screen magnification programs offer some of the basic features of screen magnification software, such as the ability to:

- adjust the degree of magnification within a given range

- track or follow cursor movement
- invert colors (reverse polarity)
- enlarge the cursor

Screen magnification software packages that fall into the freeware and shareware categories typically offer some additional features, such as:

- ability to adjust location of magnified area on screen
- cursor or pointer enhancements

Commercially available screen magnification software packages for the Windows environment have refined these features and added still others, such as the ability to

- adjust magnification in a range from 1× to 16×, including 1.25×, 1.5×, and 1.75×;
- track or follow movement or changes on the screen, including the mouse pointer, the writing cursor or caret, opening and closing windows, menus, and buttons and other controls in dialog boxes;

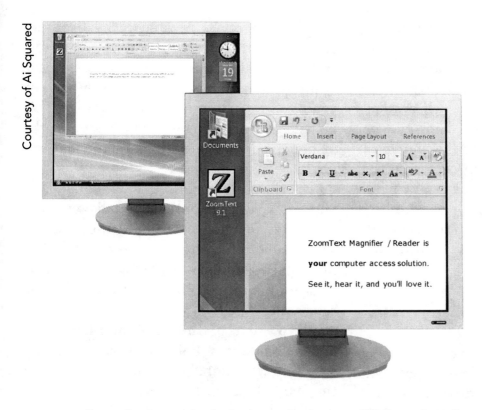

Courtesy of Ai Squared

Commercial screen magnification programs offer many features that can help students with low vision access the computer.

- set boundaries to include or exclude areas of the screen where tracking will be in effect;
- adjust the alignment of an object being tracked or followed on the screen;
- smooth colors to avoid pixilation;
- adjust polarity;
- enlarge and enhance cursors.

High-end screen magnification programs also include some basic screen-reading functions that can be useful to some users by providing auditory information about what is on the screen. (Screen-reading software is discussed in the section on auditory access later in this chapter.) These functions include the following:

- Basic screen-reading features for common screen elements, such as menus and icons with synthesized speech
- Document-reading features that provide a tool for viewing a document with each word highlighted as it is spoken with synthesized speech

High-end software that includes all these features will generally be more expensive, but the features offer significant advantages.

Adjusting Magnification

The degree to which screen magnification software can enlarge information that is displayed on a computer screen can range from 1× to 16×. The magnification can be adjusted several ways. One of the easier ways is to press a combination of keys on the keyboard—often referred to as *hot keys*—to issue a command. For example, pressing and holding the Control key and the Shift key, and then pressing the Plus key (+) on the Numpad (the display of numbers on the right side of many keyboards) might increase the magnification, while pressing Control + Shift + Minus (-) on the Numpad might decrease the magnification. These hot keys can allow users to adjust the degree of magnification quickly so that they can zoom in for a detailed view and then zoom back out to see a wider view easily. Since the amount of information displayed on the screen decreases as magnification increases, with magnification above 6× or 8×, the user may be viewing such a small amount of information that using screen magnification may no longer be the most efficient way for that person to access the computer. In such cases, the user may want to explore other options, such as auditory methods of accessing the computer, including screen-reading software (discussed later in this chapter).

Becoming Oriented to the Magnified Image

Even when using the entire screen to display a magnified image, a magnification program will only be able to display a portion of the original image regardless of whether its content is text or pictures. If, for example, a student selects a 2× magnification, the screen will only be able to display one-quarter of the original image at any one time. The student may move the display to view other portions of the original image but will not be able to see more than this. It can be challenging for users with low vision to figure out what portion of the original unmagnified image they are viewing and where it is located in the image as a whole. Determining their location in and orientation to the unmagnified image is one of the cognitive skills that students must master to use screen magnification software efficiently.

Several features and options have been added to high-end commercial software packages to assist users with this challenge. For example, some programs have a hot key command that temporarily returns the screen to an unmagnified view in which the section of the image that had been magnified is displayed in a negative image—that

is, with the colors reversed. The user can use this highlighting effect to establish the section's location and orientation within the original image and then press the hot key again to return to the magnified image. This helps the user to know what section of the display he or she is looking at and what has not yet been seen.

Another approach to this challenge is to offer a variety of options for viewing the magnified image. For example, the user can select a small rectangular area of the screen to be used to display the magnified image. The unmagnified image appears in the remaining portion of the screen. Only a small portion of the original image will appear magnified, but it will appear on the screen in its original location directly under the lens. This option simultaneously provides a view of the entire unmagnified screen along with the ability to magnify a specific part of the display. It simulates the effect one might get from viewing the screen with a handheld magnifier, which may make this option seem familiar to students and therefore easy to learn. This "lens"-type viewing mode does not lend itself to reading long text documents, but it is an excellent tool for looking at maps and other graphic information. It is helpful for many users with low vision who can see well enough to comprehend the basic layout of what is on the unmagnified screen and its major components, but need the magnification to read text and view small details. It also works well for those who wish to view the entire image and then zoom in on a specific section of the image. Another viewing option is to have the program magnify only one line of text and leave the remainder of the screen unmagnified. The user presses the Up and Down Arrow keys or uses the mouse to move the magnifier up and down on the screen. This is similar to reading with a bar magnifier. Many users find this to be a good tool for reading documents and e-mails.

Another useful feature is the ability to adjust the location and size of the rectangular viewing windows that appear on the computer's screen. Some computer applications, such as word processing or accounting software, require the user to view information located in different parts of the screen and perform specific actions. The ability to change the size of the window can facilitate those tasks. For example, editing word-processing documents requires the user to read text and make changes to it. Adjusting the size of the magnified viewing window so that it is the height of one line of text and the full width of the screen can make the editing process much easier for someone with low vision because it highlights one line of the text and makes it easier to track across the line. In contrast, a user working with an accounting program that displays multiple columns of numbers might choose to adjust the viewing window to the width of one column and the height of the full screen rather than of a horizontal line. Selecting the best viewing window size and shape will generally be a matter of personal preference and will depend on the task. Users will need to develop a general knowledge of the various options for viewing windows and then try them with different applications to determine which is best for a specific activity.

Efficient use of these features can help students to cope with the location and orientation issues caused by screen magnification. When a user chooses to use a full-screen viewing mode in which the magnified image fills the screen, maintaining orientation can become difficult. In this viewing mode, users have no reference points to help them determine if they are

viewing the top, side, middle, or bottom of the original image. When portions of the original image are left unmagnified, many users with low vision can see the screen well enough to determine their location while viewing the details in the magnified window.

On occasion, a user might wish to have multiple viewing windows open at the same time. Some programs allow the user to have more than one magnified viewing window displayed on the screen. For example, a student might put a magnified viewing window around the time display on the screen and also have a second window for the information displayed by the application that he or she is using.

Navigating with Screen Magnifiers

Regardless of which viewing option users might select, they will need to navigate, or move the magnified view around to view different parts of the unmagnified image. This can be done by using the mouse (or some other pointing device such as a trackball or joystick) or keyboard commands. Using the mouse to navigate around the screen works well for some users who wish to move quickly from one area of the screen to locate text or graphics in another part of the screen. The flexibility this provides is particularly beneficial when viewing material such as a map, where the user wishes to explore at random instead of in a straight line horizontally or vertically. Navigating with the mouse becomes more of a challenge when the user wants to read text and must move the mouse from left to right over the words. Because the mouse moves so easily, it is difficult to prevent it from moving vertically while it is moving horizontally across the text—motion that sometimes results in nausea or motion sickness (similar to the sensation felt by untrained users of video magnifiers, as mentioned in Chapter 2). Using the mouse to navigate text is usually not an efficient option for most users with low vision. Students will want to explore both mouse and keyboard navigation options to see what will work best for them; a combination of these two methods will provide the user with the most flexibility.

For users who find the mouse difficult to use, high-end screen magnification programs provide keyboard navigation commands that facilitate the task of reading text. The commands are usually executed by a combination of keys. For example, many commands use a "modifier key" (such as the Alt, Ctrl, Shift, or Caps Lock), combined with the arrow keys or one of the other traditional navigation keys (such as Home, End, Page Up, or Page Down) to move around and view another portion of the text. These commands will display text as groups of lines and words. Depending on the view being used and the magnification level selected, the user may be able to see an area only about 5 to 10 words wide and 5 to 10 lines high. Reading with keyboard commands requires that the user not only memorize the commands but also master the timing and coordination necessary to issue the command at exactly the right moment to move smoothly across the text.

Automatic *scrolling* (vertical movement) and *panning* (horizontal movement) features have been added to screen magnifiers to address the difficulty of navigating through text. These features allow a user to have the text move automatically at his or her selected speed for both horizontal and vertical movement. The scrolling of lines can be controlled so that the program moves the text up one line at a time, as it pans back and forth across the lines of text, or

the user can have the vertical movement delayed until after a specified number of lines have been panned.

Controlling Appearance and Presentation

Scrolling and panning can be combined with other common features of screen magnification software to enhance their usefulness. The ability to control the color of the text and its background can be used to display each word in turn in its reverse (or inverted) text and background color combination, highlighting each word as the program pans through the text. Synthetic speech, discussed later in this chapter, can also be provided as an auditory presentation of the text. This combination of auditory and visual information can be an invaluable tool for individuals with low vision. The ability to see and hear text simultaneously can be very useful. Many people with fluctuating low vision who access printed information visually have developed the habit of rereading letters and words to confirm their identification. When users hear the text at the same time they view it, the auditory information that is provided confirms or corrects their understanding of the word, eliminating the need to reread it (see Technology Tip: "Using Screen Magnification to Improve Reading").

Users can also select how text will be formatted on the screen. There are three popular ways for displaying the moving text. The first is for the software to pan across the text from left to right while highlighting and speaking each word, jump back to the left, delay for a preselected period of time, and then pan across the next line. At a point selected by the user, the text will scroll up a predetermined number of lines (so that the

USING SCREEN MAGNIFICATION TO IMPROVE READING

The ability of some screen magnification software to magnify text, speak it aloud, and highlight words as they are spoken allows students to use two sensory modalities for reading simultaneously. This combination of visual and auditory reading reinforces a student's understanding of the text and can make reading more efficient than when a student uses either sense alone.

Paired auditory and visual reading can also be used as an instructional tool to help individuals with low vision develop better skills in both visual reading and audio-assisted reading when these reading modalities are used independently of each other. Since screen magnification software enlarges the text on the monitor, fewer words are shown at a time, requiring additional time for the student to navigate through the text. This can have an adverse effect on reading speed for some students.

Strategies for Increasing the Visual Reading Rate of Readers with Low Vision

To help a student increase his or her visual reading rate, the instructor can use features of screen magnification software to start the student reading visually, then add speech, gradually increase the auditory reading rate, and finally decrease the magnification:

- Work with the student to help determine the ideal combination of visual features available in the screen magnification program so that the student will be able to sit in a relaxed position and at a comfortable distance and view the displayed text at the ideal size for that working distance.
- Once the student is comfortable with the visual display, add the synthetic speech and allow the student to listen and follow along visually.
- Determine, by observing the student reading the text, when he or she might be ready to increase the auditory reading rate. The amount of practice needed to become proficient with each increased reading rate will vary from individual to individual.
- After the student becomes comfortable with several increases in the auditory reading rate, try decreasing the magnification one level.
- Students who are already good readers but who wish to increase their reading speed may want to try the strategy of identifying some of the words by their size and shape, using the auditory identification of the word to reinforce what they are seeing. The student may not be able to see each letter of a word but can begin to identify the word without having to perceive all the details necessary to recognize the individual letters based instead on

(continued on next page)

TECHNOLOGY TIP *(CONTINUED)*

- the length of the word;
- the shape of the word—the arrangement of tall letters, short letters, wide letters, and letters with descenders (tails);
- the context of the word in the reading material.

As students begin to master this skill, they can attempt to apply it to printed text that is not displayed on the computer. Teachers need to be cautious in using this approach with beginning or struggling readers, however, because guessing at unknown words is not a beneficial strategy for helping students improve vocabulary or comprehension. But for students with low vision who have a solid grasp of reading, word attack skills, and automatic word identification, learning to quickly identify common words by their distinctive visual characteristics can be one way to increase reading speed.

Developing Audio-Assisted Reading Skills

Individuals who need to improve their auditory listening skills for reading can also benefit from using this combination of features to see the words they are hearing. When synthesized or computer-generated speech is difficult to understand, if a student has a visual display of the text, he or she can learn to associate the auditory stimulus with the word being displayed visually. Practice with paired visual and auditory reading can help some individuals develop more effective and efficient audio-assisted reading skills.

reading focus moves down) and then continue the panning process. Another format offers the option to view one continuous line of magnified text in a manner similar to a stock exchange "ticker." The one line of magnified text can be located anywhere on the screen, with the remainder of the screen displaying the unmagnified image of the text. The text being read aloud is highlighted in both the magnified and unmagnified view. A third option is a format that emulates a teleprompter. This display reformats each line of text so that it is presented within the space of the magnified window, and in this way the viewing window does not have to move to the right to show the end of the line and then jump back to the beginning of the next line. The text is reformatted so that a word that would otherwise be off of the right edge of the screen has been moved down one line and placed at the left edge of the screen. (This is similar to the "word wrap" feature found in word-processing software.) As the visual highlight and auditory-assisted reading pan and scroll through the text, the user is able to hear and see the highlighted words as they pass by.

Panning, scrolling, and audio-assisted reading features offer users both visual and auditory controls and adjustments to meet their individual needs. The selection of features and adjustments of options chosen by a user can be saved as a configuration file, which can be used again or transferred to other computers. Configuration files can be saved for multiple users on the same computer system, allowing each user to have the screen magnification software set for his or her ideal conditions and eliminating the need to reset the options each time the computer is used.

OTHER DEVICES THAT PROVIDE ELECTRONIC INFORMATION

As mentioned earlier in this chapter, many devices that display electronic information have small screens that do not offer the user the ability to select the font and point size of the display. For example, public information kiosks and automatic teller machines (ATMs) seldom offer the user the ability to select the size of the text being viewed (although "talking ATMs"—teller machines that allow users to listen to directions through headphones—have made these devices usable with auditory access).

E-book readers are stand-alone devices that display electronic text such as books and magazines. These devices often allow the user to adjust the point size of the text being displayed. Although these have a limited choice of fonts and point sizes, they do provide adequate access for some users. Their portability and ease of use make them attractive to many people with low vision. The addition of synthesized speech available on some of these devices and the ability to play a variety of recorded formats further increases their potential and usability for students who are blind or visually impaired. E-book readers that are designed to be accessible to people with visual impairments are often accessed auditorily and are discussed later in this chapter.

Electronic calculators are available with enlarged displays. They do not provide selectable fonts and point sizes, but simply offer a larger display of the numbers—between 3/8

and 3/4 inches high. Users will need to try out various calculators to determine if their displays are large enough and if they have all of the features and functions needed. However, optical devices can be used with calculators to access their displays. Most computers include a basic and a scientific calculator that can be accessed with the same adaptations used to access the computer in general. Talking calculators that have the added advantage of speech output to reinforce the visual display are also

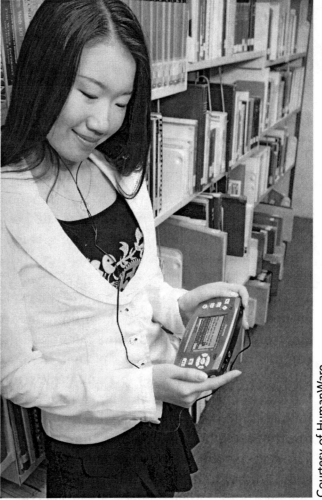

Courtesy of HumanWare

This e-book reader displays text in several fonts and point sizes, and the student can listen to the text via synthesized speech or recorded speech.

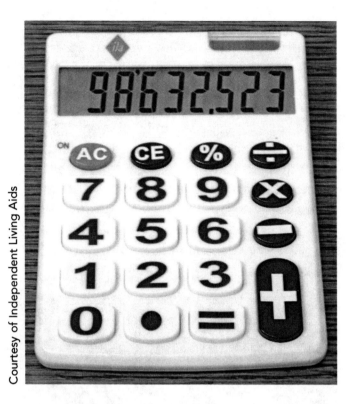

The large keys and enlarged display of some calculators make them useful for many students with low vision.

available. Users will wish to try various models to determine which one has the best features to meet their needs. Talking calculators are discussed in the section on auditory access later in this chapter.

Dictionaries, thesauruses, and other reference works are available online as an electronic alternative to print versions and can be accessed visually through a computer system with screen magnification hardware or software. There are also hand-held dictionaries, some of which have the ability to display text in more than one size. The options offered may be large enough for some individuals and might possibly be used with an optical device. These electronic dictionaries are discussed later in this chapter. All of these options have advantages and disadvantages, and can meet the needs of some individuals with low vision.

ACCESSING ELECTRONIC INFORMATION TACTILELY

Refreshable Braille
- Computers with Refreshable Braille Displays
- Accessible PDAs with Refreshable Braille Displays

Touch Tablets

For students whose primary method of reading and obtaining information is through touch, there are two basic ways to access electronic information. First, the information can be translated into braille using braille translation software and then embossed, or printed, on a braille embosser. (For more information on this technology, see Chapters 4 and 5.) This provides hard-copy braille similar to that provided in a braille book. Although braille translation software has increased the speed with which paper braille can be produced, the computer translations are not free of errors, and the process requires some production time and editing by a knowledgeable braillist. The second option for tactile access to electronic information, in contrast, provides immediate access to electronic information through the use of an electronic *refreshable braille display*.

REFRESHABLE BRAILLE

The term *refreshable* or *electronic braille display* refers to a group of devices that feature a row of plastic pins in groups of six or eight, which are raised and lowered in different combinations to represent the dots of the braille cell. These displays provide a single

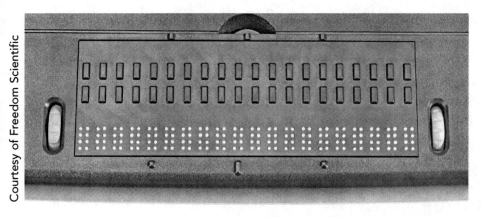

Courtesy of Freedom Scientific

This refreshable braille display can be used to tactilely access text displayed on a computer. It uses an 8-dot cell instead of the usual 6-dot cell. The bottom two dots, dots 7 and 8, are used to give additional information about the cursor location and text styles, such as bold or italics.

line of braille containing from 18 to 80 characters. Navigation features allow the user to move forward and backward through the information. Refreshable braille displays are available in two basic formats: as a peripheral device used with a computer and as a feature of a PDA.

Computers with Refreshable Braille Displays

Computer peripheral braille displays can be connected to either a desktop or notebook computer via a cable. These types of braille displays are often designed to sit in front of or underneath the standard keyboard, allowing the user to move easily between the display (for reading) and the keyboard (for writing and controlling the computer). Text that appears on the computer screen is represented in braille on the display. A user wishing to access the computer through the use of a refreshable braille display will need both the hardware device and specialized software, known as *screen-reading software*, to make it work effectively. The software directs the text to the braille display as well as to a video monitor. (For a more detailed discussion of screen-reading software, see the next section on auditory access.) Most devices will present both uncontracted and

Refreshable braille displays for computers can display either 40 or 80 characters.

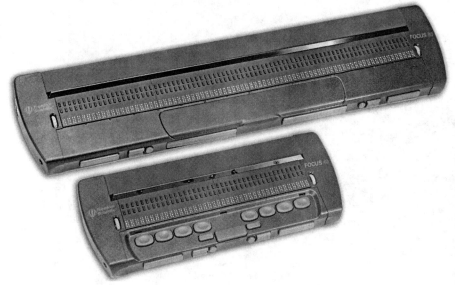

Courtesy of Freedom Scientific

contracted braille—or even computer braille—depending on how the device is configured. Because of the transmission of electronic information through devices using refreshable braille displays, the quantity of information available in a tactile format has increased enormously.

Accessible PDAs with Refreshable Braille Displays

Refreshable braille displays are also offered as a feature on some PDAs designed specifically for people with visual impairments. (Accessible PDAs are discussed in more detail later in this chapter.) These devices, also referred to as *portable notetakers* or *pocket PCs*, are available with either a six-key braille keyboard or a standard QWERTY keyboard (the typical keyboard seen on typewriters and computers, so called because of the sequence of letters on the top row of letters). They offer one line of braille, typically with 18–40 characters. A valuable feature of a braille display provided as part of a PDA is the ability to connect the device to either a desktop or notebook computer to serve as a peripheral braille display for the computer. When the PDA is connected to the computer, files or information from the Internet, as well as information stored on the computer, can be directly transferred into the device for reading via the braille display. Again, screen-reading software is required to be running on the computer when these devices are used as a braille display for the computer. Newer models of PDAs offer the ability to connect directly to the Internet, send and receive e-mail, and communicate via satellite as part of a global positioning system (GPS) for directions, as well as additional options for accessing electronic information tactilely.

Because they provide access to potentially unlimited amounts of information, accessible PDAs with refreshable braille displays are extremely valuable tools for both students and adults for several reasons. The availability of hard-copy or paper braille is significantly limited compared to the vast number of books in print. In addition, braille books need expansive storage space (for example, a high school history

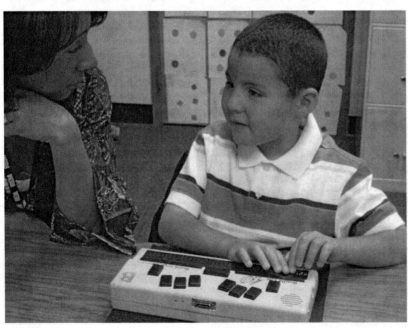

L. Penny Rosenblum

This student is reading his assignment on the refreshable braille display of his accessible PDA.

textbook in braille could fill an entire bookshelf) and, if print material is not already available in a braille version, it requires time for translation, editing, and other processing. Although paper braille will always be useful for students, especially beginning readers, as information that was previously only available in print becomes available electronically, braille readers have the potential to access hundreds and even thousands of books electronically that would ordinarily never be available in paper braille. With the appropriate technology, such as an accessible PDA with a refreshable braille display, students who read braille can gain access to vast quantities of written information in an electronic format. Providing braille readers access to electronic text, even at a young age, through the use of an accessible PDA with a refreshable braille display can increase their library from just a few books to hundreds. The impact that this access can have on the development of literacy skills for these students cannot be overstated.

TOUCH TABLETS

Some excellent instructional tools that provide tactile access to electronic information for students who are blind or visually impaired have been created by integrating tactile graphics with a computer technology known as *touch tablets*. A touch tablet is a device with a touch-sensitive surface, usually about 11 × 11½ inches, controlled by software running on a computer. The sensors in the surface send signals to the computer when it perceives a touch at various points on the tablet. Touch tablets have a wide variety of mainstream uses, from educational toys for children to drawing tools for artists and graphic designers.

Programs have been designed to take advantage of touch tablets in ways that are useful to individuals who are blind or visually impaired. These programs often use the computer to add synthesized or recorded speech to the experience. One type of program uses touch tablets for braille instruction. These programs contain a series of braille pages that can be placed over the tablet, with each page containing a lesson in braille reading that is guided by the computer software. When the student presses a graphical icon on the page, instructions for the lesson are provided in an audio format. For example, the student may be instructed to locate certain targets among the lines of dots, characters, or words embossed on the page. Pressing one of the target items sends a signal to the computer, which determines if that was the correct target and then provides spoken feedback. This type of program is proving to be an excellent tool for both youths and adults learning braille; students can also use it independently to practice and reinforce skills taught by their braille instructor.

Other programs have been developed that use a touch tablet to teach a variety of subjects through the use of tactile graphics and audio feedback. One such program provides tactile graphics of various maps. As the user examines the tactile drawing, pressing the tablet at any location on the map elicits spoken information about that location. For example, suppose a student exploring a raised-line drawing of a world map on the touch tablet becomes curious about the inverted triangle shape of India. A single press at this location might elicit a spoken message that says, "India. Country in South Central Asia." Pressing India a second time, the student might hear, "India. Largest democracy in the world." A third press might elicit, "India. Largest industry: retail, which accounts for over 10 percent of the country's GDP and around 8 percent of the employment."

A variety of educational programs and activities have been developed to take advantage of touch tablets. In addition, teachers can use this technology to create customized activities for students on any desired topic. As additional software and activities are developed, touch tablet technology has tremendous potential as an instructional tool for students who are blind or visually impaired, similar to the ways computer-based instructional tools have been used to teach specific content in general education.

ACCESSING ELECTRONIC INFORMATION AUDITORILY

Computers and Related Hardware and Software
- Speech Synthesizers
- Software Options

Other Devices
- Accessible PDAs
- E-Text and E-Text Readers
- Talking Dictionaries
- Talking Calculators
- Digital Voice Recorders

COMPUTERS AND RELATED HARDWARE AND SOFTWARE

As is evident throughout this chapter, the personal computer is the individual's key to accessing electronic information. Personal computers allow the user to input information with a keyboard, mouse, or other device. The output is usually displayed on a monitor screen, and in addition to being able to access what is displayed on the screen via the senses of vision and touch, users who are visually impaired can access it through their sense of hearing. For someone to access such information auditorily, a system is needed that processes text entered through the keyboard or displayed on the screen and speaks it aloud. Two additional components for the computer system are needed for this to take place: a *speech synthesizer* and software that directs the information input to the computer to go to the speech synthesizer as well as to the monitor.

Speech Synthesizers

The *speech synthesizer* is the part of a system that produces the sounds of oral language and combines them into synthesized speech, which can be heard through the system's speaker. Originally, speech synthesizers were separate hardware devices connected to a computer. When these systems were first developed, some people had difficulty understanding the synthesized speech because it did not sound like human speech; it sounded more like a robot voice. Users pressed manufacturers to develop synthesizers that could produce speech that would be easier to understand. This was achieved, but at a higher price; speech synthesizers ranged in price from a few hundred to several thousand dollars. High-end models provided clear, fast speech with a quick response time, while less-expensive models had poorer speech quality, and the user experienced a short delay between issuing a command and hearing the text spoken.

As computer technology improved, so did sound cards, the part of the system that produces speech. Early sound cards could not produce the high-quality sound needed for synthesized speech. But with more powerful and faster circuitry wired directly into the sound card, producing high-quality synthesized speech became possible. Programs known as *software speech synthesizers* were developed that could use the new sound cards to produce high-quality synthesized speech. This advance proved a significant boost to people seeking auditory access to electronic information because it eliminated the need to spend additional resources on a hardware speech synthesizer. However, some users still prefer to purchase a hardware speech synthesizer because they usually have a faster response time than a software synthesizer. For example, when the user issues the command to begin speaking, stop speaking, or move to a new line and speak, a hardware synthesizer will execute these commands more quickly. For many users, however the slower response time of a software synthesizer is not a big enough disadvantage to warrant the expenditure of purchasing a hardware synthesizer.

Software Options

There are several types of software that can direct the information to a speech synthesizer:

- Talking word processors
- Text readers
- Self-voicing applications
- Screen-reading software

Although screen readers offer the most features, greatest control over navigation, and maximum access to many of the items that appear on the computer screen, the other types of software can be useful in certain situations. In this section, the pros and cons of the simplest and least expensive options will be discussed first, before screen-reading software, the most popular option, is presented.

Talking Word Processors

Talking word processors are another option that can be used with a speech synthesizer to provide auditory access to information displayed on a computer's screen. They perform the same functions as a standard word processor and use synthesized speech to speak the text entered via the keyboard and read the text displayed on the screen. The text can be accessed and navigated by character, word, line, or sentence. Talking word processors generally cost less than $100.

Although this type of software can provide access to some electronic information, it does not give the user complete access to all of the information displayed on the screen. For example, some talking word processors do not read aloud all of the menus and dialog boxes displayed by the program, and of course, they cannot be used to voice other applications. These characteristics limit the value of talking word processors for students who need to access the computer auditorily. However, they can serve as an effective tool for initial keyboarding instruction and practice, because they can provide the learner with immediate auditory and visual feedback, eliminating the need for the teacher to inform the student about the accuracy of his or her keyboarding. Talking word processors are less expensive and generally easier to learn than full-featured screen readers. Another use of talking word processors for some students is as a writing tool, which will be discussed further in Chapter 4.

Text Readers

Text readers are software programs that use synthesized speech to read aloud documents that have been saved in the text format. They allow a user access to material that has already been compiled but not to information being input into the computer. These programs are available as freeware, shareware, and commercial products (see Sidebar 3.2). Most text readers are designed for individuals with reading difficulties, but some students who are visually impaired can also benefit from these programs. Users with low vision can adjust the font and point size of most documents and also listen to the text read aloud via synthesized speech. As discussed in Chapter 2, the pairing of visual and auditory information can be very helpful to some individuals.

Text readers are generally designed for reading the text from beginning to end, but most allow the user to pause or temporarily interrupt the speech and then continue reading from that point. Navigation features that help the user to move efficiently through a document (such as being able to read by characters, words, lines, and sentences) are rarely found in text readers. The other limitation of text-reading software is that it does not read aloud other screen elements that are read by dedicated screen-reading programs, such as menus, title bars, dialog boxes, and buttons. It simply reads the text in a document.

Self-Voicing Software

Unlike today's computers, the earliest "talking computers," as they were called, did not have dedicated screen-reading software—that is, a program whose function was solely to voice what was on the screen. The speech or screen-reading functions were programmed directly into specific applications, such as talking word processor programs, talking calculator programs, and talking checkbook programs. These *self-voicing programs*—that is, programs that could produce their own speech—were very useful and demonstrated how these types of tools could be beneficial to individuals who are blind or visually impaired.

Some self-voicing applications—programs that can read aloud any information displayed on a computer's screen by that particular program, including text, menu, dialog boxes, and buttons—are still useful today. These programs do not require the use of additional screen-reading software. Talking web browsers that use the computer's sound card to produce synthesized speech are an example of a self-voicing application. Some of the specialized scanning systems discussed in Chapter 2, sometimes referred to as "scan-and-read" systems, also offer self-voicing features. At first glance, self-voicing applications seem to offer great promise for accessing electronic information. Their limitation, however, is that they only allow the user to access the information provided by the specific application (for example, the web browser) but do not provide auditory access to other applications being used (such as a word processor). In addition, in order to use a self-voicing application, the user first has to make sure the computer is accessible to begin with; if not, he or she will not be able to get to the self-voicing application independently to use it. These types of applications have some use for students who have low vision and can access the computer visually because they allow the user to take advantage of the dual sensory input by accessing the information both visually and auditorily.

Specialized scanning systems are the most widely used example of self-voicing application used by students who are blind or visually impaired. In addition to allowing users to convert printed information into electronic information, these systems also have the ability to read a wide variety of electronic files. Users can open files using the software found in a specialized scanning system and have the contents of those files read aloud via synthesized speech.

Educators working with visually impaired students may wish to note that although many educational software programs tout the fact that they provide speech output, caution is indicated when considering the use of these programs for students who are blind or visually impaired. In most cases the auditory information provided by these programs is very limited and is usually not adequate for a student who is blind or visually impaired to use the program effectively. For example, an educational game may include speech, but the directions for using the game or for selecting certain options may not be spoken; rather they are only displayed as text on the screen. Most programs that offer some speech only voice parts of the text displayed on the screen but do not read aloud the menus, dialog boxes, controls, and other buttons. To make educational software easier for most students to use, many programs rely almost exclusively on the use of a mouse or some other pointing device to select items and control the program. Although some students with low vision will be able to use one or more of the screen magnification technologies described earlier to access these programs, those who need to access the information tactilely or auditorily will in all likelihood find these programs of little value.

Screen-Reading Software

Most students who need to access text auditorily, especially those who are blind, will find that they need to use a full-featured screen-reading program to obtain adequate access to information on the computer. A *screen-reading program*, or *screen reader*, is a piece of software that converts the text on the screen into electrical signals that instruct the speech synthesizer to produce the appropriate sounds. These programs are

Narrator

Narrator can read aloud menu commands, dialog box options and more.

- ☑ Announce events on screen
- ☑ Read typed characters
- ☐ Move mouse pointer to the active item
- ☐ Start Narrator minimized

[Help] [Voice...] [Exit]

Microsoft offers a basic screen reader, the Narrator, as part of its accessibility features, but most students will need additional features.

capable of voicing all of the text displayed on the screen, including such elements as menus, dialog boxes, controls, and buttons. They provide access to the information on the screen and allow users to work with applications such as word processors, spreadsheets, e-mail servers, and web browsers as well. Commercial screen readers offer the most features and flexibility for the user, but there are programs available as freeware and shareware, and even as part of the accessibility options in the Windows and Macintosh operating systems.

Controlling Speech. An important function of the screen-reading program is to provide the user with a way to control the speech and navigate through the electronic information. Screen readers allow control of such parameters as volume, rate, pitch, and tone. In addition, users can specify how much punctuation should be announced. Hearing each and every period, comma, and apostrophe indicated while reading long passages of text is distracting and decreases comprehension. Having this information becomes important to the user in other situations, however, such as when editing a word-processed document. The ability to control how much punctuation is read aloud can improve a user's efficiency to a great degree.

In addition, users can determine how numbers are voiced—as single digits, pairs, or as whole numbers. Students running applications that include telephone numbers (such as 1-555-537-0532) might prefer to hear the numbers spoken as single digits ("one five five five five three seven zero five three two"). Applications using dates (for example, June 28, 1957) can be operated more efficiently using numbers spoken as pairs ("June twenty-eight nineteen fifty-seven"), while tasks dealing with money would benefit from numbers being spoken as

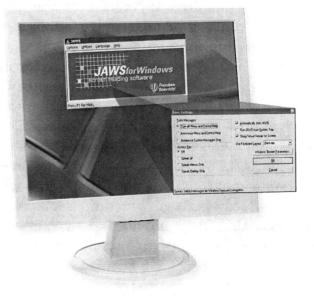

Courtesy of Freedom Scientific

Commercial screen-reading programs offer many useful features that enhance a student's ability to access electronic information provided by a computer.

whole units (so that $1,468 is spoken as "one thousand four-hundred sixty-eight dollars").

Pronunciation. Because of the complexities of the English language, speech synthesizers mispronounce many words, especially proper names. A common feature found in screen-reading software is the ability to create a dictionary for the pronunciation of words. When a word is mispronounced, the user can ignore the mispronunciation or add the word to the dictionary. The user types in the correct spelling of the mispronounced word and then types the word in phonetically until the right combination of letters and sounds produces an acceptable pronunciation of the word. This useful feature can have some unexpected applications (see "Technology Tip: When Screen Readers Speak 'Bad' Words").

Navigation. Computer users who have good vision can gather more from the screen than just the information presented by the

TECHNOLOGY TIP

WHEN SCREEN READERS SPEAK "BAD" WORDS

Professionals working with students may find that when some students begin using a computer that talks, one of the first things that they do is to make it speak profanity. Pronunciation dictionaries allow teachers to enter the correct spelling of the unacceptable words, and then have the screen reader speak some other text every time it encounters that spelling. Instead of saying the word in question, the synthesizer could be instructed to say something such as, "Please don't use that word"; "That's a bad word. You're in trouble now"; "Bleep, bleep"; or even, "I'm a nice computer. I don't talk that way."

words in the text. For example, they can see at a glance how a word is spelled or the format in which something is written. To have equal access to electronic information, users who are listening to electronic information need even more than text, punctuation, and numbers pronounced understandably; and screen-reading software provides truly equal access to material by enabling easy movement through the information and the ability to observe and interact with it. The software provides keyboard commands to navigate and read text by characters, words, and paragraphs.

For example, a user might begin by issuing a command that instructs the screen reader to start reading the text at the top of the document or web page. If the user hears something that is difficult to understand, a command can be issued to stop reading. The screen reader will usually stop very close to the last word the user heard spoken. The user can then issue a command that will instruct the screen reader to move back up one line of text and begin reading from that point. If that line contains the word that

was difficult to understand, the user can listen to that entire line again, or begin reading the line word by word until the misunderstood word is located. The misunderstood word can be spoken and repeated. If the user is still unable to determine the word, the screen reader can then speak the individual characters or spell the word. However, some letters, such as B, D, E, P, T, and V, can be difficult to identify. If the user is unable to identify some of the letters spoken, a command can be issued instructing the screen reader to use the phonetic or spelling alphabet—that is, to read aloud a word that starts with the letter to be substituted for the letter (Alpha, Bravo, Charlie, for the letters A, B, C, and so on for the rest of the alphabet). The ability to navigate easily around the screen and through the text on the screen is an essential feature of an efficient screen-reading program.

Navigating the Graphical User Interface. Information that is displayed on a computer screen is dynamic and changes in a predictable way at times and in unexpected ways at other times. For example, when a user wishes to save a document in a word processor, he or she might press Ctrl + S, which will open the Save dialog box. This is predictable. In another situation, however, such as on an unfamiliar web site, the user may move the cursor to a location on the screen and another window will open up automatically. This is unpredictable. It is the job of the screen-reading software to monitor the screen for changes and inform the user by speaking a message associated with that particular change or event, such as "Save dialogue" or "New window."

Screen-reading programs originally operated in a text-only environment and provided the user with accurate information about changes in the information being displayed. When graphics were added to the basic structure of operating systems, leading to the development of what is known as the "graphical user interface" (GUI), such as the now-familiar Macintosh or Windows environments, many users who were blind or visually impaired were unable to access the electronic information available in that format. Designers of screen-reading software have been able to develop a way for users to identify and navigate through the pertinent information displayed by a graphical user interface, but graphical environments still present the biggest challenge to both designers and users of screen readers.

Most computer applications that operate in a graphical environment accept input from a mouse or some other pointing device. Pointing devices are often not easy to use for people who are blind or visually impaired. Attempts have been made to produce pointing devices that provide tactile feedback, but they have met with limited success. Consequently, to be accessible to individuals using screen-reading software, applications must be controllable by keyboard commands. Most commonly used applications such as word processors, spreadsheets, e-mail programs, and Internet browsers offer keyboard commands, and it is a good idea for teachers to become familiar with them so that they can teach them to their students. (For a list of some of the more common keyboard commands and shortcuts, see "Keyboard Commands and Shortcuts Quick Reference.") However, many specialized software programs do not. These programs, therefore, are inaccessible for people who access electronic information through a computer using screen-reading software. (For information on screen readers for Macintosh computers, see Sidebar 3.1.)

Access to the Internet. Access to electronic information for users of screen readers has been intensified with the growth of the World Wide Web and the extensive amount of information available on the Internet. Although the major Internet browsers are accessible, many web sites are designed in such a way that some of the information is inaccessible to people using screen-reading software. Information on web pages must be encoded to indicate column location, graphics must be given a descriptive and meaningful label, and links must be identified in such a way as to indicate to the user their purpose and destination. The Web Accessibility Initiative (WAI) of the World Wide Web Consortium (W3C) (www.w3.org/WAI) has established guidelines for these and other accessibility features. Web designers can make their sites accessible by following the WAI Guidelines. Web sites that comply with these guidelines have opened a vast quantity of information to individuals using screen-reading programs. (For additional information on web accessibility, follow the Accessibility link at www.afb.org.) It is important for teachers to

KEYBOARD COMMANDS AND SHORTCUTS QUICK REFERENCE

This keyboard command reference sheet contains the most commonly used keyboard commands in Windows and some commands used in the Internet Explorer browser, but it is far from exhaustive. Different word-processing programs or applications and other browsers will have their own sets of commands. Students who use a screen reader will also need to know additional keyboard commands specific to that screen reader.

Windows Commands

- Alt key moves the focus (the portion of the screen that is currently active) to the menu bar.
- Tab key moves the focus to the next option in a dialogue box.
- Shift + Tab moves the focus to the previous option in a dialogue box.
- Up and Down arrows move the focus up or down a menu list or line of text.
- Left or Right arrows move the focus left or right on a menu, or left or right one character.
- Space bar is used to check or uncheck a check box in a dialogue box or on a web page.
- Ctrl key stops synthetic speech temporarily (clears the buffer).
- Home key moves the cursor to the beginning of a line of text.
- End key moves the cursor to the end of a line of text.
- Ctrl + Home moves the cursor to the beginning of your document or web page.
- Ctrl + End moves the cursor to the end of your document or web page.
- Shift key with any movement command will highlight text (for example, Shift + Home highlights text from the cursor to the beginning of a line).
- Alt + Tab moves to the next open application.
- Alt + Shift + Tab moves to the previous application used.
- Ctrl + A highlights all text in the document.
- Ctrl + S saves the current document.
- Ctrl + X cuts highlighted text and puts it on the Windows Clipboard.
- Ctrl + C copies highlighted text and puts it on the Windows Clipboard.
- Ctrl + V pastes text from the Windows Clipboard at the cursor location.
- Ctrl + Z undoes the last keystroke (can be repeated up to the last save).
- Ctrl + B boldfaces highlighted text.
- Ctrl + U underlines highlighted text.

(continued on next page)

TECHNOLOGY TIP *(CONTINUED)*

- Ctrl + I italicizes highlighted text.
- Ctrl + [increases the font size of highlighted text.
- Ctrl +] decreases the font size of highlighted text.
- Ctrl + E centers the line of text.
- Ctrl + L left justifies the line of text.
- Ctrl + R right justifies the line of text.
- Ctrl + 2 double-spaces highlighted text.
- Context-sensitive menu key (third key to the right of the space bar) lists suggested spellings for misspelled words when the cursor is on the misspelled word.

Internet Explorer Commands

- Tab moves from link to link.
- F6 moves to the address bar.
- Control + O opens the "open location" dialog box.
- Alt + Down arrow opens a select menu.
- Space activates a button.

The screen reader's commands do a lot of the navigating on web pages.

Source: Adapted from James Carreon and Joan Anderson, *Basic computer curriculum guide*. Fremont: California School for the Blind Technology Program.

know that despite best efforts to improve the accessibility of electronic information through the use of technology, there may still be some web sites that students will visit that are not "user friendly" to people who are visually impaired or blind.

OTHER DEVICES

In addition to computers, numerous other devices provide auditory access to electronic information. Most of these devices are stand-alone devices that can be connected to computers to transfer information. Others can receive information wirelessly from computers and accessible PDAs or from a wireless Internet connection. These devices include such items as accessible PDAs, e-text readers, talking dictionaries, talking calculators, and digital voice recorders.

Accessible PDAs

Accessible PDAs have been mentioned throughout the chapters on accessing both print and electronic information because these are such versatile and useful devices for visually impaired users who access information by touch, hearing, or both. These devices have many of the same functions as mainstream PDAs. Mainstream PDAs are essentially handheld computers, sometimes known as palmtop computers, that are often used as datebooks and address books, can usually access the Internet, may include a mobile phone and other applications, and can connect to and share data with a personal computer. (Common PDAs today include Palm Pilots, BlackBerries, and iPhones.)

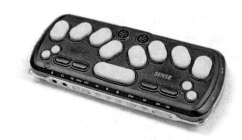

Courtesy of Independent Living Aids

Accessible PDA with a traditional six-key braille-type keyboard.

Accessible PDAs are in some ways more akin to laptop computers than standard PDAs, however, because they are larger, they have full-sized keyboards, and their primary use is usually reading and writing. In fact, they evolved from devices that are sometimes still known as electronic notetakers. These devices come with either braille or QWERTY keyboards for inputting and can provide output in refreshable braille, synthetic speech, or both. Once notetakers started to incorporate many additional features similar to those of mainstream PDAs—such as sophisticated word processors, appointment calendars, address books, e-mail capabilities, web browsers, media players, and multiple ways to connect with a personal computer and other devices—the term notetaker began to seem outdated. Hence, these multipurpose, portable devices are referred to most often as PDAs.

Accessible PDAs provide access to a wide variety of electronic information. Information can be transferred into the PDA from computers and other electronic devices. The speech output feature of these devices allows the user to hear the text contained in documents, e-mails, and web pages. Newer models have wireless access to the Internet and therefore have the capability of accessing vast amounts of information whenever the user desires.

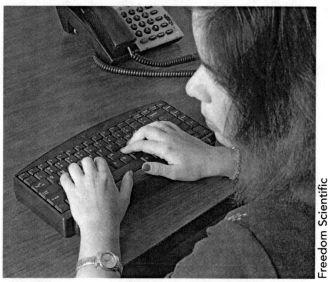

Freedom Scientific

This accessible PDA equipped with a QWERTY computer-style keyboard uses synthesized speech to enable the student to access information.

E-Text and E-Text Readers

Information that is available as an electronic text file is frequently referred to as "e-text." E-text files are most often accessed auditorily using a personal computer with screen-reading software, but several other devices have been developed that can read e-text files. E-text files can be transferred from a computer into most accessible PDAs and accessed through the onboard speech program or electronic refreshable braille display if the device is so equipped. Portable e-text readers have been developed that contain a speech synthesizer and enough

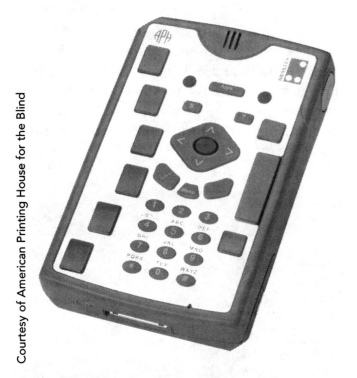

This accessible PDA has the ability to access a wide variety of e-book file types and present them to a student via synthesized speech.

memory to hold the speech program and large quantities of electronic text. These devices may vary in size, but most are about the size of a 3 × 5 inch index card and are 1–2 inches thick. E-text files can be transferred from a computer or PDA into the reader. A numeric keypad on the reader allows the user to select from multiple volumes and navigate through the text. These battery-operated devices can be used with headphones to provide a private and portable tool for accessing electronic information auditorily.

As discussed in Chapter 2 in regard to reading machines, there are times when the line between print and electronic information becomes blurred. Print information may be entered into a computer by typing the text into a word processor or some other software application and saved as an electronic file. Print documents can be scanned into a computer using an optical scanner and optical character recognition (OCR) software, and then saved as an electronic file. These two input methods have produced an enormous amount of information available as electronic text files. Many of these files are available at various web sites on the Internet. Selections include important historical documents, reference works such as dictionaries and encyclopedias, books in the public domain, and scanned documents of all types, including books, magazines, and a wide variety of other publications (see Dresner, 2004). As time goes on and more print documents are put online, the line between print and electronic information is ever harder to distinguish.

Talking Dictionaries

Electronic dictionaries are readily available on the Internet or as files stored on a CD or on a computer's hard drive. With accessible hardware and software, individuals who are blind or visually impaired can take advantage of this and other reference information. In addition, there are a variety of stand-alone talking dictionaries available for students who want to have access to a dictionary without having to use a computer or whose teacher requires them to have their own pocket dictionaries available in class. These devices allow the user to search an electronic file of text information and to hear the pronunciation and definitions of words. They are small, lightweight, and battery operated, allowing them to be used in a wide variety of settings. Their portability is just the first of a long list of features that make these devices extremely valuable.

Buyers need to be cautious, however, when selecting a talking dictionary. These devices range in price from about $50 to

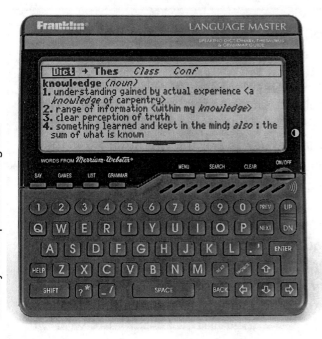

This talking dictionary has many features that make it a valuable tool.

$450, and several of the less expensive models are not that useful for individuals who are blind or visually impaired. They are designed for mainstream users to help them hear the correct pronunciation of words, so some of them speak a word only after it is typed or entered into the device and do not speak the word's definition. Other models intended for elementary students do read each letter as it is typed or entered, and pressing a command key makes the device speak the word. However, the definitions are worded simply, as appropriate for the target age group, and are typically spoken in a voice whose quality makes it difficult for many users to understand.

Models that provide more accessibility to users who cannot see the display tend to be more expensive but offer many useful features for students and adults and have proved to be great learning and reference

tools. At the time of this writing, there is only one product in this category that offers the features needed by this population, manufactured by Franklin (see the Resources section). Additional features of this model include a thesaurus and grammar guide, and more than 100,000 entries can be found in the dictionary and the thesaurus. The dictionary displays a complete entry for each word, including the traditional pronunciation guide, the word's origin and part of speech, common derivatives of the word, and multiple definitions when appropriate. The thesaurus also offers a brief definition of each word before displaying the synonyms to confirm that the word entered is in fact the word to be defined.

All the features of this talking dictionary can be accessed in several ways. The device is equipped with a visual display capable of displaying text in two sizes, the larger of which is adequate for some users with low vision. Users who cannot see the larger display can access the device through its speech output. The device echoes or speaks each letter as it is typed. When an entry is located, the unit usually reads the entire content of the entry unless instructed to stop. The arrow keys on the keyboard can be used to navigate through the definition or other text displayed. The user can have the text spoken by words and lines, or have an individual word spelled out. In addition, the user can adjust the rate of the speech to improve its understandability. Sidebar 3.3, "Uses of a Talking Dictionary," describes some additional features and uses of a full-featured, accessible talking dictionary.

Talking Calculators

Calculators are an important electronic tool for both classroom and professional use, especially in advanced mathematics

USES OF A TALKING DICTIONARY

A truly accessible and full-featured talking dictionary can do more for students than just give them the definition of a word. It can help students to determine the correct spelling of words, even when they are not sure of the exact spelling. If the word entered does not match any of the words in the device's memory, then it will display a list of words similar in spelling to the word that was entered. The user can press the arrow keys to scroll through the list and hear each word spoken or spelled until the correct word is reached. The user can then press the Enter key to see and hear the definition of that word. Words can also be looked up using "wildcards" when a student is not sure of the correct spelling. Wildcards are markers such as a question mark (?) or asterisk (*) that can be substituted for an unknown letter or a group of letters. The wildcard instructs the device to display a list of words that contain the entered letters and any characters represented by the wildcard. These features are very useful to individuals who have difficulty with words that have unusual spellings or vowels with similar sounds that are easily confused. Talking dictionaries that offer assistance with the spelling of words are a great teaching tool for students because they do not automatically correct an error. They simply offer a list of suggested spellings from which the student can choose.

Among other features offered in advanced talking dictionaries is a grammar guide. Although it does not check a writer's grammatical usage like the grammar tools found in computer-based word processors, it provides an accessible, portable guide to many of the common rules and information related to grammar and the English language. Another interesting and entertaining feature, known as Classmates, helps writers find words they may be searching for to add variety to their writing. It allows the user to search for additional words in the same category as a word that the user enters. For example, a student may be writing a story about a camping trip and wishes to name some trees to describe the physical setting. The student can enter the name of a tree he is familiar with and ask the device to display a list of words in that same classification. He or she will receive a long list of names of various trees.

Talking dictionaries also include a number of accessible versions of word games, such as hangman, word scramble, and other activities. Instructors of adults and youths find this a useful tool to help learners with lists of spelling or vocabulary words. The games have preprogrammed word lists that can be selected, but an instructor can also create customized lists of words, such as a student's list of spelling words for the week. The games alleviate the rote task of memorization when the student has to spell certain words correctly to succeed at the game.

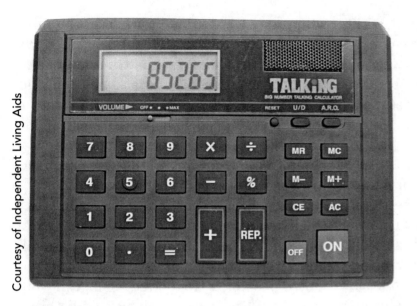

Courtesy of Independent Living Aids

Talking calculators provide students with an auditory tool they can use to complete math and science problems.

and science. Talking calculators provide auditory access to these devices by reading aloud or announcing the mathematical operations that they perform. In general, as the user presses the keys of such a calculator, they are identified via speech output, and the calculator's display is spoken as well. These calculators are available as stand-alone units, as features offered on accessible PDAs, and as software programs used on personal computers. In addition to all-purpose calculators that provide basic operations such as addition, subtraction, multiplication, and division, there are specialized models, including scientific, business, and statistical calculators.

Basic four-function calculators have been available in talking models for many years. These units have dropped dramatically in price compared to the prices at their initial entry into the market. Many also offer date and time functions. Some have enlarged displays of the numbers, allowing individuals with low vision the ability to confirm the speech output visually. Overall, talking calculators are available in a range of models and forms and at a range of

prices. Specialized calculators designed to perform scientific and higher mathematical functions, such as exponential and trigonometric functions, are now becoming available at more affordable prices, but other specialized talking calculators, such as business and statistical models, have not seen comparable decreases in price.

Some accessible PDAs and portable notetakers also offer talking scientific calculators among their features. Computer programs for performing scientific and higher-level mathematical calculations that are self-voicing applications and do not require additional screen-reading software are also now available. Other software programs that provide advanced calculator functions that are accessible with screen-reading and screen magnification software have become part of the general operating system software provided with personal computers. These programs offer basic functions and features found in scientific calculators.

Many advanced math and science classes require the use of graphing calculators, which offer even more advanced calculations, as well as the ability to graph data, and are often programmable. Students with low vision who wish access to these calculators visually may be able to do so using an optical device or a video magnifier. No device at present provides tactile access to a graphing calculator, but there is one talking scientific graphing calculator at present, the Audio Graphing Calculator manufactured by ViewPlus Technologies, that provides auditory access (see the Resources section). This self-voicing software program displays results through speech and sound, as well as by visually presenting numbers and graphs. It is intended to have capabilities comparable to a full-featured handheld scientific and statistical graphing calculator, and offers so many capabilities that it can be used for sighted students as well. The onscreen graphics are visible by students with low vision using an enlargement feature and can be listened to by using an audio-wave feature as well. Print copies can be made with any standard printer using a variety of fonts, including braille. The print copies with braille fonts can be copied onto swell paper and run through a tactile imaging machine, creating a raised-line drawing. Alternatively, embossed copies can be created by sending the graphic to a Tiger braille or graphics embosser (see the Resources section) or printed with a braille or graphics embosser (see Chapter 5; Osterhaus, 2008a, 2008b, 2000c). (For more information about talking calculators and other tools for mathematics, see Osterhaus, 2008c).

Digital Voice Recorders

People who are blind or visually impaired have long relied on cassette and later microcassette tape recorders for voice recording—for example, to record class lectures, a live reader reading books or other material, or notes to themselves and in other situations

when they wanted auditory access to information (see the section on Digital Audio Formats in Chapter 2). This method of recording could be useful to some people but had distinct disadvantages. Information could be recorded and played back at any time, but the only playback option was to listen to the recording in the same sequence in which it was recorded; it was difficult to skip to a specific part on the recording that the listener wanted to hear. Although excellent audiotape editing equipment is available, its expense makes it prohibitive for many people. Introduction of digital voice recording has greatly improved this situation. Digital voice recorders offer many new features that allow the user to produce voice recordings of auditory information.

Digital voice recorders are small, lightweight, battery powered devices that provide the user with a portable method of recording auditory information. A keypad, microphone, and speaker provide the tools to interact with the device. These recorders

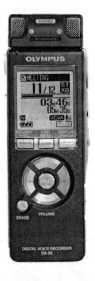

Courtesy of Independent Living Aids

Accessible digital recorders can be used for recording lectures and other presentations, but this one can also be used to access electronic information that has been saved in a compatible file format.

provide an accessible tool for taking voice-dictated notes and organizing information stored as audio voice recordings. The ability to insert bookmarks allows the user to mark certain parts of the recording that can be located easily for later review. By using the bookmark feature, the student can skip ahead to find important parts of the recording without difficulty.

SUMMARY

Much information that was previously only available in print is now available electronically, and electronic information has become commonplace in schools and in the workplace. To be successful in education and employment, people who are blind or visually impaired must therefore learn to use tools that will allow them access to this information. Students have a wide array of technology available for accessing electronic information visually, tactilely, and auditorily.

The vast majority of electronic information is computer based, and overall students can access it visually through the use of screen magnification technologies, tactilely through refreshable braille displays, and auditorily through synthesized speech. Nevertheless, some forms of electronic information remain inaccessible, and continued improvement is needed to increase accessibility to both print and electronic information to ensure that students who are blind or visually impaired are able to maximize their potential in education, employment, and daily life.

REFERENCES

Dresner, A. (2004). *Finding e-books on the Internet* (2nd ed.). Boston: National Braille Press.

International Society for Technology in Education. (2007). National educational technology standards for students: The next generation. Retrieved from www .iste.org/Content/NavigationMenu/ NETS/ForStudents/2007Standards/ NETS_for_Students_2007.htm

Osterhaus, S. A. (2008a). Suggested adaptive tools and materials for blind students in college mathematics. Unpublished manuscript. Austin: Texas School for the Blind and Visually Impaired.

Osterhaus, S. A. (2008b). Suggested adaptive tools and materials for low vision students in college mathematics. Unpublished manuscript. Austin: Texas School for the Blind and Visually Impaired.

Osterhaus, S. A. (2008c). Teaching math to visually impaired students. Texas School for the Blind and Visually Impaired, Austin. Retrieved June 25, 2008, from www.tsbvi.edu/math

4

Technologies for Producing Written Communication

<table>
<tr><td colspan="2">CHAPTER OVERVIEW</td></tr>
<tr>
<td>

Producing Written Communication Visually

- Manual Writing Tools
- Electronic Writing Tools

Producing Written Communication Tactilely

- Manual and Mechanical Braille-Writing Devices
- Electronic Braille-Writing Devices

</td>
<td>

Producing Written Communication Auditorily

- Accessible Computers with Word-Processing Software
- Accessible PDAs

</td>
</tr>
</table>

Communicating through writing can be a challenge for someone who is blind or visually impaired. Producing legible writing with the traditional tools of paper and pen or pencil can be a laborious and time-consuming task for a person with low vision, and impractical for one with no usable vision. However, a number of advances in writing technologies have greatly benefited students who are blind or visually impaired. Tools are now available that allow them to produce efficiently written communications that can easily be read by sighted classmates, teachers, and others.

This chapter will describe the variety of technologies that, by providing visual, tactile, or auditory access to information, can be used to create written materials.

Reading and writing are intricately tied together, and the skills used for one task support the skills needed for the other. Because the task of writing cannot be completely separated from reading, many tools serve multiple purposes and are discussed as both reading and writing technologies in this book. Although some devices can be used for writing as well as reading, it should be noted that different tools may be most efficient for different writing tasks—making a short note to oneself may call for the use of one method, while writing a lengthy report may call for another. Similarly, communicating with different audiences—with oneself, someone who reads braille, or a person who reads print only—may be accomplished with different techniques.

PRODUCING WRITTEN COMMUNICATION VISUALLY

Manual Writing Tools

Electronic Writing Tools
- Portable Devices
- Computers
- Laptop and Notebook Computers

A number of modified or adapted tools exist for producing written documents, from low-tech options, such as a felt-tip pen on bold-lined paper, to high-tech options, such as a desktop computer system. Many writers with low vision for whom vision is a primary reading channel find that the use of one or more of the manual and electronic optical devices discussed in Chapter 2 is helpful in the writing process.

MANUAL WRITING TOOLS

Effective writing instruments should enable users to produce writing that is legible to themselves and others. One low-tech solution is the wide variety of pens, pencils, and other writing instruments now available that offer variations in the line thickness, color, and permanence produced. Equally important to the type of line made by the pen or marker is the background on which it appears, which provides contrast for the viewer. Writers with low vision may select paper that has bold or raised lines or wider distance between lines for their use. With appropriate materials such as these, many people with low vision can learn to write efficiently and legibly for short writing tasks such as making lists or notes.

Longer writing tasks, however, may require different tools. Technology has provided these tools for many years, beginning with the manual and then electric typewriter. Although typewriters seemed much more efficient than handwriting for visually impaired users, they were still quite cumbersome. Even when equipped with large type, typewriters caused many users to bend over to read what they had typed, leading to poor posture and physical fatigue. Correcting and editing documents created on the typewriter was time consuming, tedious, and often resulted in a paper that was messy and hard to read. Better technology has been developed that offers more options for producing written communication that is readable and easier to edit.

ELECTRONIC WRITING TOOLS

Several devices are useful for individuals with low vision to accomplish longer writing tasks. These devices are the descendants of the electric typewriter, but offer many additional features that greatly increase their value as writing tools. Some of these devices require electricity, while others offer the portability provided by rechargeable battery systems.

Portable Devices

Dedicated Word Processors

Electric typewriters evolved into devices that became known as *dedicated electronic word processors*. As these systems became more sophisticated, manufacturers added features that allowed the user to review the information on the screen and edit it by inserting (adding) and deleting (removing) text. These devices usually consist of a QWERTY-style keyboard with a small four- to eight-line text display, which is usually too small to be read by most people with low vision. Models vary in features and complexity, but they all allow the user to enter and edit text, save it as an electronic file, and then transfer the information to a computer. These portable word processors have been useful for some individuals with low vision for taking notes on such occasions as attending lectures, discussions, and meetings. Even though the user may not be able to easily read the text as it is entered, once it has been transferred to an accessible computer system (as described in Chapter 3), a student can review the information and use all of the features of the computer's word-processing software to manipulate the text. The text can be edited, combined with other information, and used to create a master study guide or any other document that the student desires.

Originally, the display screen on these devices could only show text in 10- to 12-point type, but in order to make these devices compatible with popular personal digital assistants (PDAs), product designers have increased the size of the visual display screen to allow for additional lines of text. In an effort to widen the market for these devices, manufacturers have added a feature that allows the user to select the font and point size of the text displayed. Adding these features to dedicated word processors has increased their appeal to a wider variety of students, including students with low vision. These newer devices also offer features traditionally available on PDAs such as address books, calculators, and calendars; however, at this time, the font and point size in those applications cannot typically be adjusted. Newer models also have the ability to run small versions of desktop computer programs called applets. One applet that may benefit many students is a talking word-processing program (described in Chapter 3). While using this applet, students are also able to hear words and sentences spoken via synthesized speech. As explained in Chapter 3, the combination of a visual and auditory display provides additional reinforcement for understanding the text in two sensory modes and therefore increases the number of students who can benefit from this tool.

Dedicated word processors are considerably less expensive than devices with more capabilities, such as an accessible PDA.

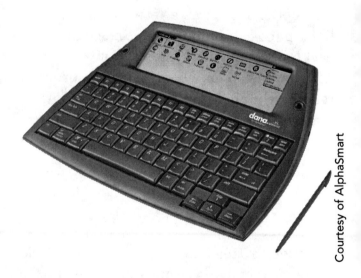

Courtesy of AlphaSmart

This dedicated word processor is an inexpensive tool for writing and note taking. It offers a limited selection of fonts and point sizes for users with low vision.

They are also easy to use. Most have a very simple filing system in which files are saved using dedicated keys such as the "F" or function keys similar to the ones found on standard computer keyboards, so that there is no need to name files to save them or to enter a file name to open a file. This allows a student to associate a key with a class, an easy way to keep files organized. For example, the student might use the "F1" file location to save notes taken in his or her first period class, "F2" for second period, and so forth. It is also simple to transfer information from the device to an accessible computer using a connecting cable. With a blank word processor document open on the computer and the file to be transferred open on the dedicated word processor, pressing one key on the unit sends the information to the computer. Some dedicated word processors are able to transfer information through a wireless connection. Although dedicated word processors do not offer the variety of valuable features found on an accessible PDA, if all a student needs is an inexpensive tool for writing, a dedicated word processor is certainly worth considering.

Accessible PDAs

The accessible PDAs discussed as tools for accessing print and electronic information in Chapters 2 and 3 are also excellent tools for completing writing tasks. In most cases these devices have familiar QWERTY keyboards for input but do not provide adequate visual access for students with low vision because their visual display is not large enough. However, they do offer auditory access that many students may find helpful when writing. Their small size makes these devices particularly easy for students to carry from class to class. Most accessible PDAs contain word-processing software

similar to that found on computers. While the features of these word processors are not as robust as those on computers, they are more than adequate for note taking and compiling information for longer reports and assignments that can be completed later on other devices, such as a computer.

Computers

Computers with word-processing software can be used by some students with low vision in two ways to produce written communications: through the use of operating system options or hardware-based screen magnification technologies. The first involves adjusting the computer's visual display properties and accessibility options, such as adjusting the font and size of the text used for different elements on the screen and choosing a different cursor or pointer, as discussed in Chapter 3. Using these adaptations along with adjustments to the particular software program can provide an effective writing tool for some students with low vision. Applications such as word processing, imaging, drawing and graphic creation, and math programs can be made accessible to some students with low vision using these adaptations. If these adaptations are not adequate by themselves, the student might wish to try them in combination with one of the hardware screen magnification technologies, such as a large monitor or flexible-arm monitor stand, or with screen-enlarging software (both discussed in Chapter 3). For some students who wish to access their computers visually, these adaptations and a word-processing program can constitute a tool for completing longer writing tasks.

Word-Processing Software

The editing features found in dedicated word processors discussed earlier in this chapter were enhanced and increased with the development of word-processing software programs for personal computers. Word-processing programs display text in various point sizes and fonts and are more sophisticated and accessible than ever before.

Adjustments to the computer's visual display properties and accessibility options may not be enough to allow some students with low vision to use the computer to access electronic information. However, some students may find that adjusting the visual display features in word-processing software allows them to use the computer more effectively as a writing tool. Students, teachers, and those performing assistive technology assessments can experiment with the settings for individual documents, as described in Sidebar 4.1, "Setting Up Word-Processing Documents for Students with Low Vision," to determine if this will be true for individual students. These specific settings may not be available in all word processors, but most will allow the student to enlarge the text in the document. However, the other screen elements of the program, such as menus,

---

SIDEBAR 4.1

SETTING UP WORD-PROCESSING DOCUMENTS FOR STUDENTS WITH LOW VISION

Adjusting the settings of a document that a student is working on in a word-processing program to enlarge the text and choosing a preferred type font can be sufficient to make the document accessible for a student with low vision. Most word-processing programs offer some options for how text is displayed on the screen similar to the ones listed here. In Microsoft Windows software (or when using Microsoft Word on a Macintosh), the following steps can be used to adjust the settings:

1. Open the View menu.
2. Select the Normal item.
3. Open the View menu again.
4. Select the Zoom option to open the Zoom dialog box.
5. Select the Page Width radio button, and choose OK. This expands the view of the page to the full width of the screen, thus enlarging the text as much as possible while still keeping all of the text in view at one time.
6. Open the Format menu.
7. Select the Font item to open the Font dialog box.
8. Choose the student's preferred font, style, and point size.
9. You may also wish to select the Character Spacing tab at the top of the dialog box and experiment with the Spacing settings. Expanded Spacing slightly increases the space between individual letters, which can be beneficial to some users.
10. Choose OK.
11. The settings selected in Steps 8 and 9 may need to be changed before printing a final copy of the document, depending on the requirements for a given assignment.

TECHNOLOGY TIP

DEALING WITH DROP-DOWN MENUS

A variety of screen elements that are used in word-processing programs, such as menus, icons, and dialog boxes, are not affected by adjustments made to improve the visibility of the document text (as described in Sidebar 4.1). Some of the adjustments discussed in Chapter 3 that can be made in the operating systems may be of assistance in this situation. Two other suggestions may help users with low vision to deal with drop-down menus when they are unable to identify visually the items being shown on menus. One involves memorizing the items in often-used menus, and the other requires learning shortcut key combinations.

With instruction and practice, a student can remember the order of the items displayed in a menu and select them accordingly. For example, he or she can learn that the twelfth item on the File menu is the Print option. To instruct the computer to print, the student can press Alt + F to open the File menu and then press the Down arrow 12 times to reach the Print option. Most students with low vision will be able to follow this process by seeing the reverse highlight on the menu items move down from one item to the next.

An easier option for many students is to learn to use the shortcut key combinations to issue the various commands, such as Ctrl + P, or Alt + F followed by the letter P to print a document. A list of common keyboard shortcut commands is found in Chapter 3.

Regardless of which approach is taken, the student will most likely discover that the editing features offered by a word processor will greatly outweigh the difficulty of learning a workaround.

icons, and dialog boxes, will not be enlarged and may not be easily viewed. Most students will be able to learn to work around this problem or can use screen magnification software (discussed in Chapter 3) as they compose text on the computer. "Technology Tip: Dealing with Drop-Down Menus" contains some suggestions. The value of this technology as a tool for writing is influenced considerably by the user's keyboarding skills (discussed in greater detail later in this section and in Chapters 7 and 8).

Word-processing software offers great value as a writing tool because of the vast array of editing and formatting features it provides. Most computer users are so accustomed to these features that we take them for granted and forget how easy it is to create and edit documents using different fonts and formats. Most word-processing programs go well beyond the basic editing features of inserting and deleting text and allowing users to copy or move text around in a document. Spell-checking, thesaurus, and grammar-checking features in the software allow users to access these resources quickly without having to leave the computer to locate an accessible version of a reference book. Writers can use these tools to assist in proofreading and produce more accurate documents. In addition, the formatting features of word processors allow users to create documents that have a more refined appearance and thus are more visually interesting to readers. Computer systems with accessible word-processing software have greatly increased the efficiency and effectiveness with which people with visual impairments can produce written communications. The development of screen magnification software and more advanced word-processing programs has allowed users with low vision to finally have a way to see text as it is being typed and has opened up the world of word processing to many who previously were unable to access it.

To make the best use of electronic tools such as computers, students need to develop proficient keyboarding skills—what used to be called touch typing—to enter text into the computer. This is an important skill for all students, but it is especially important for those who are blind or visually impaired because using a computer-based word processor can be the most efficient tool for completing longer writing tasks. Sidebar 4.2, "Teaching Keyboarding Skills," provides some suggestions for helping students to learn these important skills.

Imaging Software

Another computer-based writing tool that can be of great benefit to many students with low vision is the imaging software discussed in Chapter 2. Imaging software is not generally used as a writing tool, but it can be used effectively for the specific purpose of completing forms and worksheets. Most imaging programs have drawing tools and a text-editing feature that can be used to draw lines or place text on a scanned image, which can be very useful features for classroom activities. A common writing task for students, particularly in elementary school, is completing "matching column" worksheets in which the student must draw a line between an item in a column on one side of the page to a corresponding item on the other. Other worksheets might require the student to write text on a blank line. The text and images used in these types of materials are often too small for many students with low vision, but imaging software can assist with completing such worksheets, as explained in "Technology Tip: Using Imaging Software to Complete Worksheets."

Imaging software can also be used effectively when a student does not have access to a scanner. The forms and worksheets can be scanned by a teacher, paraeducator, or a clerical staff member and saved as an electronic file. These files can be transferred to the student's computer and the student can be taught how to locate and open them. The student can then use the same procedures described in "Technology Tip: Using Imaging Software to Complete Worksheets" to complete and print the worksheet. For this strategy to be effective, the person who scans the worksheets must use a logical and consistent file-naming and storage method that can be easily understood by the student, who in turn needs to be able to quickly and efficiently locate and open the desired files (see "Technology Tip: Creating a Logical File-Naming and Organizing System"). As with all technology, instruction and practice in the use of these tools should be provided early in students' lives so that they can become comfortable and efficient with procedures in a

TEACHING KEYBOARDING SKILLS

Computer systems and software programs are great tools for assisting students in the development of good keyboarding skills. One of the most important aspects of learning good keyboarding skills is for the learner to receive immediate feedback about the accuracy of his or her keystrokes. Text being typed into a word-processing program can be displayed at a size that is comfortable for writers with low vision to read and allows one to monitor the accuracy of the keystrokes. Immediate feedback can also be provided to students who are blind by using a talking word-processing program (see Chapter 3), which is readily available in many schools. Use of a talking word processor is also highly recommended for students with low vision. Not only does the speech increase feedback by providing a second sensory modality, but for many students it also makes the activity more interesting and increases the chances that they will continue to practice keyboarding activities and improve their skills. Feedback from the program also eliminates the need for the instructor to provide comments about accuracy and frees the instructor to assist the student by offering information about proper fingering techniques, posture, and ergonomics and by dictating interesting text to be typed.

Once the learner has received instruction about the location of the keys on the keyboard, such as the home-row keys, practice is needed to develop the neuromotor skills for touch typing. This is where computer keyboarding or typing programs can be of most benefit to students. These programs are excellent tools for providing the needed practice and reinforcement to help develop good keyboarding skills. Some mainstream typing tutors (that is, commercially available software designed for students with typical vision) can be accessed with screen magnification software, but most present difficulties for students in navigation and in locating the desired text to be typed.

Mainstream keyboarding programs are not easily accessed with screen-reading software and are of little value to students who are blind. Specialized keyboarding programs have been developed that allow the user to select the size of the text being displayed, and some also offer synthesized speech. These programs generally provide a better alternative to using screen magnification software or screen-reading software with mainstream keyboarding programs because they do not require the user to navigate around the screen to locate the targeted and typed text. Students can concentrate on the keyboarding task and not have to be concerned with the navigation commands needed to keep the targeted and typed text within view. Although these programs are excellent tools for providing the learner with drill and practice activity, they are *not* a substitute for good keyboarding instruction provided by an instructor who is knowledgeable in techniques for teaching students who are blind or have low vision.

(continued on next page)

Labeling Keys

Another useful tool for facilitating keyboarding consists of self-adhesive raised dots (often referred to as *locator dots*) that can be placed on certain keys, such as new keys to be learned or those targeted for practice. Once the student is comfortable with the location of these keys, the dots can be removed and placed on the next group of keys to be learned. When the student has learned all of the keys on the keyboard, a few stick-on dots can be placed on selected keys as basic orientation cues to the keyboard—similar to the tactile indicators found on the letters F and J on many keyboards.

Some instructors choose to use labels for the keys in large print or braille. Such key labels may be useful for very young children who are still exploring the keyboard or if a student has some type of motor impairment that will prevent him or her from learning touch typing. For students with low vision who are expected to become touch typists, however, labels are counterproductive. The larger print on the labels encourages the student to look at the keys more often and not learn to rely on the tactile and motor skills necessary to become a proficient typist. Braille labels can have the same effect on students who are blind because the student will be feeling around for individual letters instead of using muscle memory to locate the desired keys. In general, labels should be used cautiously and only in specific situations. One such situation

might be teaching prekeyboarding skills to beginning typists.

Teaching Prekeyboarding Skills

Young children are using computers at home and in classrooms at younger and younger ages. To familiarize very young students with low vision or those who are not touch typists with the keyboard, the following technique for modifying a standard keyboard can be used to break down the visually confusing keyboard with its many different keys into a more manageable display:

1. Obtain self-adhesive stickers in six bright or bold colors that will offer good contrast to dark black print; for example, fluorescent green, orange, red or pink, yellow, pastel blue, and purple.
2. Cut the stickers to fit on the keys.
3. With a medium-point permanent marker, write the characters Q, A, Z, P, semicolon, and the forward slash on the fluorescent green stickers and attach them to the corresponding keys on the keyboard.
4. Write the letters W, S, X, O, L, and the period on the fluorescent orange stickers and attach them to the corresponding keys on the keyboard.
5. Write the letters E, D, C, I, K, and the comma on the fluorescent yellow stickers and attach them to the corresponding keys on the keyboard.
6. Write the letters R, F, V, U, J, and M on the fluorescent red or pink stickers and attach them to the corresponding keys on the keyboard.

7. Write the letters *T*, *G*, and *B* on the pastel blue stickers and attach them to the corresponding keys on the keyboard.
8. Write the letters *Y*, *H*, and *N* on the pastel purple stickers and attach them to the corresponding keys on the keyboard.

Once the keyboard has been set up, students can be taught to type words that are meaningful to them using the position and colors of the letters. To locate a desired letter, instruct the student to first look on the right or left side of the keyboard; then to locate a particular color on that side of the keyboard; and then to determine whether the desired letter is the top, middle, or bottom key in that column. For letters in the blue and purple columns, simply skip the first step of looking to the right or left side of the keyboard.

For example, if a student named Tom wishes to type his name, he would be given the following instructions:

1. First find the column of keys that are colored light blue. The letter *T* is the top key in this column.
2. Look on the right side of the keyboard and find the column of keys that are orange. The letter *O* is the top key in this column.
3. Look on the right side of the keyboard and find the column of keys that are red (or pink). The letter *M* is the bottom key in this column.

Although this technique may not work with every child, the strategy may serve to minimize the "hunt and peck" system that young children often use to find the correct keys.

low-stress environment before they need to use them in the classroom.

Drawing Programs

Computer systems with word-processing software are tremendous resources for producing written communication in text, but at times information can be communicated more effectively in a graphical format, as pictures and drawings. Drawing and graphics creation programs give users with low vision an electronic way in which to create charts, graphs, maps, and drawings. Previously, students had to use paper, pencil, and mechanical drawing tools that required the individual to make precise measurements by visually matching lines imprinted on the drawing or measuring tool with lines and distances on the paper.

Although this task can be accomplished through the use of optical devices, it can be both tedious and time consuming. Now, however, simple drawing applications are found in most word processors and spreadsheet programs. Users can easily create straight and curved lines, shapes in varying thicknesses and colors, and a wide variety of graphs and charts. With full-featured drawing and graphics programs, more complicated tasks can be completed and original works of art created.

These programs offer editing features similar to those of word-processing programs. Inserting and deleting information is relatively simple. If an error is made in a drawing, the user can erase the mistake and try again. In fact, this type of software has allowed many users with low vision to

TECHNOLOGY TIP

USING IMAGING SOFTWARE TO COMPLETE WORKSHEETS

Imaging software is a useful tool in helping students with low vision to fill out worksheets. Students can be taught to place a worksheet in a scanner and use imaging software to display an image of the worksheet on the computer's monitor. Using the software's zoom feature, the student can enlarge the image until it is big enough for him or her to read the text and view the drawings or other images. The student may also need one of the cursor enhancement programs discussed in Chapter 3 to make the cursor large enough to be located efficiently.

If the task is matching an alphabet letter to a drawing of an object that begins with that letter, the student can be taught to select the line-drawing tool and place the mouse pointer on the desired letter. By clicking and holding the left mouse button, the student can drag a line from the letter to the matching drawing. When the mouse button is released, a line will be drawn between the letter and the drawing.

Once the student has used this process to complete the rest of the worksheet, he or she can select the text-editing tool and locate the blank line provided to write the student's name. Clicking on this location will produce an insertion cursor that will allow the student to type his or her name in the blank. The student can then choose the print option and print out a copy of the completed worksheet for the teacher.

Forms and worksheets that require the student to complete short-answer questions can be managed in a similar way using the text-editing tool.

---

produce graphical creations that would be practically impossible to do with mechanical drawing tools. Most drawing programs offer a "zoom in" feature that enlarges the drawing and allows the user to control it at the pixel level, the smallest level possible on a computer. This feature provides the user with the ability to make minute adjustments to the drawing to obtain precise accuracy. Drawings such as charts, graphs, or diagrams that require exact line measurement can be accomplished with tools that

allow the user to assign a precise numeric measurement to the length of a line, rather than approximating the length visually. Through the use of drawing tools and other graphical programs, individuals with low vision can produce graphics for math, science, social studies, and other classes that are both effective and visually pleasing.

Math Software and Spreadsheets

At times, written communication involves information that is best communicated in

CREATING A LOGICAL FILE-NAMING AND ORGANIZING SYSTEM

Learning to keep electronic files organized and easy to find has become an important life skill for all students. Without a logical system of storing files, a student's computer desktop or documents folder will quickly fill up with dozens of files containing documents, partially completed documents, various versions of the same document, documents created by different people (for instance, some by the student and some by teachers), and different kinds of documents (such as word-processing documents, spreadsheets, scanned images, and so forth). Students then waste precious time sorting through the folder trying to find the particular document that they need.

To prevent such chaos, files need to be organized and named in a systematic way, so that students are able to quickly locate and identify their documents. The system will vary somewhat if the computer is used by a variety of students or by only one student.

The following suggestions and examples may be helpful in designing a system that will work for a particular student. Each student should be taught to develop and use a similar method of organizing electronic materials for himself or herself.

- Create a file folder using the student's name—for example, Rita.
- Create subfolders for each class or subject in the student's folder, such as Rita\Science, Rita\English, Rita\Social Studies, and so on.
- When saving files, be sure to place them in the appropriate folder and subfolder.
- File names for class assignments should contain, in abbreviated form, such information as the subject or class, textbook chapter number, page number when appropriate, assignment type, and so forth.
- When naming files, use a system of abbreviations for subjects (for example, En for English; SS for Social Studies; Sc for Science), for sections of books and assignments (such as Ch for chapter, p for page, Ex for example, Ws for worksheet), and so forth.

Here are some examples of files named according to this system:

- A folder is created called "Rita." Within that folder is a subfolder for each of her subjects, such as Science, English, and Social Studies.
- Within the subfolder Science is a file named Rita\Science\Sc.Ch5.Ws1.
- Within the subfolder English is a file named Rita\English\En.Ch2.p27.
- Within the subfolder Social Studies is a file named Rita\Social Studies\SS.Ch7.

Your student's system does not have to be exactly like this one, but everyone working with a student needs to be aware of whatever system is being used. A laminated reference sheet of the organizational structure and all of the abbreviations can be very helpful.

numerical form. Software programs have been developed that not only help users to learn mathematical concepts but also provide tools that can be used to complete math problems and other numerical tasks. Modern spreadsheet programs allow users to manipulate and produce rows and columns of numerical information that can be displayed on the screen or printed on paper in various fonts and point sizes. Math and equation editor software can even be used to complete complicated math assignments. Individuals can use these tools to accomplish educational, employment, and personal tasks associated with numerical information.

High school students also need to be aware of online banking options that provide a tool for managing personal finances while decreasing the need to write on preprinted checks and checkbook registers. Some of these programs can be accessed using screen magnification software, screen-reading software, and refreshable braille displays, but many are not accessible. The accessibility of these types of programs needs to be determined on an individual basis.

Laptop and Notebook Computers

Accessible desktop computer systems are powerful tools for producing written communication. Their major drawback is that they require electricity and are not easily moved from place to place, especially if they have a large monitor, as discussed in Chapter 3. Laptop or notebook computers, in contrast, use battery power, so they offer portability that allows users to work in various locations. These devices offer most of the same features as desktop computers, but in a package that can easily be transported. Although notebook computers offer the user many valuable features, like any other device, they

have their shortcomings. Difficulties related to expense, weight, battery life, and startup and shutdown time can limit the usefulness of notebook computers as efficient and effective portable writing tools. For students with low vision, the smaller screen size on most laptops may make using screen magnification software more difficult as well because of the smaller amount of text that can be seen at any one time.

In summary, manual writing tools for students with low vision are adequate for short writing tasks, but for longer writing tasks students need more efficient options. The ideal tool for many students is an accessible computer system with word-processing software; the flexibility and editing capabilities of these tools allow a student with low vision to efficiently produce large quantities of written information. However, students need different writing tools for different writing tasks. Again, the point is that students who are blind or visually impaired need to be conversant in the use of many different assistive technology alternatives to take advantage of opportunities offered by their educational programs.

PRODUCING WRITTEN COMMUNICATION TACTILELY

Manual and Mechanical Braille-Writing Devices

- Slate and Stylus
- Braillewriters

Electronic Braille-Writing Devices

- Electric and Electronic Braillewriters
- Computers with Word-Processing Software
- Accessible PDAs

Many people who are visually impaired need to read and write by means of touch because they are not able to perform these tasks efficiently, or at all, by using their visual senses. As indicated in Chapter 2, braille is the preeminent instrument for tactile reading, and it is the cornerstone of writing as well. Since the days of Louis Braille, the creator of the braille alphabet, there have been various tools and strategies for writing or embossing braille. These tools fall into two categories based on how braille is produced—manual braille-writing devices and electronic braille-writing devices.

MANUAL AND MECHANICAL BRAILLE-WRITING DEVICES

Manual braille-writing devices require the user to emboss braille dots on paper physically. This action can be accomplished with a portable device known as a slate and stylus or with a mechanical device similar to a manual typewriter—a braillewriter. These devices offer portability and durability and are less expensive than their electronic counterparts.

Slate and Stylus

One of the simplest and most efficient tools for writing braille is the *slate and stylus*. This device consists of a *slate*, a flat piece of metal or plastic, which is hinged on one side to allow paper to be placed in between its two halves. The bottom half of the slate has rows and columns of empty braille cells impressed into the metal. The top half of the slate has holes corresponding to the empty braille cells on the bottom half of the slate. The writer uses a pointed device with a rounded tip, the *stylus*, to press or emboss the dots onto the paper through these holes to write braille directly onto the paper held in place within the slate.

Slates are available in a wide variety of sizes ranging from a one-line slate designed for labeling items like articles of clothing, to multiline slates and even full-page slates. These various sizes offer different advantages for the writer, depending on the

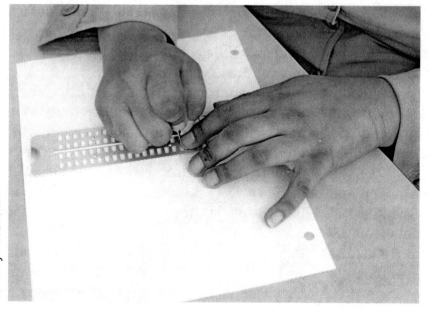

L. Penny Rosenblum

The slate and stylus is a simple and efficient tool for writing limited amounts of information in braille. This student is using a slate and stylus to write down his homework assignment.

nature and size of the writing task to be accomplished. The stylus is usually a device with a wooden or metal handle similar to a knob, but styli can vary widely in shape and size. One style, for example, allows the tip of the stylus to be unscrewed from the handle, then turned around and tucked away into the handle so that the stylus can be carried in a pocket without poking the person who carries it. The ease with which the slate and stylus can be used as a tool for labeling items and for jotting down small amounts of information such as phone numbers or addresses makes it an essential tool for students to learn and master. This device provides braille users with a simple, hand-powered tool that is portable and reliable for producing written communication tactilely in braille.

Braillewriters

Although the slate and stylus is an excellent instrument for labeling and for short writing tasks, many braille users prefer to use a mechanical or manual *braillewriter* or *brailler* for longer writing activities. The most common braillewriter allows the user to roll paper into the machine in a manner similar to the way in which paper was rolled into a manual typewriter. The device has six keys corresponding to the six dots of the braille cell. These keys are in a row from left to right, and are separated in the middle by a space bar key. On the left end of the row is a back space key and on the right end is a key to advance the paper to the next line. As the user presses combinations of the six keys, dots are embossed on the paper and then the *embossing head* (the piece of metal that actually embosses the dots) moves braille cell by braille cell to the right. The traditional Perkins Braillers can emboss 25 lines with 42 cells on an 11 × 11½ inch sheet

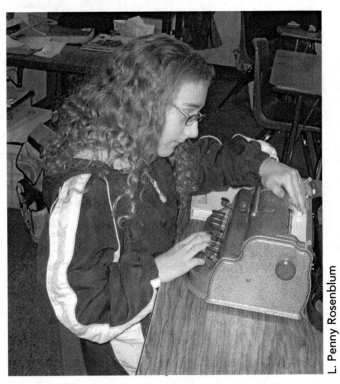

L. Penny Rosenblum

The Perkins braillewriter is a durable mechanical device for embossing braille and can be used for longer writing tasks.

of paper, while the newer Next Generation Perkins/APH Brailler only accepts 8½ × 11 paper. Using this device to write braille is usually much faster than using the slate and stylus (although some slate users become very fast). The slate and stylus is often equated with pencil and paper for print readers, while the braillewriter is compared to a manual typewriter.

One additional item to mention in this category is the Jot a Dot, a lightweight manual braillewriter designed to be portable and more affordable than other braillewriters. It is similar to other mechanical braillewriters in that the user rolls paper into the device and then uses the traditional six-key keyboard to enter characters and the device embosses the dots onto paper so they can be read tactilely by the user. However, the largest paper it can accept is only 8½ × 5½ inches, which limits braille writing to 20 cells per line. Also, the reader must move the paper forward to read what has been written and then move it back to the same line to continue writing.

Disadvantages of Manual Braillewriters

As useful as braillewriters are, they have certain disadvantages. In particular, editing or making corrections to braille that has been embossed on paper can be time consuming. Sidebar 4.3, "Making Corrections and Editing on a Manual Braillewriter," explains how this can be done, but it can be tedious when compared to the ease of making corrections on some of the electronic tools described in the next section.

Additional Options for Special Needs

The user of a manual braillewriter must have sufficient finger strength to press the keys with enough force to ensure that the dots will be clearly embossed onto the paper. For students who have trouble pressing the keys hard enough, straight or bent *extension keys* can be affixed to the braillewriter. Straight extension keys are similar to the regular keys on a braillewriter but are longer and extend several inches toward the user. This extra length provides more leverage to someone using the machine and thus reduces the finger strength needed to emboss the braille and make an imprint on the paper. Extension keys can be helpful to some users while they are developing greater finger strength, such as young students and students with certain physical impairments. Bent extension keys that bring the keys closer together toward the space bar are also available; these can be helpful for students who have trouble pressing more than one key at a time.

Some braille readers may have functional use of only one hand. These individuals can take advantage of the unimanual braillewriter, which allows the user to input braille with just one hand. After the keys on the left side of the device, representing dots 1-2-3, are pressed, these keys remain depressed while the user presses the desired keys on the right side of the device. When the user releases the keys representing dots 4-5-6 or the space bar, all keys are released and the braille character is embossed.

Braille readers who have decreased sensitivity in their fingertips have the option of using a braillewriter that embosses braille in a larger format. This large-cell braillewriter embosses the dots at approximately the same height as regular braille, but the space between the dots and between each cell or character is increased, making it easier for them to read back what they have written. This form of embossing makes the braille easier to recognize for these individuals. Extension keys can also be used with the large-cell braillewriter and the unimanual braillewriter.

ELECTRONIC BRAILLE-WRITING DEVICES

The slate and stylus was invented more than 150 years ago, and manual braillewriters have existed for a century. In fact, the model used extensively in schools today has changed little in 50 years. These manual braille devices are useful and well-loved tools with wide application. However, new technologies now available to braille readers have features that bring braille into the 21st century. Some of these tools require less physical strength on the part of the user to emboss braille. Others allow the braille reader to use computer hardware and software to create

MAKING CORRECTIONS AND EDITING ON A MANUAL BRAILLEWRITER

The braillewriter is an essential piece of equipment, particularly for young children who are developing writing skills. The ability to instantly and tactilely read back what they have written provides feedback and confirmation to students who are learning to write. As students get older and need to produce longer written pieces, the braillewriter can still be a valuable tool, particularly for first drafts, which are typically changed and revised as the student continues to work on them. Students are often taught to double or even triple space their early drafts to make room for later changes. But editing braille texts on the manual braillewriter presents some challenges.

Often a student will make an error and want to make a change in the text that was produced on the braillewriter. When the student makes an error on a braillewriter, he or she can roll the braille paper up or down until the line containing the error is over a metal plate at the back of the braillewriter, then use a *braille eraser*—a wooden or plastic device with a rounded point—to depress or flatten out the braille dots. Once the incorrect dots have been erased, the paper can be rolled back down to the correct line, the braillewriter's embossing head positioned to the proper spot, and the word or letter rebrailled. A more recent version, the Next Generation Perkins/APH brailler, has a braille eraser built onto the embossing head; to erase a character, the student must backspace twice, then press down firmly on the eraser side of the embossing head (the right side). The student can then rebraille the correct character. These correction methods work well if errors are identified quickly or if the writer makes a simple mistake like embossing the incorrect dot pattern for a braille character. However, if letters have been left out of words or unwanted characters accidentally embossed, the writer will have a more time-consuming task.

The major difficulty arises when there is insufficient space to enter the additional text or when removing the unwanted text results in extra and unnecessary spaces in the line. This situation can be handled in several ways. The writer can erase the braille that was embossed after the point at which the error appears until adequate space is achieved to make the correction. However, this solution takes time and can result in braille that is difficult to read, because after erasing or flattening braille dots and then re-embossing on the same paper, the resulting braille may not be crisp and clean. Poorly or improperly erased braille can obscure the new words that are brailled on the same spot, resulting in a messy and unreadable page. If this happens, the writer may simply have to remove the paper, insert a new sheet of paper, and emboss that page again. This is one reason that students often prefer the newer braille technologies that make editing so much easier than it has been in previous decades on the manual braillewriter.

written information in braille and in print, making it easier to write, edit, and produce desired materials.

Students have various reasons for producing written communications. At times they may wish to produce writing in braille strictly for themselves to read. Such writing can be produced with any of the braille-writing devices discussed here. At other times they will want or need to communicate with non–braille readers and produce their writing in print. This can become a challenge, especially in the classroom, when they would like to share information that they have written with classmates, family members, or teachers who do not read braille. In instances like this, either the student has to read the braille message or assignment aloud or wait until a teacher of students with visual impairments is available to interline the braille—that is, to write the print translation of the braille between the lines on the braille copy.

Neither solution is workable in the long run. Teachers who are unaccustomed to reviewing and grading written assignments auditorily often find it difficult to give students effective feedback in this way, especially on skills such as spelling and the use of paragraphs and punctuation. Waiting for the teacher of students with visual impairments has its problems as well. There may be a lengthy delay between the time a student completes an assignment and the time he or she receives relevant feedback about his or her work. Circumstances such as these can also prevent visually impaired students from receiving direct and timely instruction from the classroom teacher about the content of their writing tasks.

In addition to the educational difficulties that can be created when a student writes in braille for a non–braille-reading audience, the situation also puts the student who is blind or visually impaired in the position of a passive participant in class who must wait until material is put into other formats by someone else, instead of being an active agent who can participate in learning and classroom activities at the same time as his or her classmates. However, a number of electronic technology tools can offer solutions to these challenges.

Electric and Electronic Braillewriters

Electric Braillewriters

Some people who have difficulty using a mechanical braillewriter find that extension keys still do not provide enough leverage for them to emboss braille successfully. For these individuals, an electric braillewriter such as the electric Perkins Brailler, may be a more appropriate tool. These devices use electricity in a way similar to electric typewriters. Pressing the keys on an electric braillewriter requires significantly less finger strength than that required on a manual braillewriter.

Despite these significant advantages, electric braillewriters generally cost 25–30 percent more than manual models and are also not as durable. Their electronic components are not rugged enough to stand up to much of the physical abuse that they receive when being transported to different locations within a school, for example. Although electric braillewriters can make it physically easier for students to emboss the braille, despite being electrically powered they still do not include advanced editing features and can only produce documents in braille, unlike electronic braillewriters.

Mountbatten Brailler

The Mountbatten Brailler, a type of electronic braillewriter that became available in the late 1990s, offers many features that give it flexibility as a writing tool (D'Andrea, 2005a, 2005b). Some of its features solve the challenge of providing timely feedback from non–braille-reading teachers for the student who uses braille. One of its helpful features is the well-designed arrangement of the keys on the keyboard. Traditional braillewriters have their keys parallel to the fingers of the user, and long assignments completed on the traditional braillewriter can therefore lead to physical fatigue in the fingers, hands, wrists, arms, shoulders, and back of the user. The Mountbatten Brailler has its keys angled slightly toward the middle of the device. This allows the user's hands to be held in a more comfortable position when brailling, resulting

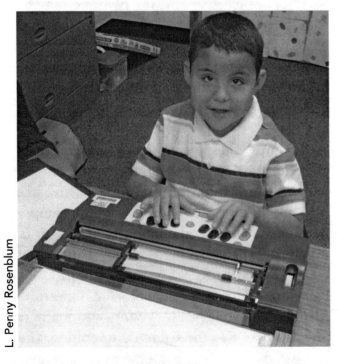

L. Penny Rosenblum

The electronic Mountbatten Brailler offers many useful features for writing and editing that are not available on mechanical braillewriters.

in less physical fatigue when longer writing tasks are being completed.

The Mountbatten Brailler can be used like any manual or electric braillewriter to emboss braille onto standard braille paper. However on this brailler, the impact of the embossing head can be adjusted so that varying weights of paper can be used with the device. This adjustability means that inexpensive notebook paper or printer paper can be used for writings that the reader will only need to read once or twice and then discard, such as early drafts of stories and reports. Then with a simple adjustment, the braillewriter can be configured to emboss on heavier weight paper for longer lasting documents.

One particularly helpful feature of this device is its ability to erase errors. The embossing head can be placed one character to the right of the mistake. When the user holds down the backspace key and presses the keys for the correct dots needed, the device will erase the unwanted dots and emboss the correct ones. This capability makes the simple editing of braille documents much easier than the methods described previously for use with manual braillers.

In addition, an onboard speech synthesizer allows the user to hear characters announced as they are entered. Other editing features are also available on some models that allow the user to review the text and make necessary changes using synthesized speech. The text is entered into an electronic file and not embossed immediately. If an error is found, the user can insert missing text or remove unwanted text. Once the user has reviewed and corrected the text in the file, a command can be issued to the electronic braillewriter to emboss the file. This ability to edit text before it is embossed greatly increases the user's efficiency when producing written communication tactilely. And because the text can be saved in an electronic file, the user can emboss additional copies if needed.

Other features extend this braillewriter's ability to produce written communications. The electronic memory of the device contains both a forward and a backward braille translator (see Chapter 3). Because of this feature, the device can be connected to a printer and have text that was entered as braille "back translated" into print and produced on paper, which provides the user with the ability to create both braille and print documents almost simultaneously. The forward braille translation feature allows a print-reading student, teacher, parent, or paraeducator to communicate in writing directly with a braille reader. Connecting a standard QWERTY computer keyboard to the electronic braillewriter provides the non–braille reader—for example, a classroom teacher or paraeducator—with the opportunity to type text into a file being saved in the device's

memory. The unit can translate the document into braille and then emboss it. The addition of a small four-line visual display (known as the Mimic) allows the non–braille reader to view the text being entered. An example such as the one in Sidebar 4.4, "Using the Mountbatten Brailler in the Classroom: An Example," illustrates how these features maximize the potential of using the Mountbatten Brailler and responds to some of the challenges inherent in communicating with others in braille.

As exciting and useful as these features are, caution must be used when considering the braille translation feature of the device, which may easily be misconstrued as having the potential to meet the braille production needs of a typical braille reader. There are several reasons why this is not true. First, the braille translator in the device is not 100 percent accurate and can make translation errors. The person entering the text must know how to format the braille properly if he or she wishes to produce anything more than very simple documents. In

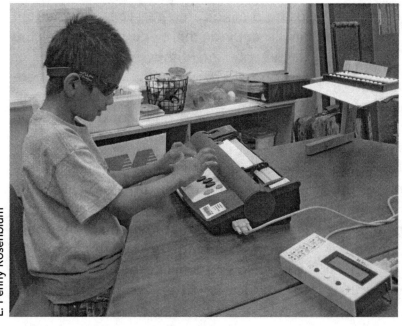

L. Penny Rosenblum

The Mimic, at lower right in this photo, provides a four-line visual display of what is being typed on the QWERTY keyboard attached to the Mountbatten, allowing classroom teachers, parents, or others who don't read braille to create simple braille documents.

USING THE MOUNTBATTEN BRAILLER IN THE CLASSROOM: AN EXAMPLE

William, a fifth-grade student who has light perception only and reads and writes in braille, has been reading the book *Bridge to Terabithia* with his classmates. Their language arts teacher, Ms. Tokada, has assigned them to write an essay in class about the book's theme. Ms. Tokada wrote the essay question on the blackboard for the students. Then she connected a standard computer keyboard to William's Mountbatten Brailler, along with the device's small visual display, the Mimic, and typed the essay question on the keyboard. Ms. Tokada could read on the display screen what she had typed and make any necessary corrections. William chose to read the essay question in braille, so he entered the command on the device instructing it to emboss the text that Ms. Tokada had entered. The Mountbatten Brailler embossed the text on plain notebook paper, and William read the assignment. He then opened a new file on the device and started to enter the text using the braille keyboard to complete the assignment. When he had finished, William issued the command to emboss the document in braille so that he could review and proofread it. As he read it through, William found a few errors that he wanted to correct. He issued the commands to have the device speak the text and to move to the desired locations in the document. After making all of the edits and changes, William embossed the document again and reviewed the final draft. Finding no additional errors and pleased with this edited version of his paper, William issued the command to the Mountbatten to print the document on the attached printer. Ms. Tokada collected and read William's work along with that of the rest of the class.

Feedback to a student about an assignment can be provided in several ways. Since both Ms. Tokada and William had an accessible copy of the document, Ms. Tokada could direct William verbally to specific locations in the document that they could then review and discuss together. A second option would be for Ms. Tokada to connect the keyboard to the Mountbatten, type comments referring to specific paragraphs and sentences, and then have the device emboss a copy. William could read these comments, locate the indicated passages in either the braille copy or the electronic copy of the document, and either make changes or respond verbally to the teacher's feedback. Upon completion of the changes, both a braille and print copy could again be produced.

The efficient use of a tool such as the Mountbatten Brailler gives educators the opportunity to apply the established learning theory that immediate feedback increases learning. An electronic braille-writer allows a braille user such as William to produce a written assignment, submit it to the teacher, and receive feedback at the same time as other students. The numerous features of the electronic braillewriter make it an extremely valuable tool for individuals who wish to produce written communications tactilely and solve some of the problems they might have in communicating with others who do not read braille themselves. Most braille readers could benefit greatly from this tool. Unfortunately, it is currently five to six times the cost of a manual braillewriter, but as technological advances decrease the price of their component parts, electronic braillewriters may become more affordable.

addition, the device was primarily designed as a personal brailler, not to emboss large documents on a routine basis. It was not designed to withstand heavy-duty use and can break down more often if it is used in this way. (For additional information on producing documents in braille, see Chapter 5.)

Regardless of these concerns, the device can still be an extremely efficient writing tool for some individuals and has proved useful in classrooms because of its advanced features (Holbrook, Wadsworth, & Bartlett, 2003; Cooper & Nichols, 2007).

Computers with Word-Processing Software

Another electronic tool that can be used to produce written communications in both braille and print is an accessible computer system with the appropriate hardware and software. As described in Chapter 3, the basis of the system is a desktop or laptop computer with word-processing software and a printer, along with some additional software and hardware to make the computer accessible. Screen-reading software is needed for the user to access the computer

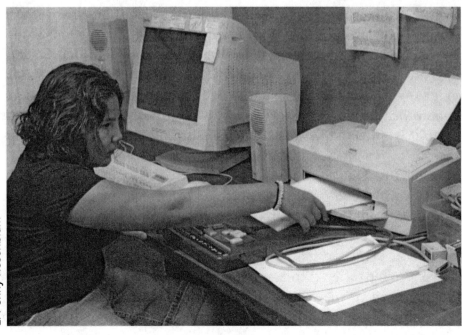

When her accessible PDA is connected to a printer, this student can make a print copy of her work for her classroom teacher.

L. Penny Rosenblum

either auditorily or tactilely. If the user wishes to access the computer's output tactilely, a refreshable braille display is also needed. With these tools, a braille reader can create, edit, proofread, and revise documents that can be produced in print.

If the braille reader wishes to produce a written document in braille, braille translation software and a braille embosser will be needed to complete the task. Braille translation software running on the computer converts the text in a word-processing document into the braille code and then sends it to the braille embosser or printer connected to the computer, which will produce hard-copy braille. (For a detailed explanation of this software and hardware, see Chapter 5.)

Accessible PDAs

Accessible PDAs (discussed in Chapter 3) are another tool that can be used to produce written documents in print or braille. Many users prefer these tools to an accessible laptop computer because they weigh less, have longer battery life, and turn on immediately for the user (rather than taking a while for the system to boot up, as with computers). These devices are available with either braille or QWERTY keyboards. Text can be entered into these devices using onboard word-processing software. The output is available to the user through synthesized speech or a built-in refreshable braille display. Many of these devices can be connected directly to a printer or embosser to produce a written document in print or braille. Units that do not have this capability can be connected to an accessible computer, and the user can transfer the file to the computer and then produce the document in print or braille. Accessible PDAs have proved efficient and effective for producing both print and braille documents because the user can

review and edit the text before committing it to paper.

Writing tools for students who access information tactilely are available as manual and electronic devices. Some of these tools are appropriate for short writing tasks, whereas others are more appropriate for longer writing assignments. To complete their writing tasks efficiently and effectively, students will need access to a variety of writing tools—a "toolbox full of tools"—to be successful.

PRODUCING WRITTEN COMMUNICATION AUDITORILY

Accessible Computers with Word-Processing Software

Accessible PDAs

Students who are blind or visually impaired who access information auditorily can also use technology to assist them in producing written communication. In the past, there were a limited number of options for writing. Years ago, the most frequently available alternative was dictating the information to a scribe who would write it down. Doing so was time consuming and labor intensive, however, and kept the writer dependent on outside help. With the advent of recording devices such as tape recorders and dictation machines, a writer could speak information into a microphone connected to a device and record it. A scribe or typist could then listen to the recording and write or type it to produce a written document, or the writer might transcribe it him- or herself. Although allowing more independence, these options have limited effectiveness for some writers, but more advanced tools have been developed that are more efficient for completing writing tasks. These include accessible computers with word-processing software and accessible PDAs.

ACCESSIBLE COMPUTERS WITH WORD-PROCESSING SOFTWARE

Accessible computers with word-processing software (discussed earlier in this chapter under electronic braille-writing devices for producing writing tactilely) provide the most powerful writing tool for students who are blind or visually impaired, regardless of the modality—vision, hearing, or touch—with which they choose to access information. Dedicated talking word processors (described in Chapter 3) can meet the needs of some writers. These are limited programs that do not give the user complete access to all of the information displayed on the screen. However, some of these programs are self-voicing and provide enough speech output to be used by writers who cannot access a computer screen visually. These writers, particularly younger students, find talking word processors to be valuable for completing many writing tasks. Other talking word processors do not voice everything on the screen or have keyboard commands for all functions and options. Although this lack of total access restricts the use of these programs, they can still be helpful to some writers who are blind or visually impaired.

As a student's writing needs increase, they can be met by a more robust word processor accessed through the use of screen-reading software (as discussed in Chapter 3). Most modern word processors are easily accessed with a screen reader. Users can produce high-quality written documents of any length, and the ability to edit text makes this alternative extremely empowering. The user can enter text as fast as he or she can type without having to worry about errors. Once his or her thoughts have been put into words, the navigation features of the screen reader and the editing features of the word processor allow the person to insert any missing text or delete text that is unwanted. The ease and speed with which a writer can correct errors and make revisions makes this a technique that can greatly increase the quantity and quality of the written tasks that can be accomplished by someone who is blind or visually impaired.

Formatting and proofreading features built into word-processing software allow the user to produce documents that are visually pleasing and organized for ease of reading. Search-and-replace options assist the writer in locating specific text in the document and in replacing an unwanted string of words with different text in multiple locations within the document. Proofreading tools such as spell check, grammar check, and a thesaurus offer an unprecedented boost to independent writing for people who are blind or visually impaired. These tools are available no matter how the student is accessing the computer—that is, visually with screen magnification, tactilely with refreshable braille, or auditorily with a screen reader.

ACCESSIBLE PDAS

Accessible PDAs (also known as portable notetakers) were described in Chapter 3 in reference to their function as tools for accessing electronic information, and some of their advantages were mentioned earlier in this chapter in regard to writing with tactile access. The presence of built-in talking word-processing software makes these devices excellent resources for producing written communication. Users can choose from models that offer QWERTY or braille keyboards. The talking word processors lets the writer hear each letter as it is entered if he or she chooses. The ability to navigate through the text and hear the entire document, a paragraph, a sentence, a word, or even a character read aloud provides the user a way to maximize the use of the system's editing features. Users can easily locate, identify, and move to errors in the text and take advantage of the editing features that allow the writer to insert missing text or delete unwanted material. Manipulating blocks of text by moving, deleting, or copying them is a powerful feature of these devices that greatly assists the writer in editing, revising, and rewriting. Most accessible PDAs also offer a spell-checking feature. When the writer has completed his or her work, it can be saved as a file to review later or transfer to a computer. To produce a print copy of the document, the user only needs to connect the device to a printer and issue the appropriate command to print the document. (Additional features of accessible PDAs are described in more detail in Chapter 3.)

SUMMARY

Technology offers a wide variety of tools that can be used to write by people who are blind or visually impaired. These tools allow the user to complete writing tasks visually, tactilely, or auditorily. There are manual and electronic tools that can be used to accomplish a variety of tasks, some of which are appropriate for short writing activities and others for longer ones. No single tool can meet all of the writing needs of a student who is blind or visually impaired. A recurring theme throughout this book has been that students with visual impairments need to be comfortable, skilled, and knowledgeable concerning a range of options that they can use to perform the tasks we all do while living and working in society today. It will take knowledge and flexibility in understanding the use of many different tools in order to successfully complete writing tasks that are part of an educational program.

REFERENCES

Cooper, H. L., & Nichols, S. K. (2007). Technology and early braille literacy: Using the Mountbatten Pro Brailler in primary-grade classrooms. *Journal of Visual Impairment & Blindness, 101*(1), 22–31.

D'Andrea, F. M. (2005a). More than a Perkins Brailler: A review of the Mountbatten Brailler; Part 1. *Access World, 6*(1). Retrieved from www.afb.org/afbpress/Pub.asp?DocID=aw060106

D'Andrea, F. M. (2005b). More than a Perkins Brailler: A review of the Mountbatten Brailler; Part 2. *Access World, 6*(2). Retrieved from www.afb.org/afbpress/Pub.asp?DocID=aw060208

D'Andrea, F. M. (2005c). The Mountbatten Pro: More than just an electronic brailler; Technology note. *Journal of Visual Impairment & Blindness, 99*(2), 115–117.

Holbrook, M. C., Wadsworth, A., & Bartlett, M. (2003). Teachers' perceptions of using the Mountbatten Brailler with young children. *Journal of Visual Impairment & Blindness, 97*(10), 646–654.

5

Technologies for Producing Materials in Alternate Formats

Before students who are visually impaired can read and access information using many of the methods described in this book, they need to have the material in an accessible format that they can use. Making sure that students obtain their textbooks and other educational materials in a format that they can access at the same time as their sighted classmates has been an ongoing concern for educators of students with visual impairments. Both technological and legal developments are revolutionizing this process.

With the passage of the 2004 reauthorization of the Individuals with Disabilities Education Act (IDEA), the provision of textbooks and instructional materials in accessible formats for students who are blind or print disabled in a timely manner is legally mandated. (See Sidebar 5.1, "Textbooks on Time: NIMAS and NIMAC" and Appendix A at the end of this book for more information.) Although textbooks may be available in braille, large print, and recorded audio from commercial producers who specialize in alternate formats, other educational material—such as worksheets, games, and supplementary materials—is not equally available. Also, on those occasions when textbooks and other materials do not arrive on time, accessible versions need to be produced by the local education agency (LEA) or the teacher of students who are visually impaired.

Technology provides excellent tools for producing alternate formats for an individual with a visual impairment. Depending on which sensory channel the student uses

---

SIDEBAR 5.1

TEXTBOOKS ON TIME: NIMAS AND NIMAC

Making sure that students who use textbooks in alternate formats receive these books at the same time that their sighted peers receive regular print books has been a long-term goal of educators of visually impaired students, which was inscribed in Goal Seven of the *National Agenda for Children and Youth with Visual Impairments* (Corn, Hatlen, Huebner, Ryan, & Siller, 1995; Huebner, Merk-Adam, Stryker, & Wolffe, 2004). This seemingly simple concept became a multiyear national project involving a consortium of interested parties, including educators, consumers, publishers, and accessible media producers. It culminated in the incorporation of this concept into IDEA and the creation of a process for textbook publishers to make files of their books available for conversion into accessible formats.

The National Instructional Materials Accessibility Standard (NIMAS; see http://nimas.cast.org) was developed to guide publishers in producing electronic files of their textbooks, which are deposited and maintained at the National Instructional Materials Accessibility Center (NIMAC; www.nimac.us/), housed at the American Printing House for the Blind. However, these deposited files are just the source files that provide the content to be converted into accessible formats; they are not designed to be distributed to teachers, individual schools, students, or parents, and they generally do not contain descriptions of images, tables, or charts and graphs.

In states that join the program, the state educational agency designates a small number of authorized users who have access to the textbook files—usually the state instructional resource centers. (If states do not coordinate with NIMAC, they will still be required to ensure that students with print disabilities receive high-quality accessible materials in a timely manner.) These authorized users engage accessible media producers (AMPs), who use the types of technology described in this chapter to prepare the files in the appropriate format for the production of a braille, large-print, or auditory version. The books are then provided to the student in the desired format. Most teachers or students who seek accessible materials will go through the same agencies and channels they have used in the past to acquire their textbooks. (For additional information, see Renfranz, Taboada, and Weatherd, 2008.)

most effectively for particular tasks or ongoing learning, information can be converted into the appropriate medium: a visual format such as large print; a tactile format such as braille; or an auditory format such as a recording. Technology also offers the option of storing information electronically and allowing the student to choose which sensory modality to use to access the information. School system personnel need to use specific hardware and software to convert information into the alternate formats used effectively by students who are blind or visually impaired. This chapter explores the various tools and techniques available to them.

PRODUCING MATERIALS IN A VISUAL FORMAT

Materials Enlarged on a Photocopying Machine

Commercially Produced Large Print

Computer-Based Large-Print Production

Producing or obtaining accessible print materials for people with low vision can be accomplished in various ways, including purchasing commercially produced large-print books and materials, enlarging materials on a photocopying machine, and using a computer system to produce customized large print. As with most of the assistive technology options considered in this book, each of these production techniques may be particularly appropriate—or inappropriate—for certain individual students, depending on the student's needs. Each technique will have advantages and disadvantages for students.

(See Chapter 2 for additional information about accessing materials visually.)

MATERIALS ENLARGED ON A PHOTOCOPYING MACHINE

Photocopying machines are widely used for providing materials in an enlarged format. They can enlarge an image approximately 130–150 percent. Although this magnitude of enlargement increases the size of the printed text, it is difficult to determine the exact point size that results. It may therefore be difficult to predict the enlargement setting needed for a given student. If, for example, a student prefers or reads effectively with 20-point type, and a teacher is using a photocopier to enlarge the text of a paperback novel for English class, the teacher will have to guess how much to enlarge the book to produce the text in the student's preferred size.

Several considerations need to be addressed when using a photocopier to produce enlarged materials:

- The copy needs to be made from the original document if at all possible. If photocopies of the original document are used, they will often have variations in ink density as well as smudges and distortions at the boundaries between the text and the background. A copy of a copy will often be difficult to read.
- The original should have crisp, clean text.
- Care should be taken to fit the complete enlarged image on the page. Doing so can become a process of trial and error, depending on the size of the paper being used for the copy.

Some copiers have settings for commonly used paper sizes, such as 8½ × 14 inches and 11 × 17 inches.

In general, using photocopiers to enlarge materials has several drawbacks. Typically, they cannot provide enough enlargement for most individuals with low vision, who may still need to use an optical device to read the text effectively. Even if the main text is large enough, smaller print used in such elements as photo captions, mathematical subscripts and superscripts, graphs, and footnotes is often too small to read. Photographs often do not copy clearly, and unless a school has a color copier, any colored areas (on a graph or a map, for example) will become a mass of gray, with the different colors difficult to distinguish.

To further increase the size of the text, it is possible to make an enlarged copy of the first enlargement. This process can be repeated until the text is large enough for a student to read. However, making enlargements of enlargements greatly increases the difficulty of getting all of the material on one page, and also makes the print fuzzier and harder to read, even if the original was clear. The use of 11 × 17 inch paper can help to fit enlarged text onto a single page, but it is often inconvenient for the reader to handle because it is larger than standard notebook paper and therefore difficult to keep in a notebook. Repeatedly enlarging a single print page to reach the level of enlargement needed by some readers often results in multiple pages of enlarged print that have text overlapping or repeating from page to page, unless someone takes the time to cut and tape together portions of the text. If that is not done, a reader may finish an enlarged page and find that when he or she begins reading at the top of the next page, several lines repeat from the page before. This repetition can be confusing for some readers and a waste of time.

Overall, using a photocopying machine is often the most readily available method for providing enlarged print, but it is usually the least desirable. It bears repeating that this production method should be used only as a "stopgap" approach until better solutions can be determined. Too often, however, this method is the only option considered and denies the student the opportunity to receive information in the most appropriate format. Nevertheless, students who wish to access information visually do not have to rely solely on this production method because other technologies can be used to produce materials in large print.

COMMERCIALLY PRODUCED LARGE PRINT

Books in large print can be obtained from publishers who specialize in this medium. (For listings of such publishers, see the *AFB Directory of Services for Blind and Visually Impaired Persons in the United States or Canada* [2005], also available online at www.afb.org/services.asp.) The American Printing House for the Blind (APH) has been a traditional provider of large-print textbooks for students with visual impairments, but some commercial publishers now specialize in books in large print (see the Resources section at the back of this book for more information about such sources). Some publishers also have more popular titles available in large print. Although these titles are competitively priced with their standard-print counterparts, commercially produced textbooks in large print are still quite expensive. The selection of available

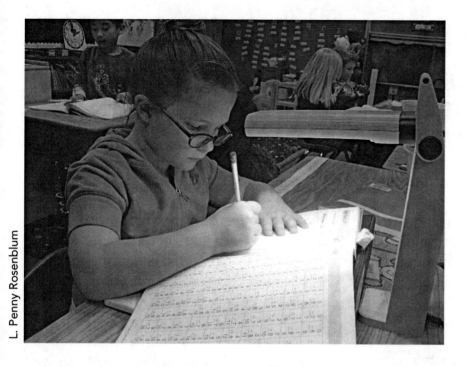

L. Penny Rosenblum

Textbooks and other titles can be obtained in large print from publishers who specialize in this medium.

titles is more limited than it is for standard-size print books, but it is increasing as some publishers see a market for large print among the aging population.

COMPUTER-BASED LARGE-PRINT PRODUCTION

Even if all of the books that students require were available from commercial producers of large print, the needs of individuals with low vision who wish to access print information visually would not be met because much of the information that students need to read is not in book format. Students might read this material by using some of the tools for accessing print information visually that are described in Chapter 2, such as low vision devices or video magnifiers. There are times, however, when a student needs, or prefers to have, a large-print copy. In these situations, some of the computer-based technologies introduced in previous chapters can be used to produce large-print versions of materials.

If the print information is already available in an electronic format—say, as a word-processing document—it is easy to modify the text in a compatible word-processing program so that it can be printed out in the student's preferred font and point size. Graphics can be enlarged using the program's drawing tool. The resulting document might need to be reformatted, especially if there are blank lines for answers to questions, as might be found on a worksheet. If the material is not available electronically, then it can be scanned and a file created using a computer system equipped with a scanner and optical character recognition (OCR) software. (For more information on these devices and software, see "Scanning and OCR Systems" in Chapter 2.) Sidebar 5.2, "Using a Computer to Produce Large-Print Materials," provides two examples that explain this process in more detail.

This method of producing large-print materials using a computer, scanner, and word processor—which might be described

USING A COMPUTER TO PRODUCE LARGE-PRINT MATERIALS

As the following examples illustrate, print materials can be produced with relative care in a large-print format, tailored to a student's preferences for size and font, using a computer and scanner equipped with optical character recognition (OCR) software.

Example 1

Ms. Mendez, a third-grade teacher, wants to conduct part of her science lesson outside in the park. She is going to have her students take with them a four-page packet of materials stapled together and clipped to a clipboard. The pages contain text, graphics, and questions with blank lines on which to write the answers. Ms. Mendez knows that she has two students in her class who have low vision but who access their materials visually. Rachel uses a video magnifier for reading, while Dimitri prefers to use a stand magnifier.

Ms. Mendez knows that Rachel cannot take the video magnifier outside and that Dimitri would find it difficult to manipulate the stand magnifier, the clipboard, and his bold-line marker with no desk to place them on. In addition, Rachel prefers print materials in Verdana bold 24-point font and Dimitri prefers 16 point APHont. How can she meet the needs of these two students and conduct her outdoor lesson?

Ms. Mendez contacts Mr. Polonsky, the teacher of students with visual impairments who serves these students, several days before the lesson to explain what materials she needs to have adapted. Together they will decide to make the necessary adaptations for the two students and who will do it. In this case, Mr. Polonsky has trained Alecia, a clerical staff person in the school's media center to assist in the production of materials in large print.

Alecia first needs to check with Ms. Mendez to see if her materials packet is available as an electronic file. Many teachers at the school use a computer word-processing program to create classroom materials. Usually Ms. Mendez does have such a file, which saves time. (If she has the electronic file, Alecia can skip to Step 4 below.) In this case, however, she does not, so Alecia needs to scan the document as described in Steps 1, 2, and 3 of the following procedure:

1. Obtain a good, clean copy of the document and take it to a computer system that is equipped with a scanner, OCR software, word-processing software, and a color printer.
2. Scan the document into the computer, run the OCR software to transform it into text, save it as a file, and then open it in the word-processing program.
3. Execute the spell-checking feature of the program and then proofread the document to locate and correct any scanning errors.
4. Execute the "select all" command for the program to highlight all of the text and then choose Verdana bold 24-point font to change the text to Rachel's preferred font.

5. Select the graphics in the document and use the program's drawing tools to enlarge the images.
6. Check the blank lines where the answers should be written, as they may not have scanned correctly, and insert new blank lines if necessary.
7. Check to see if any reformatting needs to be done and make the appropriate adjustments. Most likely the blank lines will need to be adjusted.
8. Insert a line of dashes and page numbers to indicate where the original print pages break.
9. Save the file and print it on the color printer.
10. Execute the "select all" command again and choose APHont 16-point font to prepare the same worksheet for Dimitri.
11. Check to see if any reformatting needs to be done and make the appropriate adjustments. Most likely the blank lines will need to be adjusted.
12. Save the file under a different name and print it on the color printer.
13. Staple the pages together and give them to Ms. Mendez.

Example 2

A student interning at an insurance company receives a three-page report that will be discussed at an upcoming meeting. The intern will need to be able to read and refer to the information in the report during the meeting. He would prefer to have the information available in large print, rather than using another method to access it. To produce a large-print copy of this report, the intern, or someone who works with him, might follow these steps:

1. Check with the writer of the report to determine if it is available as an electronic file. If it is, skip to Step 7. If not, continue to Step 2.
2. Obtain a good, clean print copy of the document and take it to a computer system equipped with an optical scanner, OCR software, a word-processing program, and a printer.
3. Place the document in the scanner and run the scanning program that came with the scanner.
4. After the document has been scanned, have the OCR software perform the recognition process and save its results as a file.
5. Once the recognition process is complete, open the file in a word-processing program.
6. Execute the spell-checking feature of the program, and then proofread the document to check for scanning recognition errors.
7. Execute the "select all" command for the program and then choose the desired font and point size.
8. Review the document to determine if any of the text needs to be reformatted and make any necessary adjustments.
9. Insert a line of dashes and page numbers to indicate where the regular print pages break.
10. Save the file and then print it. The intern will now have a print copy of the report in his preferred font and point size.

as "making your own"—has many advantages over using a photocopying machine to enlarge a document. The text can be produced in the reader's desired font and point size, and the graphics can be enlarged in a way that maintains color and clarity. Probably the most significant advantage is the ability to produce the materials on standard-sized paper. The quality of the print and the graphics in materials created with a computer and scanner will usually be much better as well.

Making your own materials has some advantages over using commercial large-print books as well. The materials are usually a great deal less expensive, and this methodology can provide materials that are not available from large-print publishers. Professionally produced large-print books may be bound better and be more durable than materials produced through the use of scanners and a computer, but many of the needed titles and supplemental materials (such as workbooks, study guides, and worksheets) may not be readily available to students. Many materials needed on a day-to-day basis simply have to be created because there is no other way to obtain them efficiently. Most school systems and businesses have access to the hardware and software required to complete their production. If the necessary equipment is not already available, it can be purchased for a reasonable price. Moreover, the cost of the equipment can be minor compared to the expense of purchasing large-print books for several students. The only additional cost is for a staff member (often a paraeducator) who will create the materials as part of his or her job.

Many large-print books are only available in 18- or 24-point type (although this is changing as customized books are becoming more common); many students will function better with point sizes other than 18 or 24 point. In addition, the same document can easily be produced in different sizes and fonts for multiple individuals who need access to the same information. The printout can be on 8½ × 11 inch paper, which will fit into notebooks, file folders, and other standard binding options. Color graphics can be scanned and integrated into the final document, but there may be times when the user will prefer to view them with an optical device in their original format.

The flexibility inherent in using technology to produce materials in large print also allows you to accommodate students in other ways. Individual users do not always want all of their materials in the same font and point size. Sometimes a student may prefer a larger or smaller point size depending on the task and the location in which it is to be completed. For example, Jeremy may prefer to use the class's regular textbook with an optical device for English class, but want to use 20-point type on a tabletop reading stand when reading material from a math textbook. He may also find it more efficient to read materials other than textbooks, such as an information packet, in a 24-point or larger font, while keeping the worksheet with accompanying questions in smaller type. In that way, he can read the information packet in the larger point size on one sheet of paper and then write on the question-and-answer sheet without having to move his head and body physically to view and work with two sets of the materials. If the reading material is printed in a larger point size, Jeremy can keep the question-and-answer sheet directly in front of him on the table and glance over at the reading material on the other page when necessary. If the reading materials were not printed in a larger point size, he might need to move his head and body, or pick up the material and bring it closer to his eyes. Thus, the ability to create materials tailored to a student's individual needs enhances the efficiency and effectiveness of the student's efforts.

PRODUCING MATERIALS IN A TACTILE FORMAT

Who Produces Braille?

Tools for Producing Braille

- Manual, Mechanical, and Electronic Braille Production Tools
- Braille Translation Software
- Braille Embossers
- Interlining

Tactile Graphics

- Collage
- Tooling
- Capsule Paper and Fuser
- Computer-Assisted Tactile Graphics

Producing educational materials for students who are blind or visually impaired in tactile format generally means providing braille with tactile graphics. The ultimate goal is to supply the information that students need for their studies in their preferred alternate format at the same time that the sighted students in their classes are receiving their textbooks and other materials. Historically, however, transcribing print into braille and embossing (printing) in braille have been time consuming and expensive, and the resulting books themselves have been bulky and difficult to handle. Improvements in the technology of braille production have enhanced the ability to produce high-quality braille and tactile graphics efficiently in larger quantities and at quicker speeds. In addition, as noted earlier, requirements in the most recent reauthorization of IDEA request textbook publishers to provide files of their core curriculum materials in the specialized file format (NIMAS) that facilitates production of alternate media, including braille, and have a more efficient system of braille production created.

As described in Chapter 4, braille and tactile graphics can be produced manually (collage), mechanically (tooling), and electronically (computer generated). Which method is most efficient depends largely on how much writing is being done and the quantity of material that needs to be produced. Some individuals who read braille limit their braille production to personal communications, such as notes and lists, and to information storage of such items as addresses or recipes. For these tasks, manual and mechanical devices, such as the slate and stylus or mechanical braillewriter, are often all that are needed. Those who wish to produce braille documents of moderate length that may only be used for a limited time—such as a study guide for an English course—often find both mechanical (braillewriter) and electronic (computer-based) production methods to be adequate. Producing lengthy documents such as braille textbooks requires tools that provide efficiency, speed, accuracy, and the ability to make multiple copies, such as braille translation computer programs, braille embossers, and commercial plate embossers.

WHO PRODUCES BRAILLE?

Braille books, particularly textbooks and other lengthy volumes, are most often produced commercially. The American Printing

House for the Blind (APH) is probably the largest braille textbook producer in the United States and has a long history of producing textbooks for the K–12 education market. However, during the last half of the 20th century, as larger numbers of braille readers began to be educated in regular public schools, the variety of titles that needed to be available in braille increased significantly. Educators began looking for additional sources of braille textbooks.

Traditionally, braille volunteers—groups of individuals dedicated to producing materials in braille, often as a community service—have been one of the more widely used alternatives to commercial production. Members of these groups became braille transcribers by completing training and becoming certified through the National Library Service for the Blind and Physically Handicapped (part of the U.S. Library of Congress) in Washington, DC, and usually provided braille textbooks for students at little or no cost. But this pool of transcribers has been shrinking as retiring volunteers have not been replaced by new ones. Other sources of braille production were needed.

Since the 1970s, educators, along with the assistance of several national organizations, have been establishing instructional materials centers (IMCs; also known as instructional resource centers [IRCs]) around the country to share braille textbooks and create educational materials, including tactile graphics, to distribute to students who need them. Most states have an IRC or IMC that acquires books from APH, volunteer or paid transcribers, and other commercial producers. Innovative thinkers began to tap into a labor force that had not been previously used: prisoners

serving long-term sentences. Numerous states have established prison braille programs in which inmates learn to be braille transcribers.

The increasing demand for braille materials has also led to the development of small-scale private production companies and a growing number of individual transcribers using technology to produce a wide variety of materials in braille on a contractual basis. These providers usually contract with individual school districts or state agencies to produce braille and serve as a valuable resource in providing the materials necessary for students to receive an appropriate education.

A final source of braille production is personnel and staff in the education field—teachers of students with visual impairments, paraeducators, and other staff who have been trained to produce braille materials for students in public school. These individuals do not usually produce textbooks, but in some cases they produce sections of textbooks while waiting for the books to be provided by one of the large-scale production sources. Although many of these personnel may not be certified transcribers, it is critical that they receive sufficient training to accurately and efficiently produce the needed materials.

Through the use of all of these resources, significant strides have been made in the provision of braille textbooks to braille readers in a timely manner and the more widespread availability of materials in braille. What is required to make this happen is appropriate staff training and access to the necessary production tools that are described in the section that follows.

TOOLS FOR PRODUCING BRAILLE

Manual, Mechanical, and Electronic Braille Production Tools

Low-tech manual and mechanical devices for producing braille—the slate and stylus and the manual braillewriter—provide durable and relatively inexpensive options. These tools can be thought of as the "pen-and-paper method" of braille production. They are not efficient for larger production tasks, but can be appropriate for short jobs that need to be completed on the spot. Electronic braillewriters offer some advantages in editing capabilities and reduction of manual labor. (For more information about these devices, see Chapter 4.)

However, while these devices offer portable and affordable means of producing braille, they lack the advanced editing features and embossing speeds needed for large-scale braille production and publishing, and they are not appropriate to use for producing multiple copies or long documents. For these jobs, braille transcribers need high-tech tools in the form of computer software and hardware, and high-speed embossers.

Braille Translation Software

Braille translation software provides an efficient and time-saving method that can be used by a transcriber to prepare and transcribe documents for braille production. Braille translators are much like word-processing software, and in fact, some translators also offer a word processor or text editor as a basic component of the program. The editor component of these programs can accept text entered directly from the keyboard, open or import files from scanned documents, or open files from the Internet and other e-text sources. Once the text has been opened in the program, the user can

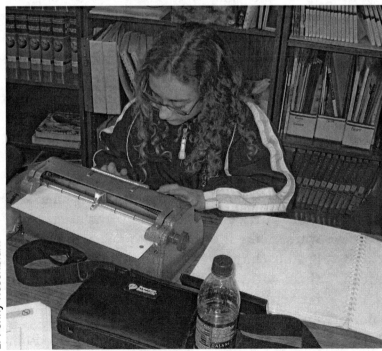

Mechanical devices for producing braille, such as this braillewriter, are useful for short jobs that need to be completed on the spot, but larger production tasks require a braille embosser.

manipulate the text in several ways. Text that has been scanned using OCR software will often have formatting and recognition errors. The text can be easily changed using commands for inserting and deleting. Although this kind of editing is an important feature for producing braille quickly and efficiently, it is only the first step.

More powerful features of braille translation software allow the user to establish the formatting of the braille when it is embossed. In order to correctly convey the meaning of the printed information, it is essential that indentations, paragraphs, columns, and tables be formatted correctly according to the rules and guidelines established by the Braille Authority of North America (BANA). Braille that is not properly formatted makes it difficult for the reader to grasp the layout of the material, which is usually fundamental to comprehension. Trained transcribers who are knowledgeable about proper braille formatting can use the numerous features of the braille translation software to ensure that headings, lists, outlines, poems, foreign language texts, and even mathematical and scientific notations are appropriately formatted.

Once the text is properly laid out, the program translates it into the appropriate braille code. The translated document can be displayed on the computer screen in what is referred to as "sim braille." Sim braille, short for "simulated braille," is a visual display of the braille dots arranged in patterns that are identical to the text that will be embossed and can be viewed on the computer screen or printed in ink with a regular printer. Trained transcribers and teachers of visually impaired students use sim braille to proofread the translation and the formatting of text visually before embossing it. When errors are located, the user can apply the program's six-key braille editor mode to make corrections. This helpful feature allows the transcriber to use the computer's standard QWERTY keyboard to input braille. In this mode, the *F*, *D*, and *S* keys represent the dots 1, 2, and 3 of the braille cell, and dots 4, 5, and 6 are represented by the letters *J*, *K*, and *L*. The transcriber can press down several computer keys at the same time to create braille letters as is done on a mechanical braillewriter. The six-key editor mode allows the trained transcriber to produce complicated documents manually but with the added benefit of the editing capabilities of a computer word processor.

Production of math and science materials in braille has also benefited from new technologies. Mathematics and science materials (such as chemistry) are transcribed into a different braille code from standard literature, which uses what is referred to as "literary braille." This math and science code is called the Nemeth Braille Code for Mathematics and Science Notation (1972). Programs exist that can assist a qualified braille transcriber in producing materials in Nemeth Code. Although these tools are more complicated to use than the literary braille translation programs that are available, educators who put the time and effort into mastering them are able to produce braille materials that will allow students who read braille to fully participate in higher level math and science classes.

The technologies discussed in this section, particularly braille translation software, make it easier and quicker to produce braille than ever before. When discussing them with administrators who are unfamiliar with the production of braille and the needs of braille readers, it is extremely important to be clear about the need for properly trained personnel to use them. It is not uncommon for people to think that all that is needed to meet the braille production needs of a braille-reading student is to purchase a braille translation program and a braille embosser. It may seem that a clerical or support staff member can produce braille without much training, simply by opening an electronic version of the desired material in the braille translation software, choosing the "translate" command, turning on the embosser, and selecting "emboss." In fact, braille produced this way–often referred to as "quick and dirty" braille—is likely to have many errors and be difficult for a student to read. All of the characters and words might be there, but the intent and meaning of the text may not be clear because of improper formatting or errors in the transcription.

Translation software is a wonderful tool, but it is not foolproof and errors will be made. If a staff member lacks knowledge of braille, he or she will not be able to proofread documents to determine if the information is correct. The expertise of a certified braille transcriber or a teacher of students with visual impairments who is knowledgeable about braille formatting is needed to ensure that a braille document is correct and formatted properly. Print materials that are improperly formatted and full of errors would not be tolerated for students in the classroom, and the same high standards need to be applied to braille materials. Extensive training is needed for any staff member who is hired to produce braille for students. In short, braille production technology does not eliminate the need for certified braille transcribers.

Braille Embossers

Although braille translation software enables a transcriber to edit and format documents, it is hardware in the form of a braille embosser that actually produces the paper copy of a braille document. Current braille embossers use continuous tractor- or pin-feed paper in one long, continuous fan-folded stack similar to that used by dot matrix printers. After embossing, the pages need to be torn apart along their perforations. By giving the user the ability to produce longer documents without having to insert each page into the embosser, the use of continuous tractor-feed paper has greatly increased the efficiency of the braille production process.

Thanks to the use of braille translation software and continuous tractor-feed paper, the production of braille on various sizes of paper is now feasible. Transcribers currently have the ability to produce braille on 8½ × 11 inch paper for braille readers who prefer documents that can be stored in standard notebooks, folders, and envelopes. However, the same document can be produced just as easily on 11½ × 11 inch paper for readers who prefer the fluidity of reading a longer line before needing to locate the beginning of the next line. These technologies provide the braille transcriber and the braille reader with tools that assist in the efficient production and use of braille.

Braille embossers designed to perform light braille-production duties are known as personal braille embossers. These comparatively lightweight embossers are transportable and are best suited for individual use. The embossing speeds of 10–15 characters per second that they offer are adequate for short- to medium-length documents. Documents of greater length, which require the embosser to emboss continuously for long periods of time, overtax the capabilities of these machines; using a personal embosser in this way will greatly increase the number of repairs that the device might require and significantly decrease its life-span. A personal braille embosser is probably capable of meeting the needs of several beginning braille readers or one experienced braille reader in middle school or high school for supplemental braille materials.

Embossers with increased speeds have been designed to operate at 25–60 characters per second and to emboss continuously for longer periods of time. Durability and speed are further enhanced by interpoint embossers, which can emboss simultaneously on both sides of the paper. Interpoint braille saves a significant amount of paper and makes longer braille documents less bulky and easier for students to carry and store. This type of braille embosser would be necessary to meet the needs of several braille readers of varying experience levels and abilities in an educational setting.

Commercial braille producers require embossers with even higher speed and output. Embossers designed to operate at more than 100 characters per second for extended periods of time have greatly increased the number of commercial braille producers, but are prohibitively expensive for many smaller producers. Large-scale braille publishers are also beginning to use computer hardware and software to program and control the presses and plates used to emboss multiple volumes of large texts. The use of braille translation software and braille embossing hardware has dramatically increased the production of braille.

Interlining

There are many situations in which it is useful to have the print translation or equivalent of braille available on the same page as the braille. For example, general education classroom teachers working with students who use braille may find it difficult to help a student find a particular section or passage of text in braille. The printing of text above embossed braille on the same page is referred to as *interlining*.

There are several methods for interlining braille. Embossers that are hybrids of a traditional braille embosser and an ink-jet printer are capable of embossing braille and printing text on the same page. These devices are more expensive than the average braille embosser, but in some cases can be worth the extra expense.

Another approach to addressing the need for print and braille is a system that connects a braille embosser and a standard dot matrix printer. First, the tractor- or pin-feed braille paper is fed through the dot matrix printer and the text is printed on the page. The print is arranged on widely spaced lines, leaving room for the braille to be embossed. The same paper is then loaded into the braille embosser and the program will emboss the braille in the appropriate location on the page. Materials produced in this manner can be read simultaneously by the student tactilely and the teacher visually.

The sim braille display option mentioned earlier, which is offered by most braille translation programs, can allow a sighted instructor and a braille reader to read the same information simultaneously without the need to print and emboss at the same time. The sim braille document can be printed with ink on paper; selecting the "interline" option in the print dialog box prints the document with a line of print text above each line of the sim braille. A teacher can refer to this printed page and see the print text translation for each line of the braille copy while the braille reader reads a separate embossed braille version. This allows the teacher or student to refer to specific lines or words on a line, thus facilitating communication.

TACTILE GRAPHICS

When preparing educational materials to be read in a tactile format, simply describing the accompanying pictures, photographs, maps, and charts is not always sufficient to convey the information depicted visually and graphically. As described in Chapter 2, there are a number of ways to create tactile graphics to represent visual graphics, and many educators will find these materials essential for their students' understanding of graphically presented information. Tactile graphics such as maps, charts and diagrams, and information for tests need to be of high quality and be able to be used over and over again. (For ideas on creating quick, if less permanent, tactile graphics in the classroom, see "Technology Tip: Inexpensive Tactile Graphics on the Fly.")

Commercially produced tactile graphics are becoming more available, and many of the volunteer braillists mentioned previously also provide tactile graphics for textbooks and other educational materials. However, the production of commercial-quality tactile graphics is often time consuming, and if a commercial or other producer has not already created a needed graphic, teachers will need to allow adequate lead time to create custom orders for their students with braille producers. In addition, there will be numerous occasions when students need access to graphical information used in the classroom that is not part of the regular textbook and may not be available commercially. It will be the responsibility of the educational system to provide students with a tactile graphic. To provide this service, someone on staff, or

hired on a consulting basis, who is familiar with the methods and the tools needed to produce tactile graphics will be needed to provide the materials that students need.

Producing effective, high-quality tactile graphics requires both specialized tools and specialized training. It is not simply a matter of reproducing a print graphic in a tactile format; in fact, in many cases a direct *reproduction* will be of very little value in communicating the pertinent information to the student. Rather, a *representation* of the information will usually be more effective.

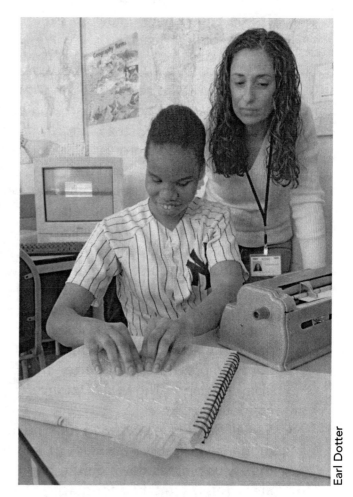

Some tactile graphics are available commercially, like this tactile atlas, but if a required graphic is not already available, someone who knows how to produce tactile graphics will need to create one.

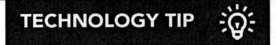

INEXPENSIVE TACTILE GRAPHICS ON THE FLY

Sometimes a subject or concept comes up unexpectedly in class that could be illustrated by a quick tactile diagram. There is no time to use one of the methods for producing high-quality, reusable tactile graphics described in this chapter. Luckily, there are several easy, low-cost, and rapid ways to create a tactile graphic that is meant to be ephemeral. These "on the fly" graphics are not necessarily intended to be saved or reused; they are meant to demonstrate a new concept quickly to a student in a "teachable moment." (See the Resources section at the end of this book for sources of the products described here; many are sold by the American Printing House for the Blind [APH] or Exceptional Teaching.)

- *Screen Board.* A particularly easy method of creating a quick tactile graphic is to use ordinary wire screen used in window screens to raise a texture on a regular piece of paper. A screen board can be made by cutting a piece of window screen and affixing it to a piece of sturdy cardboard or plywood, and securing it with duct tape. When a regular piece of paper is put on the board (not thick paper such as braille paper) and a student or teacher draws with a crayon on the paper, the texture of the screen comes out on the paper where the crayon has pressed it into the screen and can be felt with the fingers. This is an extremely quick way to draw basic shapes and outlines. For example, if the kindergarten teacher has given all of the students a worksheet with basic shapes on it for the children to color, it's easy to use a screen board to outline the shapes for the child with visual impairments to feel so he or she may participate in this activity.
- *Swail Dot Inverter.* Another easy way to create simple graphics is with the Swail Dot Inverter from APH. This device is a metal stylus with a recessed tip. When paper is placed on the rubber sheet that comes with the set, the teacher or student can press the dot inverter into the paper, creating a tactile dot that is raised from the paper. The Swail Dot Inverter can also be used to outline a shape on a handout quickly.
- *Sewell Raised Line Drawing Kit.* The Sewell Raised Line Drawing Kit comes with a rubberized clip board, a stack of thin plastic textured sheets, and a stylus. When the stylus presses down on the plastic pages on the board, a tactile line is created. This is a method for quickly making images that probably will not be reused, such as a geometry diagram that the teacher draws on the board as an example of acute and obtuse angles.

- *Quick-Draw Paper.* APH is the source for Quick-Draw Paper, a thick one-time-use paper that creates quick graphics. When the teacher or student uses a water-based marker, the paper swells up to create a tactile line. APH also sells a Textured Paper collection—a selection of brightly colored paper of varying textures that can be cut out and affixed to a background to create textured shapes, lines, and illustrations.
- *Wheatley Tactile Diagramming Kit.* APH also offers the reusable Wheatley Tactile Diagramming Kit (also referred to as the "Picture Maker"). The kit comes with a felt board to which the teacher or student can attach Velcro-backed shapes and thin lines to create a variety of pictures and diagrams.
- *Wikki Stix.* This is another reusable method for making quick diagrams. Wikki Stix are thin, waxy, bendable sticks that come in a multitude of colors. They stick to paper or to each other and can be used to make shapes, outlines, and other tactile graphics. They peel off the paper and can be re-used as needed.

There will always be a need to create high-quality tactile graphics using collage, tooling, and other methods. But for a quick "in the moment" diagram or outline, the tools described here can do the trick!

Thus, the person who creates tactile graphics needs to understand both the significance of the information conveyed by a print graphic and the most appropriate way to represent that information. One rule of thumb might be, "If it *looks* really good, it is probably not an effective tactile graphic." Graphics that look good to the eye often have too much detail and tactilely seem cluttered to the student. Thinking that the essence of tactile graphics is the line-for-line duplication of a print graphic is an easily made mistake that highlights the need for extensive training. However, with appropriate training and tools and a little research, teachers of students with visual impairments can learn to produce some of the tactile graphics that their students need. Teachers generally will not have time to produce all of the tactile graphics needed by students, so funding is needed to obtain the majority of tactile graphics from commercial producers or through the state's IMC. (For an in-depth treatment of tactile graphics, see Edman, 1992.)

Several types of tactile graphics and production methods were introduced in Chapter 2. Different types of graphics may require different production methods and production tools. The first two methods described here, *collage* and *tooling*, use relatively low-tech methods to produce tactile graphics, whereas *capsule paper and fusing* and *computer-assisted graphics* use more high-tech tools.

Collage

Tactile graphics made with the collage method use materials of varying textures to represent the components of a print graphic: areas, lines, and point symbols used to designate specific locations on a map or coordinates on a graph. The collage method relies more on a wide variety of textured materials than on specialized tools. The materials are often those found at craft and hobby stores, such as the following examples:

- *Area textures*: braille paper, cardboard, disposable cleaning cloths (such as HandiWipes), textured paper, fine sandpaper, needlepoint backing, fabric
- *Line textures*: string, wire, candlewick, carpet thread, puff paint
- *Point symbols*: cork, felt, paper circles created by a hole puncher, balsa wood cutouts, foam shapes, basic cardboard shapes, small metal rings

Common items used to make collages, such as scissors, tweezers, needle-nose pliers, and a utility knife or craft-type blade, are tools that teachers may have available for other tasks. Individuals using the collage method to produce tactile graphics will also find a variety of glues and spray adhesives to be very useful. Laminating sheets sold in office supply stores and self-adhering plastic sheets can serve as excellent labeling materials. Sufficient funds will need to be available to ensure that staff has the necessary materials.

The collage method is often used to create a master tactile graphic that is then copied onto special plastic sheets using a vacuum form process known as thermoforming. The thermoform machine can be thought of as a copying machine for braille and tactile graphics. Multiple copies of braille pages and some tactile graphics can be made with the machine and transferred onto a special thin plastic page. This special thermoform "paper" represents a tactile copy of the shapes and textures on the original graphic. Thus, instead of having to create multiple copies of a tactile map by hand, for example, the teacher can make one map and give each student a copy of it reproduced via thermoform. Tactile graphics produced using the collage method and the tooling method (described in the following section), particularly those tooled onto aluminum sheets, can be reproduced successfully using a thermoform machine (Hasty, 2008).

Tooling

Tooling is a production method that uses special tools to press or imprint points,

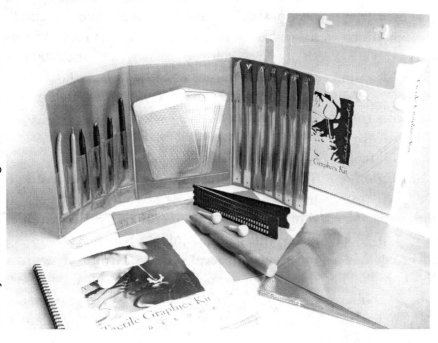

Producing effective, high-quality tactile graphics requires specialized training as well as specialized tools, such as this Tactile Graphics Kit from the American Printing House for the Blind.

lines, and textures onto the back side of paper and other media to produce a raised image. Tooling is used on various materials, including braille paper, overhead projector sheets, report covers, file folders, heavy-duty foil, cardboard, and other thick paper and plastic sheets. Some of the tools needed for this production method are commonly found objects, while others are designed specifically for this purpose. Sewing tools such as crochet hooks, tracing wheels for use with tracing paper, large needles, leather tooling wheels and other supplies, paper embossing and stenciling supplies, popsicle sticks, and tongue depressors are some of the items used that are readily available at fabric, craft, or hobby stores. A rubber pad is important when using the tooling method because it provides a flexible backing that allows the tool to imprint or emboss the paper without tearing it.

APH offers a Tactile Graphics Kit that includes a variety of tools, aluminum foil squares for creating "thermoformable" designs, and a rubber pad to place underneath the paper while tooling (see the Resources section). While these tools and others can be used by skilled producers to create effective tactile graphics, many are used in combination with collage and other production methods.

Capsule Paper and Fuser

Capsule paper is a special paper coated with thermally formed microcapsules that respond to light energy by swelling up when heated. Graphical information can be drawn on the paper with certain markers. The graphic may also be transferred by photocopying it directly onto the capsule paper or printing directly on the paper with some inkjet printers. The capsule paper can then be fed through a special machine called a *fuser*, which uses light and heat to produce a raised line, surface, or texture where the ink appears on the page. Several different brands of fusers and papers are available, and teachers may wish to experiment with samples of each before making a decision about which system to purchase. Using capsule paper and a fuser is one of the quickest production methods, especially for simple graphics that do not require a great deal of labeling, but the images do not usually have the fine tactile detail that can be obtained with other methods.

Drawings made on capsule paper can also be raised through the use of a Thermo-pen (see the Resources section), which does not apply ink but uses heat to raise the surface of the paper wherever the pen is applied. The teacher can draw or trace over an image printed or photocopied onto the paper. This system can be used by a science or math teacher to quickly produce a tactile graphic to explain a concept being discussed in class. Students can also use capsule paper and the Thermo-pen to create original drawings that can be felt on paper.

Computer-Assisted Tactile Graphics

In computer-assisted tactile graphics, computer software is used to create a graphic image in an electronic format, and either a braille embosser that has graphic capabilities or capsule paper and fuser are used to create the tactile version of the graphic.

Creating the Image

Several strategies can be used to acquire a graphic. One of the easier strategies is to locate a file that already contains the image that is needed. There are several depositories of files that have already been prepared for production as tactile graphics (see the Resources section). Although the exact image that is needed may not be found, one that contains most of the information that needs to be conveyed is in all likelihood available, which will still save a great deal of time. The image can be customized with one of the graphics or drawing programs available for most computers. For example, if a student needs a tactile graphic of a paramecium that matches the one in his or her textbook and the exact graphic cannot be found ready-made, the teacher can use one that is similar and add or delete features until the graphic closely matches what the student's classmates are using.

If an existing file with a usable approximation of a graphic that needs to be duplicated cannot be located, the original print graphic can be scanned into a computer using imaging software (*not* OCR software, which is used for text; see Chapter 2) and saved as an electronic image file. This file can then be opened with a drawing or graphics program that can be used to edit the graphic. Some of the original graphic may need to be removed to eliminate tactile clutter in the final representation, while some additional information may need to be added to clarify meaning.

Simple graphics can be created from scratch on a computer in a graphics or drawing program, using a mouse or the keyboard to control the program's drawing tools. This method is usually adequate for simple shapes, some graphs, and basic diagrams. Since drawing with a computer mouse can be tricky, especially for more complicated designs, some people prefer to use a drawing or graphics tablet connected to the computer to prepare tactile graphics. This tablet is a device containing a flat surface that is sensitive to touch. The user presses a drawing stylus (a pen-like instrument with a rounded tip) on the surface of the tablet and moves it around. The resulting drawing can then be seen on the monitor. Another strategy is to tape the original graphic to the tablet and trace over it to create the electronic file of the image.

An additional option for inputting graphical information is the use of graphics drawn on an electronic whiteboard (described in Chapter 2). Some teachers use this tool for classroom presentations and draw graphics to illustrate the topic under discussion. Whiteboards are often used in math classes, particularly geometry. Images on an electronic whiteboard can be saved to a computer and quickly embossed on an appropriately equipped braille embosser. The embossed tactile graphic will not be ideal in most cases, but in general it will be sufficient for students to understand the basic ideas discussed by the instructor. A braille reader in high school, provided with the appropriate tools, can be taught to produce this kind of tactile graphic and have access to the information within a matter of minutes. Or, a knowledgeable tactile graphics transcriber can use a drawing program to modify the drawing to enhance its effectiveness and provide an even more informative product. The drawing can also be printed onto capsule paper and a raised drawing can be created with a fuser.

Producing the Tactile Graphic

Regardless of which method a producer uses to obtain a graphic image in electronic format, some sort of device will be needed to produce the tactile version for the student. There are two tools currently available that can produce a tactile graphic from an electronic file.

An electronic file of a graphical image can be printed or photocopied onto capsule paper. This page can then be fed through the fuser to raise the image. This production method works well with some types of graphical information but does not provide a means by which the producer can use variation in the height of the raised lines, surfaces, and points to differentiate various elements of the graphical information.

In addition, many braille embossers have the capability of producing a tactile graphic through the use of embossed dots. Some can emboss dots of variable height, and others offer variable spacing between dots. This production method offers many interesting features that make it attractive to producers. However, there is generally a limited number of textures available to create the tactile graphics, which restricts the usefulness of this method for conveying certain types of graphical information, such as three-dimensional images and drawings with overlapping areas. (A thermoform machine can also be used to make additional copies of the tactile graphic produced by braille embossers.)

Tactile graphic production can be an interesting and enjoyable activity for teachers and others who are trained to produce tactile graphics for students. Each of the production methods has strengths and weaknesses, so teachers should vary the method depending on the subject matter. For example, in a social studies class, a basic map of the United States might be provided as part of an atlas that has been produced with a braille embosser, while a bar graph of population of the country by regions might be easier to convey using a graphic created with capsule paper and a fuser. Producers will frequently wish to use a combination of production methods to create the most effective tactile graphic for conveying pertinent information. Having a wide array of production tools, trained and knowledgeable producers, and ample time to prepare graphics are key to providing effective tactile graphics to students who are blind or visually impaired.

PRODUCING MATERIALS IN AN AUDITORY FORMAT

Recording

Editing

Production and Duplication

Playback Equipment

It is much easier today than ever before to find educational materials in auditory formats for blind or visually impaired students whose primary learning channel is their sense of hearing or who use auditory materials to supplement other learning media. A wide array of textbooks and leisure reading is available from organizations such as Recording for the Blind and Dyslexic and BookShare.org (see the Resources section). But there are times when ready-made audio recordings are not available. In such cases, teachers can make their own auditory materials using the methods and strategies described here. In addition, teachers can create training materials for students to become more skilled and productive in using auditory recordings and synthesized speech effectively. Students also need to learn effective strategies for recording information such as classroom lectures and discussions.

A variety of tools and technologies can be used to produce materials in an auditory format. Analog and digital recordings can be easily produced with relatively inexpensive equipment, and auditory materials can be created as well via synthesized speech in various electronic formats using the methods and equipment described in Chapter 3.

The most widely used production methods and formats for producing auditory information are audio recordings and electronic or computer-based productions. Information can be read aloud and recorded as either analog or digital recordings (see Chapter 2) by individuals, volunteers, or production companies. The technology and equipment used for recording, editing, and playback of auditory information has evolved rapidly in recent years for both commercial producers and individuals making their own recordings.

RECORDING

The basic equipment needed to record information read or spoken aloud is a microphone and a recording device. Professional recordings are made in state-of-the-art recording studios using soundproof recording booths equipped with highly sensitive microphones, sound-absorbing walls, and top-quality analog and digital recorders. Advances in general electronics and mainstream technology have brought down the cost of audio books and other recordings, making them available to a wider number of listeners. These improvements in affordable recording equipment and media have also made it possible for low-volume producers and individuals to make usable recordings outside a professional studio.

Audio recorders are available that can be used to produce an analog or digital recording. Modified accessible tape players and recorders (discussed in Chapter 2) are often used by individuals and volunteers to record a reader, a speaker, or classroom lesson or to dictate information the user wishes to record for his or her own use. Most of these recorders have an internal microphone, but the use of an external microphone will make a significant difference in the quality of the recording and make it easier for the listener to understand what is being said. Inexpensive, high-quality external microphones are available that allow the user to take advantage of the higher quality recording capabilities of today's recorders (see Sidebar 5.3, "Using Microphones to Get the Best Recording").

Although analog cassette tape recorders are being phased out quickly, some individuals still find them useful for recording and listening to books and other information. Cassette tape recorders/players are still available to users through the National Library Service (NLS), APH, and commercial suppliers of products for people who are blind or visually impaired. Even though NLS is in the process of implementing a new digital format for their books, at the time of this writing they are still providing books on cassette. The four-track and slow-speed recording features of these adapted analog recorders will help individuals to maximize the amount of information that can be recorded onto one tape. Another valuable, often-overlooked feature of these recorders is tone indexing. When an individual who is recording a reader or speaker encounters information or a certain passage that he or she would like to review later, the tone indexing button on the recorder can be used to insert a tone in the recording that marks the spot for later review. (For more information on tone

USING MICROPHONES TO GET THE BEST RECORDING

Low-cost but high-quality external microphones can help students and teachers to produce higher quality recordings, which will make it easier for the listener to absorb the information presented. Microphones are available in either omnidirectional or unidirectional models, and many offer a remote On/Off switch on the microphone. *Omnidirectional* microphones pick up sounds from all directions and would be well suited to provide good recordings of small groups gathered around meeting tables. *Unidirectional* microphones perform best when recording a single speaker or reader, because they will only pick up sounds made directly in front of the mike and do not pick up other surrounding or background noise.

One of the more significant advances in microphone technology is the development of wireless microphones, which are available in two basic types: handheld microphones and lapel microphones. Wireless handheld microphones are often passed around in large meetings to group members who wish to make comments or ask questions so that everyone's voices are picked up in the recording. They are also frequently used by lecturers who want the freedom to move around on stage. Lapel microphones that fasten to the speaker's clothing have become very popular, allowing hands-free movement and providing good recordings of lectures and other presentations. Both types of microphones work in similar ways. The wireless handheld microphone has a transmitter embedded in its case. The sounds picked up by the microphone are turned into electrical signals, which the transmitter sends to a receiver connected to the recording device. The lapel microphone is clipped to a speaker's clothing near his or her mouth. A wire connects the microphone to a small box containing the transmitter, which can be placed in a pocket or clipped to a belt.

Either type of wireless microphone provides two important advantages over traditional wired microphones. A wireless handheld or lapel microphone used by a teacher will produce a much higher quality recording than a traditional stationary microphone placed on the teacher's desk. Recordings made using a wireless microphone eliminate unwanted background noises and provide a recording that makes it much easier for the listener to attend to the teacher's voice and absorb the information being conveyed. Teachers will appreciate the fact that they can lecture and move about as usual without tripping over a wire or worrying that important information is not being picked up by the student.

A second benefit of using a wireless microphone is that the listener can keep the recording device within easy reach to monitor the recording, even when the microphone is near the speaker. This allows the listener to mark important parts of the recording, either by inserting an electronic bookmark in a digital recording or using the tone indexing feature of an analog cassette recorder (discussed in Chapter 2).

indexing and other features of adapted cassette recorders, see Chapter 2.)

Newer digital recorders offer some advantages over older analog tape recorders in both recording and playback capabilities. These recorders create electronic files that can be saved on a variety of memory storage devices, such as a flash drive, memory card, or CD, thereby affording much greater storage capacity than did older cassette tapes that were used with analog recorders. The user can store more information in less space, and these files can also be used on personal computers and personal digital assistants (PDA). Additional devices that can play and support these files continue to be developed. Digital recorders also offer a bookmarking feature that allows the user to move to specific locations within a recording, which is much easier than tone indexing on analog recorders.

Some laptop computers can also be used to create digital recordings. Laptops often come with built-in microphones, or an external microphone can be added at little cost. Easy-to-use software allows the student to record and edit lectures and presentations and play them back later. For students who already bring a laptop to class, being able to make a recording with their computers means one less piece of equipment to carry and keep track of.

EDITING

The editing of auditory information, once it has been recorded, has also been heavily affected by the development of technology. Professional producers have extensive electronic editing tools for both analog and digital recordings. For individuals, accessible digital recording software provides a tool to edit audio information recorded in digital formats and create customized audio files. Segments from one or several digital recordings can be combined into a final product that contains only the segments of the recordings that the user wants to keep.

For example, in the following scenario one student working on a group project uses a variety of devices effectively:

Jamilla is blind and will use several assistive technology devices to complete her contributions to her group assignment. The students choose to break up the assignment into various topics, research them individually, and then report back to the group. When the students report on their research, Jamilla decides to record all of the reports for later review using a digital recorder. She chooses to place an omnidirectional microphone in the center of the meeting table. In addition, she passes around a wireless handheld microphone to individual speakers who are giving a report or talking for several minutes. As she listens to the other presentations, Jamilla embeds digital markers in the recording to indicate important points that she will want to come back to later. After the meeting, she can open the file containing the digital recording on an accessible personal computer running a digital sound-editing program. She can listen to the recording at a much faster speed than the one at which it was recorded to locate both marked and unmarked passages that could be cut and pasted into a summary file of the important parts of the meeting. When she is finished, Jamilla has produced a digital recording of the important information from the meeting, which can be listened to on her choice of one of the digital playback devices discussed later in the section on "Playback Equipment," all of which provide high-quality auditory output.

PRODUCTION AND DUPLICATION

The third area of audio recording that continues to improve is in the tools available to produce and duplicate recordings. High-speed and high-capacity tape and CD duplicating machines allow commercial producers to provide a larger collection of materials and a more cost-effective service. CD burners on personal computers make it possible for individuals and low-volume producers to create multiple copies when necessary. Digital recordings in electronic files can now be reproduced or transferred to multiple users easily.

PLAYBACK EQUIPMENT

The fourth area of audio recording in which technology has had a tremendous impact is the development of playback equipment—such as digital recorders, MP3 players, accessible PDAs, and other devices that were discussed in Chapter 2—that can take advantage of improvements in the other three areas of the recording process. Digital recordings that allow easier navigation through the recorded information and the ability to increase the playback rate without pitch or quality distortion have increased the usability of this medium for accessing information.

Technology in audio production is changing so rapidly that educators or school districts that need to produce a lot of high-quality auditory materials for their students will need to consult experts in this field in order to take advantage of these advances. However, access to the latest high-tech recording equipment is not absolutely necessary for producing information in an audio format that can be useful to students. Even with their disadvantages, adapted cassette recorders can be used to teach students how to acquire information from an audio source. Digital recordings and synthesized speech can also be used to help students learn to access audio information more efficiently.

SUMMARY

Many tools are now available that improve the efficiency with which information and materials can be produced in alternate formats. Educators can use computers to produce printed text in a wide range of fonts and point sizes to meet the needs of a variety of students with low vision. Braille translation software and braille embossers can be used by qualified braille transcribers to produce much greater quantities of braille than was ever possible with previous production methods. Technology has also provided an array of tools for the production of tactile graphics, greatly increasing their availability to students. In addition, advances in audio recording, editing, and playback equipment have given educators and students many options for producing auditory information. All of these tools have made a dramatic difference in the quantity and quality of materials available to students who are blind or visually impaired.

REFERENCES

AFB. (2005). *AFB directory of services for blind and visually impaired people in the United States and Canada.* New York: AFB Press.

Corn, A. L., Hatlen, P., Huebner, K. M., Ryan, F., & Siller, M. A. (1995). *The national agenda for the education of children and youths with visual impairments, including those with multiple disabilities.* New York: AFB Press.

Edman, P. K. (1992). *Tactile graphics.* New York: AFB Press.

Hasty, L. (2008). *Tactile graphics.* Retrieved May 7, 2008, from www.tactilegraphics .org

Huebner, K. M., Merk-Adam, B., Stryker, D., & Wolffe, K. (2004). *The national agenda for the education of children and youths with visual impairments, including those with multiple disabilities* (Rev. ed.). New York: AFB Press.

Nemeth braille code for mathematics and science notation (Rev. ed.). (1972). Louisville, KY: American Printing House for the Blind.

Renfranz, P. Taboada, S., & Weatherd, J. (2008). Progress and stalemates: The complexities of creating a textbooks-on-time system for blind students. *The Braille Monitor 51*(7). Retrieved from www.nfb.org/images/nfb/Publications/bm/bm08/bm0807/bm080706.htm

The Assistive Technology Assessment Process

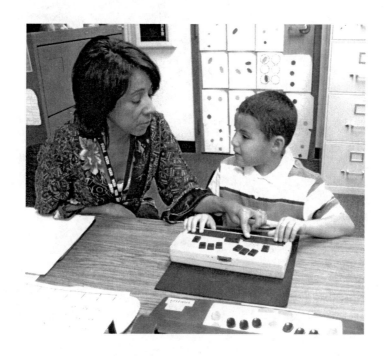

6

Getting Ready for the Assessment

Students who are blind or visually impaired are a heterogeneous group; they do not fall neatly into categories and packages. Each child has unique needs and strengths, likes and dislikes, and a unique place in school, home, and community. Some students can function independently with little assistance. Some need a great deal of support to make educational and aspirational progress—that is, to reach life goals. Some need initial support, which is gradually withdrawn over time as the student begins to succeed. There are no "one-size-fits-all" solutions when it comes to students with visual disabilities.

The need to individualize instruction and solutions for visually impaired students means that creating a student's Individualized Education Program (IEP), of which assistive technology is a part, is of paramount importance for a student to meet with success. The IEP is a legal document that contains a statement describing a student's current levels of performance as well as the goals and objectives for the coming year. It is most successful when it draws on input from all of the people who interact with the student: family members and guardians, classroom teachers, teachers of students with visual impairments, and orientation and mobility instructors, as well as specialists as needed, such as occupational therapists, physical therapists, speech and language pathologists, and others. This input should be obtained from formal and informal assessment information, such as observation checklists, standardized and criterion-referenced tests, classroom work samples and portfolios,

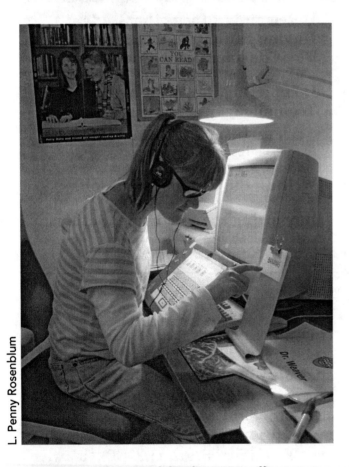

L. Penny Rosenblum

Students who are blind or visually impaired are a heterogeneous group. Some students can function independently with little assistance. Some need a great deal of support. There are no "one-size-fits-all" solutions when it comes to students with visual disabilities.

progress monitoring systems (such as graphs and data charts), interviews (for example, with family members and caretakers), and other forms of documentation.

IEPs should *not* be generic—that is, they should not be based on generalizations about what a child *might* need—and should not be written without careful consideration of all of the information at hand about the student. Rather, they should be unique, customized documents that present a true picture of the individual child. The "I" for "individualized" in IEP is what makes special education truly special.

The need to individualize services and instruction applies to *all* aspects of the student's educational plan, including the provision of assistive technology devices and instruction. It is the IEP team's responsibility—with feedback from all team members—to determine the student's current needs and which individual adaptations, modifications, or assistive technology tools will best meet those needs. The administration of an assistive technology assessment is essential to provide the team with the necessary information to make this determination. Moreover, an assessment of this kind is mandated by law (see Appendix A, "It's the Law: Q&A About Assistive Technology and Special Education" at the back of this book).

One of the purposes of this book is to provide professionals with a guide that can be used to conduct an assistive technology assessment. Chapter 7 describes in detail the assessment and how to conduct it. However, there is a lot to do beforehand to prepare for conducting the assessment itself. The major steps for completing an assistive technology assessment are the following:

1. Selecting appropriate specialists to serve as the members of the

assessment team and deciding who will coordinate or chair the assessment team

2. Gathering the necessary background information on the student
3. Determining the tasks that the student is having difficulty accomplishing (using a form such as the Considerations Checklist discussed later in this chapter)
4. Completing the assistive technology assessment (addressed in Chapter 7)
5. Writing the recommendations (addressed in Chapter 8)
6. Having the IEP team review the recommendations, write assistive technology goals, implement the goals and objectives (addressed in Chapter 9), and follow up

A group known as the QIAT (Quality Indicators for Assistive Technology Services) Consortium has developed a list of statements (see Sidebar 6.1, "Quality Indicators for Assistive Technology Services") that, if put into practice, would help to ensure the provision of high-quality assistive technology services. It would be helpful for the IEP team to keep these principles in mind throughout the process of preparing for and completing an assistive technology assessment.

It is important to note that although the steps outlined in this chapter represent the major components and essential structure of a comprehensive assessment, the assessment process itself is not standardized and may vary widely across the United States. Each state—in fact, each school district—may have its own procedures and protocol, depending on the individual circumstances and considerations at hand. It is therefore essential for professionals involved in assessing students to keep the following key points in mind:

- Be aware of the requirements, procedures, and protocols, if any, that exist in your school district, locality, or state that relate to student assessments in general and assistive technology assessments in particular.
- The assistive technology assessment is a customized examination of an individual student, and its outcomes—recommendations and follow-up—need to be customized for the student as well. There are few shortcuts to getting to know a student's needs and abilities in depth, in order to arrive at effective technology solutions that are enabling for a student.
- A team approach is essential to assessing students with disabilities, and it is critical that individuals who are specialists in any such disabilities play a major role in the assessment.
- Communication, coordination of effort, and respectful consultation among team members are basic ingredients in a successful assessment process.

SELECTING THE TEAM

As already indicated, students with visual impairments have unique needs. Careful assessment of the student's current levels of performance in all areas is essential, including considerations for the use of assistive technology. The first step in completing the assistive technology assessment is consulting with the IEP team and selecting a coordinator for the assessment team and effective team members. In some school districts, the IEP team will be able to make a referral to an assistive technology specialist or an assistive technology team that is

QUALITY INDICATORS FOR ASSISTIVE TECHNOLOGY SERVICES

Considerations for Assistive Technology Needs: Quality Indicators

Consideration of the need for assistive technology devices and services is an integral part of the educational process identified by IDEA for referral, evaluation, and development of the IEP. Although assistive technology is considered at all stages of the process, the indicators outlined below are specific to the consideration of assistive technology in the development of the IEP as mandated by IDEA. In most instances, the indicators are also appropriate for the consideration of assistive technology for students who qualify for services under other legislation (e.g., Section 504 of the Rehabilitation Act of 1973 and the Americans with Disabilities Act). They specify critical guiding principles to be followed during assistive technology assessments.

1. Assistive technology devices and services are considered for all students with disabilities regardless of type or severity of disability.

Intent: Consideration of assistive technology need is required by IDEA and is based on the unique educational needs of the student. Students are not excluded from consideration of assistive technology for any reason (e.g., type of disability, age, administrative concerns, etc.).

2. During the development of the Individualized Education Program (IEP), the IEP team consistently uses a collaborative decision-making process that supports systematic consideration of each student's possible need for assistive technology devices and services.

Intent: A collaborative process that ensures that all IEP teams effectively consider the assistive technology of students is defined, communicated, and consistently used throughout the agency. Processes may vary from agency to agency to most effectively address student needs under local conditions.

3. IEP team members have the collective knowledge and skills needed to make informed assistive technology decisions and seek assistance when needed.

Intent: IEP team members combine their knowledge and skills to determine if assistive technology devices and services are needed to remove barriers to student performance. When the assistive technology needs are beyond the knowledge and scope of the IEP team, additional resources and support are sought.

4. Decisions regarding the need for assistive technology devices and services are *based on the student's IEP goals and objectives, access to curricular and extracurricular activities, and progress in the general education curriculum.*

Intent: As the IEP team determines the tasks that the student needs to complete and develops the goals and objectives, the team considers whether assistive technology is required to accomplish those tasks.

5. The IEP team *gathers and analyzes data* about the student, customary environments, educational goals, and tasks when considering a student's need for assistive technology devices and services.

Intent: The IEP team shares and discusses information about the student's present levels of achievement in relationship to the environments and tries to determine if the student requires assistive technology devices and services to participate actively, work on expected tasks, and make progress toward mastery of educational goals.

6. When assistive technology is needed, the IEP team *explores a range* of assistive technology devices, services, and other supports that address identified needs.

Intent: The IEP team considers various supports and services that address the educational needs of the student and may include no-tech, low-tech, mid-tech, and/or high-tech solutions and devices. IEP team members do not limit their thinking to only those devices and services currently available within the district.

7. The assistive technology consideration process and *results are documented in the IEP* and include a rationale for the decision and supporting evidence.

Intent: Even though IEP documentation may include a checkbox verifying that assistive technology has been considered, the reasons for the decisions and recommendations should be clearly stated. Supporting evidence may include the results of assistive technology assessments, data from device trials, differences in achievement with and without assistive technology, student preferences for competing devices, and teacher observations, among others.

Common Errors

1. Assistive technology is considered for students with severe disabilities only.
2. No one on the IEP team is knowledgeable regarding assistive technology.
3. The team does not use a consistent process based on data about the student, environment, and tasks to make decisions.
4. Consideration of assistive technology is limited to those items that are familiar to team members or are available in the district.
5. Team members fail to consider access to the curriculum and IEP goals in determining if assistive technology is required in order for the student to receive free, appropriate public education.
6. If assistive technology is not needed, the team fails to document the basis of its decisions.

Source: Adapted from QIAT Consortium. (2007). *Quality indicators for assistive technology services.* (Rev. ed.). Retrieved June 6, 2008, from www.qiat.org

already in place. Teachers will need to follow their school district's guidelines regarding how assistive technology assessments are conducted. The team needs to contain members who collectively are knowledgeable about the student's educational needs and abilities, vision loss, any other conditions the student may have, mainstream educational technology, and assistive technology relevant to the student's visual and other conditions.

If the administration of the assessment is to be successful, a good deal of time will be required for the coordinator to organize the assessment team, obtain the necessary background information, prepare materials, become familiar with the technology necessary for the assessment, conduct the assessment, analyze the results, and make decisions about recommendations. The time and effort required to complete the assessment may seem demanding, but the importance of this process is readily understandable and the activity is justified when all parties realize the impact that the appropriate technology can have on the life of the student. As indicated in Chapter 1, by enabling a student to use his or her primary sensory channel effectively and by supporting the student's performance of critical tasks, appropriate assistive technology is in fact what allows a student to learn, obtain information, participate in school, and be an active member of society and the world. In addition, performing a thorough assessment and taking adequate time from the very beginning saves money in the long run by ensuring that the assessment is done well so that the right equipment is ordered for each student.

If a particular school system does not have its own assistive technology department, the responsibility for coordinating the assessment may fall to the teacher of students with visual impairments or an assistive technology (AT) specialist. If a local AT specialist is not available, one may be available from the state from a statewide assistive technology project (see the Resources section). In some cases, a private contractor who is skilled in the area of technology for students with visual impairments can be hired, if someone is available in your area. (See the *AFB Directory of Services for Blind and Visually Impaired Persons in the United States and Canada*, 2005, which is also available online at www.afb.org/services.asp.) Any of these individuals may have the skills necessary to administer numerous sections of the assistive technology assessment and, because of their specialized knowledge, will serve as consultants to other specialists in completing other sections of the assessment. If the assistive technology specialist does not have specific experience with students who have visual impairments (which is not unusual given that visual impairment is a low incidence disability), a close partnership between the teacher of students with visual impairments and the assistive technology specialist is helpful.

Another route the IEP team may take is to name an assessment team coordinator who organizes the assessment and ensures that it is administered appropriately but assigns the job of carrying it out to specialists who have expertise both with that child and with the parts of the test evaluation in their specific area. For example, if the student is visually impaired and also has cerebral palsy, the assessment coordinator may arrange for the physical therapist to work closely with the teacher of students with visual impairments to ensure that the student is sitting in comfortable and supported seating that will maximize his or her ability to function.

Regardless of which approach is taken by the IEP team, it is important that the assessment team consist of members who collectively possess the skills necessary to conduct the assessment. If an assistive technology specialist is available, that person should be included in the assessment team, even if such a specialist has not previously been part of the IEP team. Optimally, the team should contain members who are knowledgeable in the areas listed in Sidebar 6.2, "Knowledge Requirements for Members of the Assistive Technology Team," that are relevant to the student's disability.

Students with multiple disabilities often have complex and challenging needs, and careful assessment from knowledgeable specialists is imperative. A multidisciplinary team is vital for all students and essential for students with visual and additional disabilities. Although Chapters 2–5 of this book focus primarily on hardware and software assistive technology for students with visual impairments, it is important to know that there are numerous exciting and innovative assistive technology devices available for students with limited motor control, communication difficulties, and severe cognitive disabilities (Copeland & Keefe, 2007; Downing, 2005). The sheer number and variety of these devices make it impossible to add them all to this book, but the Resources section at the back of this book lists helpful books and web sites that give more information about assistive technology for students with multiple disabilities. It takes trained, experienced team members to assess students with complex motor, speech, and cognitive needs, and each team member will provide information essential for a holistic picture of the student and his or her needs.

GATHERING BACKGROUND INFORMATION

Medical Eye Examination

Learning Media Assessment

Clinical Low Vision Examination

Functional Low Vision Assessment

General Medical, Psychological, and Academic Evaluations

Formal and Informal Teacher Assessment and Observations

Acquiring the necessary parental permission for the evaluation and gathering the background information is typically spearheaded by the assessment team coordinator. Unless the student is new to the school system, the IEP team may itself have enough knowledge of the student to select the needed specialized members of the assessment team. However, information from the student's permanent records combined with functional data from formal and informal teacher evaluations and observations are critical to the assistive technology assessment process. Any information about the student's use of assistive technology in the past should be included, along with a list of questions and concerns compiled from everyone involved with the student.

Although much of the background information about the student that is needed to complete the assistive technology assessment may be found in the student's permanent

SIDEBAR 6.2

KNOWLEDGE REQUIREMENTS FOR MEMBERS OF THE ASSISTIVE TECHNOLOGY TEAM

For the assessment team to be most effective, members of the team should have some knowledge of the following:

- The student personally and his or her needs and preferences
- The student's eye condition and how it affects his or her functioning
- Any additional disabilities or medical conditions affecting the student and medications that have been prescribed for the student and their possible effects
- Basic computer operations and hardware
- Basic computer software, such as word processors and Internet browsers
- Use of manual and electronic braille writing devices
- Optical devices that the student might be using and the proper use of these devices
- Electronic video-magnification systems and how they are used by students with low vision
- Screen-magnification software
- Screen-reading software
- Personal digital assistants (PDAs) with braille keyboards and braille displays
- PDAs with QWERTY keyboards
- Digital recorders/players
- Additional tools, such as talking or large-print calculators and dictionaries
- Alternative input devices for students with motor impairments
- Alternative and augmentative communication devices
- Hardware and software designed for students with cognitive disabilities

record, certain necessary information may not be available. For example, information about the student's preferred literacy medium or media may not be available, so a formal learning media assessment (Koenig & Holbrook, 1995) may need to be completed before administering the assessment. If the suggested information is not available in the reports, then the team will need to obtain this data before continuing with the assessment. At minimum, the information from the following assessments will be necessary to ensure the AT assessment team has the background information to make good recommendations:

- medical eye examination
- learning media assessment
- clinical low vision evaluation
- functional low vision evaluation
- general medical, psychological, and academic evaluations
- formal and informal teacher assessment and observations

Figure 6.1 presents an example of a form that some assessment teams might use to summarize some of the essential background information about the student that is gathered by the team that might be useful to have while conducting the assessment or to give to other professionals called in to consult. The sample form shown here has been completed for a 10th-grade student with low vision named Bill Alonso, whose IEP team is preparing for an assistive technology assessment. (A blank version of this form appears in Appendix D at the back of this book.) The information gathered might vary considerably for different students.

MEDICAL EYE EXAMINATION

The results of the medical eye examination, usually conducted by an ophthalmologist, are often referred to as the "eye report." A medical eye evaluation is generally required of all students who receive services from a teacher of students with visual impairments. There are several key pieces of information to glean from the report that are relevant to assistive technology. The student's visual acuities are important, especially if there is a discrepancy between his or her near and distance vision. But the person conducting the assessment should also check for information about possible visual field loss, as this will be essential when determining where in the student's field of view to present information during the assessment. For example, the student may have more usable vision in the lower-left quadrant of one eye than when viewing something presented at center. A critical item to look for is a statement about the stability of the student's visual impairment.

Unstable visual impairments require a detailed assessment of the student's changing needs for assistive technology in the future.

LEARNING MEDIA ASSESSMENT

The results of a learning media assessment, described more fully in Chapter 1, will guide the assessment toward exploration of technologies that can best assist the student by allowing him or her to access information through his or her primary and secondary literacy media. Special care should be taken to note the student's ability to use literacy tools in addition to the regular classroom materials, such as braille, print, or auditory information. The learning media assessment and functional vision evaluation will offer information about the student's preferred font size, comfortable reading distance, location of materials for optimum viewing, lighting preferences, and issues related to visual fatigue that are prerequisite information for completing the assistive technology assessment.

CLINICAL LOW VISION EXAMINATION

A clinical low vision examination can be an invaluable component in developing an effective assistive technology plan for students with low vision. Optical devices, both near and distance, are one type of assistive technology that can benefit many students, and these need to be prescribed by a qualified low vision specialist. The proper prescription and use of low vision devices can, in certain cases, meet the needs of some users through the use of less-expensive "low-tech" alternatives.

Figure 6.1 Sample Completed Background Information for Assistive Technology Assessment for Bill Alonso

---

Background Information for Assistive Technology Assessment

Student's Name: _Bill Alonso_   Birthdate: _4/18/1993_   Grade: _10_

Name of parent(s)/guardian(s): _George Alonso and Barbara Callen_

School: _Morningside High School_

Teacher of students with visual impairments: _Samantha Higgins_

Referred by: _Samantha Higgins_   Reason for Referral: _Difficulty completing assignments_

Initial or Ongoing Assessment (Ⓘ) O

Additional Disabilities: Y / Ⓝ Describe: _____

Current medication(s): _none_

Reported/observed visual side effects: _____

Eye Report Summary (see Eye Report)

Dr.: _Sarah Johnson_   O.D.   Date of last examination: _3/18/08_

Eye condition: _congenital cataracts_

Prognosis: _stable_

Visual Acuity

| | Distance | | Near | |
	Without Correction	With Correction	Without Correction	With Correction
OD	_____	_____	_____	_____
OS	_____	_____	_____	_____
OU	_____	_____	_____	_____

Field Restriction(s): Y / N   Degrees: _____   Location: _____

Recommendations

Eyeglasses   ❑ Wear/Use Constantly   ❑ Wear/Use as Needed

Contact Lenses

    For distance?   Y / N   ❑ Wear/Use Constantly   ❑ Wear/Use as Needed

    For near?   Y / N   ❑ Wear/Use Constantly   ❑ Wear/Use as Needed

Low Vision Device(s) (specify): _4x stand magnifier_

Other: _____

Information from Learning Media Assessment

Primary learning channel: ☑ visual   ☐ tactile   ☐ auditory

Secondary learning channel: ☐ visual   ☑ tactile   ☐ auditory

Other: _____

Other current accommodations and technology _Dark pencil and bold-lined paper for_ _writing; some large-print books_ _____

_____

Reading Preferences (if reported):

Preferred visual format without device (specify): _____

Point size: _____   Font: _____   Distance: _____

Approximate reading rate: _____ wpm

Preferred visual format with device (specify): _____

Point size: _____   Font: _____   Distance: _____

Approximate reading rate: _____ wpm

Lighting preferences: _____

Braille: approximate reading rate: _____ wpm oral   _____ wpm silent

Experiences visual/physical fatigue after reading ____ minutes

Relevant information from functional low vision assessment: _____

_____

_____

Relevant information from medical, psychological, and academic evaluations: _____

_____

_____

Relevant information from teachers' observations and assessments: _____

_____

_____

Additional comments: _____

_____

_____

FUNCTIONAL LOW VISION ASSESSMENT

A functional low vision assessment, conducted by a teacher of students with visual impairments, provides information about how the student uses his or her vision for everyday tasks, both academic and nonacademic. The report of this assessment typically includes facts and observations about such basic visual skills as tracking and scanning, figure/ground discrimination, awareness of spatial relationships, recognition and discrimination of forms and form constancy, and the ability to understand how symbols are used to represent objects and ideas. Information of this type will be extremely important for assessments of students with multiple disabilities as it may suggest the type of assistive technology that might be most useful, and how materials may be displayed. (For information about conducting a functional low vision evaluation, see Anthony, 2000.)

GENERAL MEDICAL, PSYCHOLOGICAL, AND ACADEMIC EVALUATIONS

Medical, psychological, and academic evaluations provide necessary information about a student's motor, auditory, cognitive, behavioral, and academic functioning. Details contained in these assessment reports can provide helpful clues to understanding the student's ability to complete tasks when the information is related to functional behaviors, so the team will want to read them very carefully. For example, a report might mention the student's abilities in understanding of cause and effect, receptive language, memory, sequencing in tasks with multiple steps, and problem solving. All of these skills can be helpful for the assistive technology assessment team to consider as this information may suggest the pace or intensity of instruction necessary for learning to use particular devices. (Instruction in the use of assistive technology devices is discussed in more detail in Chapter 9.) The team or assessment coordinator should not hesitate to confer with the administrators of these evaluations for help in interpreting the data in the reports and determining if appropriate accommodations have already been made for the student's visual impairment, in order to ensure that what has been documented is accurate and reflective of the student's actual needs.

FORMAL AND INFORMAL TEACHER ASSESSMENT AND OBSERVATIONS

All teachers ought be tracking their students' progress in their individualized programs; monitoring progress is the basis for updating and changing IEP goals from year to year. The assistive technology assessment team will need to review and discuss any formal or informal assessments that have been conducted, such as informal reading inventories, criterion referenced tests (such as end-of-chapter tests or tests based on grade-level standards), progress monitoring data from assessments required by the school, and running records completed during individual sessions with a student. Teachers' observations are also valid and important. This information will be vital to determining the tasks with which the student is having difficulty, which is the next step of the assessment process. All areas of the core curriculum and the expanded core curriculum (see Sidebar

6.3, "The Core Curriculum and the Expanded Core Curriculum") need to be considered.

DETERMINING TASKS THE STUDENT IS HAVING DIFFICULTY ACCOMPLISHING: THE CONSIDERATIONS CHECKLIST

In this part of the assessment process, the team determines the tasks that the student is having difficulty completing. In general, when a student is unable to perform an activity efficiently, it is often an indication that the circumstances warrant an examination of some kind. Whether the student is in need of additional instruction, assistive devices, or other support, exploring the situation is important. Only by identifying areas of strength and need can appropriate solutions be recommended. In essence, this activity is a prelude to a formal assistive technology assessment and it alerts the team to tasks that need to be addressed. Various team members need to provide information about the student's performance in all areas of

---

SIDEBAR 6.3

THE CORE CURRICULUM AND THE EXPANDED CORE CURRICULUM

In considering the tasks with which a student may need additional assistance and where assistive technology might be useful, the assistive technology assessment team needs to consider all aspects of both the core curriculum and the expanded core curriculum—the unique skills that the student needs to learn as a result of his or her visual impairment.

The Core Curriculum

- English language arts and other languages, to the greatest extent possible
- Mathematics
- Science
- Health and physical education
- Fine arts
- Social studies and history
- Economics and business education
- Vocational education

The Expanded Core Curriculum

- Compensatory or functional academic skills, including communication modes
- Orientation and mobility
- Social interaction skills
- Independent living skills
- Recreation and leisure skills
- Career education
- Use of assistive technology
- Sensory efficiency skills
- Self-determination

Source: Phil Hatlen. (1996, Spring). Core curriculum for blind and visually impaired children, including those with additional impairments. *RE:view*, *28*, 25–32.

functioning and in all of the places that the student learns—including school, home, and community—for the examination to be complete.

To assist with this process, team members can use a considerations checklist. In some school districts, submitting such a form is necessary to obtain a formal assessment for a student. A sample considerations checklist completed for Bill Alonso, who was introduced earlier in this chapter, is shown in Figure 6.2, and a blank copy appears in Appendix D at the end of this book. The considerations checklist can be completed by interviewing family members and people who work with the student regularly and by observing the student carrying out typical classroom activities. The subjects listed on the form prompt the assessment team to identify the tasks required to complete assignments in each area and then make a determination about the student's ability to complete each task independently or using any current accommodations or assistive technology, or whether additional assistive technology or services would be needed. A checklist such as this can help the team to collect information and document progress in essential areas like reading, writing, spelling, mathematics, oral communication, daily living skills, recreation and leisure, prevocational or vocational skills, and mobility.

The considerations checklist in this chapter is provided as an example that the team can use; other similar forms can also be found on the Internet and are available from other sources, such as state assistive technology projects. Some school systems have their own required forms. In general, the assessment team should use whichever form best fits their needs. Regardless of the form used, the important principle on which

to focus is that all aspects of the student's educational program and all learning environments need to be considered.

The sample form shown here captures a great deal of information about all aspects of the student's learning program and environments and offers an example of how this information can be efficiently collected. Typically assessment team members who are well acquainted with the student would fill in the form. The student's current level of performance is indicated with special note of tasks that are difficult for the student to perform, such as taking notes in class, reading his or her own handwriting, or seeing the chalkboard from a distance. Information about all of the student's natural environments is noted, including special education settings, general classroom settings, home, and community (meaning such locations as job sites and after-school care).

On the form, assessment team members note activities in which the student engages on a regular basis and the environment in which the student performs each one. In addition, information is collected on how the student currently accomplishes the task with standard classroom tools that children without disabilities use, noting which tasks can be completed independently. For example, if the student can write legibly on regular lined paper and read back his or her handwriting without difficulty, the evaluator would check the box provided to indicate that this task can be done independently and write in "loose leaf paper, pencil, pen" (or whatever implements the student generally uses). It is important to note that even if tasks are currently being completed independently, they might be performed more efficiently with modifications, accommodations, or assistive technology.

Figure 6.2   Sample Completed Assistive Technology Considerations Checklist for Bill Alonso

ASSISTIVE TECHNOLOGY CONSIDERATIONS CHECKLIST

Student: <u>Bill Alonso</u>   School: <u>Morningside High School</u>

DIRECTIONS

1. Complete the student information section below to provide information on the student's needs, abilities, and difficulties as well as environments and barriers to success.
2. Please check (❑) the instructional or access areas in Column A that are appropriate for the student. Please leave blank any areas that are not relevant to the student. Specify all relevant tasks (for example, copying notes from board, responding to teacher questions, and so on) within each area in the space provided. Check the settings in which the task is required. GEC: General Education Classroom; SEC: Special Education Classroom; COM: Community; and HOM: Home.
3. In Column B, specify the standard classroom tools (low technology to high technology) used by the student to complete relevant tasks identified in Column A. Place a check (❑) in the boxes in Column B if the student is able to independently complete the tasks with standard classroom tools. For areas in which the student can complete the tasks independently, it will not be necessary to complete Columns C or D.
4. In Column C, specify the accommodations/modifications and assistive technology solutions that are currently being utilized. Place a check (✔) in the boxes in Column C if the student can adequately complete the tasks specified in Column A using the identified accommodations/modifications and assistive technology solutions.
5. Complete Column D if the student cannot adequately complete the task with accommodations/modifications and assistive technology solutions specified in Column C.

Student needs, abilities, and difficulties: <u>Bill is having difficulty completing tasks requiring reading and writing in the time allotted. This is true for all subjects, including math.</u>

Student environments:

☑ General Education Classroom (List all classes): _____

❑ Special Education Classroom (List all classes): _____

❑ Community (List all settings): _____

❑ Home: _____

Barriers to student performance and achievement: <u>Bill's low vision makes it difficult for him to complete reading and writing tasks using regular print materials and read what is written on the chalkboard.</u>

Source: Reprinted with permission from the Georgia Project for Assistive Technology, Georgia Department of Education, Atlanta.

(continued on next page)

Figure 6.2 (continued)

A. Instructional or Access Areas	B. Independent with Standard Classroom Tools	C. Completes Tasks with Accommodations/ Modifications and/or Assistive Technology Solutions Currently in Place		D. Additional Solutions/Services Needed, Including Assistive Technology
		Accommodations/ Modifications	Assistive Technology Solutions	
☑ Writing ☐ GEC ☐ SEC ☐ COM ☐ HOM	Bill can use a standard pencil and paper for writing but it is very laborious for him and often the result is illegible.	Bill is allowed additional time for completing some writing assignments.	Dark pencil and bold-lined paper	Tools for completing longer writing tasks
☑ Spelling ☑ GEC ☐ SEC ☐ COM ☐ HOM	Bill exhibits numerous spelling errors in his writing and is very slow at locating words in the dictionary using his prescribed optical device.		Bill uses a 4x stand magnifier but it is not adequate to improve his speed.	Accessible talking dictionary Writing tools with spell check
☑ Reading ☑ GEC ☐ SEC ☑ COM ☑ HOM	Bill's reading is on grade level but his rate is very slow.	Bill is allowed extra time to complete many reading tasks.	Bill uses 4x stand magnifier and some large-print books but they are not adequate to make him an efficient, independent reader.	Tools for reading text more efficiently and for reading from the board
☑ Math ☑ GEC ☐ SEC ☐ COM ☐ HOM	Bill is functioning on grade level in math, but he has difficulty following explanations on the board	Bill sits close to board but this is not helping	Bill tried using a hand-held telescope but found it too time consuming to switch between reading on board, writing on paper, and relocating target on board.	Tools for reading from board.
☑ Study/ Organizational Skills ☑ GEC ☐ SEC ☐ COM ☐ HOM	Bill has difficulty keeping materials together (some accessible, some not) when preparing to study for exams.	Uses notebook organizer and separate file folders.		Tools for combining information from multiple sources into one master study guide.
☑ Listening ☑ GEC ☐ SEC ☐ COM ☐ HOM	Bill has excellent listening skills in class	Bill has tried using some recorded books but finds them ineffective.		Bill needs additional training in the use of recorded information and the technology to access this type of information.
☑ Oral Communication ☑ GEC ☐ SEC ☐ COM ☐ HOM	Bill's teachers report that he has good oral communication skills.			
☐ Aids to Daily Living ☐ GEC ☐ SEC ☐ COM ☐ HOM				

A. Instructional or Access Areas	B. Independent with Standard Classroom Tools	C. Completes Tasks with Accommodations/ Modifications and/or Assistive Technology Solutions Currently in Place		D. Additional Solutions/Services Needed, Including Assistive Technology
		Accommodations/ Modifications	Assistive Technology Solutions	
❑ Recreation and Leisure ❑ GEC ❑ SEC ❑ COM ❑ HOM				
❑ Prevocational/ Vocational ❑ GEC ❑ SEC ❑ COM ❑ HOM				
❑ Seating, Positioning, and Mobility ❑ GEC ❑ SEC ❑ COM ❑ HOM				
❑ Other (specify): ❑ GEC ❑ SEC ❑ COM ❑ HOM				

Consideration Outcomes:

❑ Student independently accomplishes tasks in all instructional areas using standard classroom tools. No assistive technology is required.

❑ Student accomplishes tasks in all instructional areas with accommodations and modifications. No assistive technology is required.

❑ Student accomplishes tasks in all instructional areas with currently available assistive technology. Assistive technology is required.

☑ Student does not accomplish tasks in all instructional access areas. Additional solutions including assistive technology may be required.

Specify any assistive technology services required by this student.

Requesting an assistive technology assessment to determine what assistive technology may be of
most benefit to Bill

Consideration Checklist Completed by:
Samantha Higgins

Position:
Teacher of Visually Impaired Students

Date:
9/15/2008

For each task that the student has difficulty doing unassisted, information is noted on whether the task is currently completed with accommodations or modifications or with assistive technology. (An accommodation allows the student to do the same activity or learn the same content as his or her classmates with changes to the process, such as putting a story into braille. A modification alters the task itself, because the activity is deemed inappropriate for a particular student—for example, requiring a totally blind kindergarten student to match colors on a worksheet [Bolt & Thurlow, 2006]). This documents which solutions are being tried now with the student. If he or she is already using some type of assistive technology, specific information should be provided about what is being used and its effectiveness. For example, Bill, the student whose considerations checklist is shown in Figure 6.2, is reading some large-print books and using an optical device—a 4× magnifier—but the checklist indicates that these accommodations are not sufficient to make him an independent, efficient reader.

Tasks that are difficult for a student to complete even with current modifications and accommodations may require additional solutions, and it is particularly important to note these tasks. Even if a student is currently using modifications and assistive technology, the student may not be working to his or her optimal level. As students grow and change, the tools that they need will also change. In addition, a particular tool may work in one environment—say, the classroom—but not be practical in another—such as a community setting. Or perhaps the student had appropriate tools for elementary school, where he or she stayed in the same class all

day, but will need different options for middle school when changing classes. Thus, how the student's performance might be improved with additional tools should also be considered and indicated on the form. For example, as noted earlier, a student may use large-print books and optical devices with regular print books, but the team may determine that the student is not able to keep up with required reading in class using these accommodations, is not able to complete homework independently, or gets fatigued quickly while reading. Thus, the IEP team may request an assistive technology evaluation because the current solutions are not meeting the student's needs and additional assistive technology tools might be helpful. The considerations checklist is a useful place to capture all of this information prior to the actual assessment so that the assessment team has a clear picture of how the student is functioning in school and why the assessment has been requested.

When considering a student's current functioning, additional information about the tasks required in the targeted subject areas should be noted, such as the settings in which they occur and the time it takes for the student to do the tasks. Since there is a variety of technology tools to choose from for any given activity, it is helpful to know the magnitude of a task and if it is to be completed in class, the media center, the computer lab, at home, or somewhere else. For example, a seventh-grade student with low vision may be having difficulty reading most regular print materials. The student's teacher prefers to give short reading assignments in class and have longer ones completed at home. The class is periodically assigned to read stories of about eight pages at home and then respond to discussion questions in small groups the next day in school. Given these circumstances, the recommendation made after the assessment might be to offer the student a choice of assistive technology for each task, such as large-print or audio books for the longer homework reading task and a magnifier for the brief task of reading the discussion questions in class. Thus, it is important to note the quantity of material to be read and the settings in which reading will take place. The more details that can be provided on the considerations checklist, the better the assessment can address the student's needs.

COMPLETING THE ASSISTIVE TECHNOLOGY ASSESSMENT

Gathering the Materials

The Testing Environment

The information recorded on an assistive technology considerations checklist, combined with the background information collected on a student, will help the team to complete the applicable sections of the assistive technology assessment and determine if input from additional specialists is needed. Chapter 7 will go into considerable detail on the assessment process itself and the use of a comprehensive assessment form. Completing the applicable sections of the assessment will help the team to determine which technologies will assist the student in critical tasks, such as accessing print and electronic information and producing written communication. In addition,

it will provide information about the student's need for materials produced in alternate formats.

GATHERING THE MATERIALS

The results of the student's learning media assessment should guide the coordinator of the assessment team regarding the appropriate media—visual, tactile, or auditory—in which to prepare materials for the student. The assistive technology assessment should investigate the student's potential to use tools with both primary and secondary learning media. The materials may require reading samples and other materials on the student's independent reading level in various fonts and point sizes, in braille, as an audio recording, and as electronic files that can be used on a computer or an accessible personal digital assistant (PDA). The assessment will also require access to all of the different types of equipment on which the student needs to be assessed.

The assessment form in Chapter 7 includes a great number of tools that can be considered for each student, and it would not be unexpected to find that a local school system lacks access to a number of the technologies listed. The first step is to determine which specific items needed for the assessment are not available in the local school system, including both hardware and software. It may be surprising how many of the technologies listed are readily available somewhere in the school system (such as scanners) or are inexpensive and easy to obtain (such as OCR software), even if a few are not easy to find (such as refreshable braille displays). The items in the assessment may actually help the team or AT specialist to create a list of tools that should be generally available when conducting assessments on students with visual impairments. Sidebar 6.4, "Wait! I Don't Have One of *Those!*" considers a variety of approaches that the assessment team can explore to obtain other technologies that it may be missing.

Lack of access to certain technologies—particularly high-tech devices—should not stop or delay the assessment team from conducting the parts of the assessment that can be completed with available resources. The assessment team can complete the parts of the assessment checklist that can be evaluated with the available resources while pursuing other options for obtaining the equipment that is not currently available.

THE TESTING ENVIRONMENT

The testing environment is an important factor in a successful assessment. When conducting any assessment, the comfort of the student should be paramount. In many schools, finding a quiet, well-lit room with adequate space will be a formidable task in itself. (Some factors to consider in setting up the assessment conditions are suggested in Sidebar 6.5, "Setting up the Assessment Environment.") While pulling the student out of class to conduct part of the assessment may be necessary, assessment team members need to consider the usual classroom environment and what kinds of tasks the student is required to perform there. Therefore, it may be informative to complete part of the assessment in the student's regular classroom. Ultimately, the student will be using any assigned assistive technology devices in natural environments (classroom, home, or community), so any solutions discussed as a result of the evaluation will have to be chosen with this in mind. For example, if the student is in a crowded classroom out in a trailer with few electrical outlets, a video magnifier with a 28-inch screen attached to a computer system and requiring electrical cords to be draped across the room may not be the most practical solution to the student's needs.

It may not be necessary to investigate every device or technology suggested by the items on the assistive technology assessment form provided in the following chapter, but it is important that each area be addressed. For example, students who are braille readers may not need to be evaluated for the use of screen magnification software, but a brief explanation such as "has no usable vision" or "cannot maintain focus" will remind the team why this particular area is not being addressed directly.

An often-overlooked issue during the assistive technology assessment phase is the local school district's or the state's technology plan, guidelines, or curriculum. How will students who are blind or visually impaired participate in this plan and access the technology instruction being offered? It is imperative that the teacher of visually impaired students and the IEP team are attentive to this area. For example, many schools require students to take keyboarding and other computer classes. The team will need to think ahead about how the student with visual impairments will participate in these classes. Identifying the tasks required to participate in the school's technology curriculum will be fundamental to the assistive technology assessment and its recommendations. Finding solutions or acceptable alternatives for how the student will access networked computers and keyboarding classes may take additional time. Addressing these issues in the assistive

WAIT! I DON'T HAVE ONE OF *THOSE!*

When an assessment team begins to explore the materials needed for a comprehensive technology assessment, the members may have to exercise some ingenuity to obtain access to all of the technologies with which a student needs to be evaluated. The assessment team can try the following suggestions to obtain the various tools it needs.

Use Demonstration Software

Some of the software listed in the assessment form may be specialized enough that the school system does not have it installed on any computers. For example, the local school system may not have a licensed copy of a screen magnification or screen-reading program. Most companies that sell these types of programs offer trial or demonstration versions of their products. These "demo" versions may not have all of the features and options of a fully licensed version but are quite adequate for allowing the evaluator to determine if the student has the basic skills necessary to use this type of technology.

The assessment coordinator will also need to consult with the school system's technology department about installing demonstration software and configuring a computer system for the evaluation. Also, if the evaluator needs to try out the demo software to become familiar with the program prior to the assessment, it is important to determine whether the demo version only operates for a limited time period. If so, the assessment coordinator will need to take this into consideration when planning for and conducting the AT assessment. In most cases such details can be managed to ensure a successful assessment—it just takes some advance planning.

Borrow from Other Agencies

Obtaining hardware that is not available in the local school system may require more creative solutions. The first option to investigate is whether there is a statewide assistive technology program through the department of education that would be able to loan the local school system the equipment or assist in the assessment. Many states have such programs that can loan equipment for assessment and even for trial periods with students.

If such a program is not available, a neighboring school system or the state specialized school for students who are blind may be willing to loan the technology for assessment purposes. If this is not possible, then they may be open to the student and the evaluator using the equipment at a specified location within the district or at the specialized school. This might be an excellent alternative in some cases, particularly if the school's teacher of visually impaired students can attend and assist with the evaluation of the specific technology.

Many states have assistive technology demonstration and training centers where the needed technologies might be available (see the Resources section). These resources can be very helpful because

(continued on next page)

these centers have personnel who may have greater experience with the technology than the evaluator does. In some cases, the demonstration sites even have sample workstations set up, so students can try several pieces of equipment set up as if in a classroom or a work site. Although using these resources may require transporting the student and the evaluator to the site, which presents some hurdles and expense, its value can greatly outweigh these concerns. Purchasing technology that does not meet a student's needs is considerably more expensive than the cost of the transportation to a site that has the needed technology. An appropriate evaluation of the student's use of the technology can actually save money.

Two other resources to investigate are local colleges or universities and the local office of the state vocational rehabilitation system. Many institutions of higher education provide support services for students with disabilities, which at times include various types of assistive technology. Vocational rehabilitation agencies often provide assistive technology to their clients and may have a demonstration or training site available. Agency personnel might also be able to put the assessment team coordinator in touch with clients who use assistive technology and would be willing to work with the team on a limited basis.

Another way to connect with adult technology users is to contact the two major blind consumer organizations, the American Council of the Blind (www.acb.org) and the National Federation of the Blind (www.nfb.org) (see the Resources section). These organizations can assist in locating individuals who might be willing to let an evaluator use a piece of technology for assessment purposes.

Make Use of Vendors

The final option for locating assistive technology to be used for evaluations is to contact representatives of companies that manufacture assistive technology for people who are blind or visually impaired. Vendors can be valuable resources, as they are knowledgeable about the products that they sell. Although vendors can be an excellent resource, several words of caution are necessary. Vendors are generally trained to demonstrate products in a way that highlights the product's positive features, which may not be the approach that yields the best information for determining the potential of the technology to meet the student's needs. For example, the vendor may downplay the need for a particular feature that is not available on his or her product but that feature might be valuable for the student, or the vendor might enthusiastically endorse a feature or device that is of less importance.

If the assessment team does decide to use vendors to provide some of the technologies for the assessment, the team coordinator will need to have a frank conversation with the vendor explaining that the purpose of the vendor's visit is to facilitate the evaluation. The coordinator can offer the vendor another opportunity to present the products and promise to invite a wider audience who might be interested in purchasing them.

It is essential for the coordinator to clearly identify the functions that the vendor should demonstrate at the assessment. The explanation will need to be specific and detailed in accordance with the assessment form provided in Chapter 7. The evaluator may wish to ask the vendor for additional input, but the evaluator does not necessarily have to concur with all of the vendor's suggestions. During the assessment process the evaluator will not want the vendor to demonstrate and explain all of the features available with the hardware or software, because they might cause confusion for the student without contributing any additional information to the assessment process. Using vendors to provide access to technologies for assessment can be a valuable tool, but the assessment team needs to be cautious about the interaction of vendors with the student.

technology assessment can initiate an assistive technology solution.

WRITING THE RECOMMENDATIONS

Once the data from each section of an assessment has been collected, the person completing each section will also need to make appropriate recommendations and write a document providing the rationale and justifications for them. The coordinator of the assessment team will then combine all of this information into a report for the IEP team. This topic will be discussed in detail in Chapter 8.

REVIEWING THE RECOMMENDATIONS IN THE IEP TEAM

Once the recommendations have been compiled, the coordinator of the assessment team will present the team's findings to the IEP team. The IEP team should then review the recommendations and begin their implementation. This is one of the most important steps of all, because the reason an assessment is conducted is to implement solutions to help a student accomplish tasks that are difficult for him or her. Chapter 9 will provide more details on this crucial part of the process.

SUMMARY

Conducting an assistive technology assessment is not a process that can be followed like a recipe in a cookbook. Each student will be different, and each solution will be unique. Just because two students have the same eye condition, are at the same grade level, or are in the same school does not mean that the same assistive technology tools will fit the needs of both. Since many devices are expensive and require considerable instruction time before a student can use them efficiently, assessments need to be done carefully and thoughtfully so that valuable resources are not wasted in the rush to provide a solution that ends up being the wrong one. It is not uncommon for expensive devices to be ordered only to then sit in closets unused because the necessary

SETTING UP THE ASSESSMENT ENVIRONMENT

In many schools, finding a place to do an assistive technology assessment can be difficult, because any available space is often scheduled by specialists and volunteers who work with groups or individual students outside the classroom. The assessment team will need to plan ahead to find a room suitable for conducting the assessment. The following elements should be given careful consideration when deciding on the location for the assessment and when preparing the assessment environment. Although the "perfect" room may not be available, the best assessment results will be obtained in an environment that contains as many of these elements as possible.

- *Auditory environment.* The assessment environment needs to be free of auditory distractions. Many of the technologies used in the assessment produce sounds that might be difficult for the student to comprehend if there is background noise in the environment. The sounds produced by these devices might also be distracting to other students, so it is recommended that the assessment not take place in the student's regular classroom. Speakers on laptop computers may not provide adequate volume for conducting many of the auditory access items in the assessment. Therefore, the examiner will need to have external speakers and a good quality set of headphones available.
- *Lighting.* An empty classroom similar to the student's regular classroom might be a good choice for the assessment, because it is likely to have similar or identical natural and artificial lighting conditions. The evaluator should also have available the lighting options discussed in this chapter.
- *Access to electrical outlets.* The assessment room should offer the examiner easy access to electrical outlets.
- *Ergonomic furniture.* Any tables or chairs used during the assessment should be appropriately sized for the student and allow equipment to be placed at the correct height and position for him or her to use.
- *Temperature.* The temperature in the room needs to be comfortable for the student.
- *Assessment materials.* The examiner will need to gather age- and academically appropriate material in various formats: print, large print, braille, and auditory materials, as well. Findings from the learning media assessment and the other background information discussed in Chapter 6 will guide the examiner in selecting these materials. Specific suggestions for materials needed in the assessment are offered in the guidelines for various items provided throughout Chapter 7.

planning was not done beforehand. Taking the time to create an effective assessment team, carefully reviewing documents, and filling out a considerations checklist prior to the start of the assessment will help to ensure that the final assessment and recommendations are in fact helpful for the individual student.

REFERENCES

AFB directory of services for blind and visually impaired persons in the United States and Canada (2005). New York: AFB Press.

Anthony, T. (2000). Performing a functional low vision assessment. In F. M. D'Andrea & C. Farrenkopf (Eds.), *Looking to learn* (pp. 32–83). New York: AFB Press.

Bolt, S. E., & Thurlow, M. L. (2006). *Item-level effects of the read-aloud accommodation for students with reading disabilities* (Synthesis report 65). Minneapolis: University of Minnesota, National Center on Educational Outcomes. Retrieved January 8, 2008, from http://education.umn.edu/NCEO/OnlinePubs/Synthesis65/

Copeland, S. R, & Keefe, E. B. (2007). *Effective literacy instruction for students with moderate or severe disabilities.* Baltimore: Paul Brookes.

Downing, J. E. (2005). Teaching literacy to students with significant disabilities. Thousand Oaks, CA: Sage Publications.

Koenig, A. J., & Holbrook, M. C. (1995). *Learning media assessment* (2nd ed.). Austin: Texas School for the Blind and Visually Impaired.

QIAT Consortium. (2005). *Quality indicators for assistive technology services.* Retrieved November 14, 2006, from www.qiat.org

7

Performing an Assistive Technology Assessment

There is no question about the critical importance of an assistive technology assessment for a student who is blind or visually impaired. But how does one go about conducting an assessment? The preceding chapter explained how to prepare for this important process. In beginning the assessment itself, and throughout the process, it is vital to keep the main focus in mind: The purpose of the assessment is to determine the ways in which the student needs to be supported by assistive technology, based on his or her sensory and other characteristics, and which devices and techniques are most appropriate in providing this support. Maintaining this focus will provide overall structure to the activities of the assessment team and will determine the questions to be asked and the information to be gathered.

ASSESSMENT: KEY QUESTIONS

As described in Chapter 6, as the members of the assessment team begin evaluating a student, they need to answer certain essential questions that will guide the actual assessment:

- What information needs to be gathered in order to obtain a complete picture of the student and how he or she functions?
- What essential tasks does the student need to perform?
- How does the student perform these tasks?
- Are there supports that would help the student perform these tasks more efficiently?

By adhering to the primary purpose of the assessment, the individuals involved will be able to identify the sources of information they need to consult and the tasks to select in order to determine the ways in which the student may benefit from assistive technology supports. The team should remember to consider all the environments in which the student interacts (that is, school, home, and community). The team should also be proactive and attempt to consider future needs. For example, if the student is doing well in fifth grade, the team needs to consider how his or her needs may change after the transition into middle school.

In beginning the assessment, the team to be assembled needs to include a teacher of students with visual impairments, as well as other professionals knowledgeable about the student's additional disabilities, if any, and assistive technology. In addition, a coordinator of the team needs to be selected. The background information—the student's

medical and educational records, learning media assessment and functional vision assessment reports, Individualized Education Program (IEP) materials, and other relevant data—need to be assembled and reviewed by the team members involved. The assessment sessions need to be planned, with times, tasks, necessary testing equipment and materials, and appropriate environments determined, as discussed in Chapter 6.

As these varied and complex activities proceed, it is helpful to keep careful records throughout the process, both to record important notations and decisions concerning the student and to serve as a communication medium among members of the assessment team. For this reason, an Assistive Technology Assessment Checklist for Students with Visual Impairments has been included in this book. This form is far more than a list of items to check off to indicate progress or enter a notation. It is a tool that can help an assessment team structure its activities and be aware of the many elements to be considered during an assessment, and it can act as a central repository for information on a student's needs and performance. Sections of the assessment form are presented in this chapter as they are discussed, and a sample completed form for Bill Alonso, the student whom we met in Chapter 6, appears as Appendix 7A to this chapter, as a example of how the form might be completed. (There is an additional example in Appendix C to this book.) A complete blank copy of the assessment checklist appears in Appendix D, as well.

FORM AND PROCESS: AN OVERVIEW

Once the assessment team has made the preparations for conducting an assessment described in Chapter 6—including reviewing the student's background information and previous assessments and determining the strategies and sensory media that the student prefers to use for various educational tasks—the team can begin to organize its activities. Reviewing the Assistive Technology Assessment Checklist can help in this process. By deciding which sections need to be completed for the particular student being assessed, the team can determine what devices and additional materials are needed to complete these sections, and make any necessary preparations.

The results of the student's learning media assessment should guide the coordinator of the assessment team regarding the appropriate medium—visual, tactile, or auditory—in which to prepare materials for the student. (Chapter 5 offers suggestions on producing materials in various alternative formats.) Overall, the assistive technology assessment should investigate the student's potential to use tools with his or her primary and secondary learning media. Among the other factors to consider in determining which sections of the assessment are necessary for any individual student are the responses to the key questions listed at the beginning of this chapter. The wide variety of items included in the Assistive Technology Assessment Checklist is intended to prompt the assessment team to consider areas that may be relevant to a student and ensure that potentially useful technologies are not overlooked.

Remember also that the assistive technology assessment is an ongoing process. Teachers will need to periodically monitor the student's progress in completing educational tasks and determine whether new adaptations, modifications, or assistive technologies might be able to support the student in completing these tasks and whether existing technologies and strategies need to be modified or changed. The assessment checklist is a tool that can be used to initiate this process or support its continuation; that is, certain sections may be completed during an initial assessment session, while others may be spread out over several weeks or even months, depending on the student and his or her needs. Not all sections of the assessment form will be appropriate for every student or need to be completed every time an assessment is undertaken or in the order listed on the form. The team will need to decide which sections of the checklist need to be completed and assemble the materials that are suggested for those sections. It is also important to indicate on the cover sheet and in each section the specific dates on which each section was completed, because doing so documents the student's performance, abilities, and needs at a given time. It is important to keep in mind that completing the form is not the aim of the assistive technology assessment; the form is simply a guide or an outline of the elements that should be considered in the process.

The checklist included in this book outlines three broad areas to be covered when a student is assessed: Accessing Print, Accessing Electronic Information, and Communicating through Writing (see Figure 7.1). When a student is able to perform the tasks described by an item, the examiner should mark that item, for example with a check or an X. Some items will require the examiner to circle a choice; enter specific numbers, letters, or words; or write a comment. All items not assessed should be marked NA, to indicate "not attempted" (or "not applicable"); otherwise it might be assumed that the student currently cannot perform the task. As indicated in Chapter 6, if a student is not being evaluated on a particular section of the checklist, it is helpful to note briefly why that area is not being addressed, by noting, for example, "has no usable vision." Throughout the assessment process, notes and observations can be documented in the comments sections of the form to record the student's needs and abilities and to serve as data to support the recommendations that will be made.

The assessment team and the individual examiners working with a student will need to decide what criteria they wish to use in deciding whether a student is able to perform a given task. The criteria may be different for different tasks. Since the objective of the assessment technology assessment is to determine which tools may be beneficial to a particular student in accomplishing a particular task, in some cases the criteria will simply be whether the student has the visual, tactile, auditory, cognitive, and physical abilities necessary to use a given tool to accomplish the task in question. Therefore, determining a specific level for completing a

Figure 7.1 Assistive Technology Assessment Checklist Coversheet

---

ASSISTIVE TECHNOLOGY ASSESSMENT CHECKLIST
FOR STUDENTS WITH VISUAL IMPAIRMENTS

Student's Name _____   Person Completing Checklist _____
Student's Grade _____   Position _____
Student's Date of Birth _____   Date(s) of assessment _____

This document is a summary of information collected during the above-named student's assistive technology evaluation. Information for this assessment was obtained from the student's learning media assessment, the clinical low vision evaluation, the functional low vision evaluation, and from observation and assessment of the student's use of specific devices, as outlined below.
The assessment covers three main areas:

- **Section I: Accessing Print**, which covers how the student uses visual, tactile, and/or auditory tools to access textbooks, workbooks, assigned novels, and other printed information generally used in the classroom, including information presented on chalkboards or whiteboards
- **Section II: Accessing Electronic Information**, which covers how the student uses visual, tactile, and/or auditory tools to obtain information from electronic means, such as computers, electronic dictionaries and similar devices, digital books, and electronic braille devices
- **Section III: Communication through Writing**, which includes manuscript (print) and cursive writing, braille writing, and the use of electronic writing tools

The assessment sections of this document are followed by a recommendations section. The notations made will become part of the final written report detailing the rationale for each recommendation submitted to the student's Individualized Education Program team.

Directions: Indicate in the space provided the date each section is completed. All items not assessed should be marked NA.

task—for example, completing a task with 80 percent accuracy—may not be necessary. (The assessment form will suggest a criteria level for some items.) In general, it is reasonable not to expect students to perform each task independently, but only after demonstration and instruction from the examiner.

Team members will find it helpful to consider ahead of time the potential benefit of a particular device or technology to the student. The information provided in Chapters 2–5 will help the assessment team understand which technologies can be helpful in accomplishing particular tasks. If a particular type of technology seems to be promising for a given student, the team can learn more about it, if they choose, by reading about it online, contacting the company that sells it, or by contacting their state technology assistance program (see the Resources section). It is also important to explore with the student whether he or she would be willing to use the technology in different situations, such as in a regular classroom, while working alone with the teacher of students with visual impairments, or while completing assignments at home. Otherwise, a device that seems perfect for a student may wind up sitting unused in the proverbial drawer or closet.

Before beginning an assessment, the team needs to consult appropriate individuals on such issues as how to position the student physically, if the student has additional disabilities, and how to communicate effectively with the student, if the student has a disability affecting his or her ability to communicate. If a student's native language is not English, it is also important to engage a speaker of that language as an interpreter or examiner if he or she has the appropriate skills. Determining ahead of time and making provision for such factors as the student's need for environmental modifications, such as the reduction of glare, or tendency to fatigue quickly, will help ensure an assessment that accurately determines the student's true needs and abilities.

As has been stressed throughout this book, there is a wide variety of tools that can be used to help students who are blind or have low vision access print and electronic information, produce written communication, and produce materials in alternate formats. Like all of us, individuals with visual impairments need and can choose to use different formats or media for different tasks at different times. Therefore, when completing an assistive technology assessment, it is important to remember that students will use a combination of formats, tools, and techniques to accomplish their educational activities. The objective of the assistive technology assessment, then, is to select the most efficient format for dealing with different types of information under different circumstances and choose the tools that are best suited for completing each task. The sections that follow describe the procedures for completing each subsection of an assessment and the checklist and may suggest different approaches to obtaining information about a student.

CONSIDERATIONS FOR STUDENTS WITH ADDITIONAL DISABILITIES

The examiner will need to carefully select appropriate materials and methods when assessing students with visual impairment and additional disabilities. The basic assessment structure provided in this chapter can be used with these students, but particular consideration must be given to the tasks the student needs to accomplish. If the teacher of students with visual impairments is conducting the initial assistive technology assessment, he or she will most likely want to enlist the assistance of other team members to conduct an evaluation in the areas of seating and positioning, computer access, mobility, communication, possible work site modifications, devices for daily living, modification of the home environment, and adaptation or modification of recreation and leisure activities. At the same time, the teacher of students with visual impairments can greatly assist these specialists by supplying support and suggestions related to the student's visual functioning.

The team will need to gather information about the method that the student will use to access information displayed by computers and other technology devices. Information from the student's learning media assessment can guide the team in determining if the student will access information visually, tactilely, or auditorily. Collaborative assessment with other team members can also help to determine the input and output method appropriate for the student to interact with the computer as a tool for learning and productivity. A wide variety of input devices are available and can be tried. The team will need to assess the student's ability to interact with the computer through the use of such input devices as switches, alternative and adaptive keyboards, touch windows and touch pads, and speech recognition systems. In addition, information will need to be gathered on the methods and devices the student can use most efficiently when interacting with his or her environment and various other pieces of technology.

Some students who access information visually may not have the motor or cognitive skills to manipulate optical devices, screen magnification software, and other technologies designed for individuals with low vision. If students are unable to use the devices that will help them access print or electronic information, the team will need to locate devices and technologies that do not require vision or can be used without these other devices. Access issues and the complexity of many assistive technology devices may limit the usefulness of computers and other technologies as productivity tools for other students, as well. In these cases, data gathered from a separate computer access assessment (an evaluation conducted to determine a method of accessing a computer for someone who cannot use standard means) performed by an assistive technology specialist can help the team in making decisions about what technologies can best meet the needs of the student.

SECTION I: ACCESSING PRINT

Visual Access

- Regular Print
- Enlarged Print Produced on a Photocopier
- Large Print
- Nonoptical Devices
- Optical Devices
- Video Magnifiers (CCTVs)
- Specialized Scanning Systems for Accessing Print Information Visually
- Visual and Physical Fatigue

Tactile Access and Braille

- Tactile Graphics
- Braille Reading Rate
- Refreshable Braille Display

Auditory Access

- Live Readers and Recorded Information
- Specialized Scanning Systems for Accessing Print Information Auditorily

Reading Rates

Accessing Information Presented at a Distance

As noted earlier, an assistive technology assessment should examine students' needs based on both their primary and secondary sensory channels as identified by a learning media assessment. Chapter 2 describes the range of technologies that can assist a student who is blind or visually impaired to access print using vision, touch, or hearing. In exploring a student's ability to access print visually, it is important to expose the student to both regular and large print and to determine which assistive technology devices, including nonoptical and optical devices, will enable the student to access print information most effectively. Again, the Assistive Technology Assessment Checklist outlines the process and can be used as a guide.

VISUAL ACCESS

Regular Print

Materials Needed

- Reading passages written at the student's independent reading level (that is, material that the student can read without assistance or instruction) in 12-point sans serif type font. It may be easiest to use samples from an informal reading inventory, such as the Johns *Basic Reading Inventory* (Johns, 2008).
- Retractable tape measure or a sewing tape measure
- Stopwatch

Many students will have prescribed spectacles (eyeglasses) or contact lenses. Reports from an ophthalmologic examination and clinical low vision evaluation should have provided the examiner with information about the student's use of prescription lenses. If the student uses such lenses, his or her ability to read print both with and without them should be explored during this part of the assessment. Through the use of these lenses, some students may be able to read print found in textbooks and other supplemental materials without additional adaptations or devices. Others may be able to read regular print materials either with or without their prescribed eyeglasses or contact lenses or other adaptations to complete short reading tasks. Students can be assessed on a few items without their prescribed eyeglasses or contact lenses, since information about the student's ability to function without them can be valuable in the event that the eyeglasses become broken or unavailable. For example, the teacher can determine the student's preferred font and point size to gain an idea of how large materials would need to be made if the student needed to read them without eyeglasses or contact lenses.

For this assessment, regular print is defined as 12-point text. The two major factors to consider in determining if the student is able to function effectively with regular print materials, and under what conditions, are the student's working distance and working duration. *Working distance* refers to how close the student needs to hold materials being viewed; that is, the distance between the eye and the object or text. It is important to determine the student's working distance for reading regular print both with and without the use of spectacles or contact lenses. *Working duration* refers to the amount of time the student can read before experiencing significant visual or physical fatigue. The examiner can ask the student, teacher, or parent for the approximate length of time the student can work with this type of print before experiencing fatigue. A student may be able to read regular print with prescribed eyeglasses or contact lenses, but may experience visual or physical fatigue more quickly than when using some of the other options discussed in this section. (See the later section on "Visual and Physical Fatigue.")

It is a good idea to acquaint the student with whatever tape measure or other measuring device will be used in some parts of the assessment, since the student will be coming into close contact with it. The examiner can explain that it will be used frequently during the session to measure how far the student likes to hold objects from his or her eyes while looking at them. If you first demonstrate how to use the tape measure with the examiner as the subject, that will help to alleviate any fear a young student might have. It may put the student at ease to be allowed to measure a few things with the tape measure and pull out a retractable tape and allow it to recoil into its case. (Care should be taken that the student does not pull the tape out so far that it might damage something or injure the student when it recoils.) Depending on the student's interest, additional time with the

tape measure can even be offered as a reward for completing requested tasks.

Procedure

- To complete the first item on the checklist (see Figure 7.2), present the student with a reading passage containing a few paragraphs in a 12-point sans serif type font (such as Arial, APHont, Tahoma, or Verdana) on the student's independent reading level. If the student is wearing eyeglasses, ask the student to remove them and begin reading the text aloud. If the student uses contact lenses, it may not be practical to have the student remove them to conduct this first step. Information on the student's working distance and reading rate without lenses may be available from the background information described in Chapter 6.

- If the student is able to read the 12-point print, observe him or her for a sentence or two and then ask the student to remain still and measure the working distance between the student's eyes and the page. The measure does not have to be extremely precise; it will be used primarily to make comparisons with other measures taken later in the assessment.

- Using the stopwatch, the examiner should also take an approximate measure of the student's oral reading rate to determine if the student is reading fast enough with this size print to accomplish educational tasks efficiently. Again, this does not have to be an extremely precise measure. An approximate measure of how many words per minute the student can read can be obtained by having the student read aloud a passage on his or her independent reading level for three minutes and then dividing the total number of words read by three. (See Koenig, Holbrook, Corn, DePriest, Erin, & Presley, 2000, pp. 130–131, for a more detailed discussion of reading rate and reading efficiency.) More precise information about the student's reading rate on different types of materials should be available from the teacher of students with visual impairments as part of regular progress monitoring of the student's progress in language arts.

- Repeat these measurements with the student wearing his or her prescribed eyeglasses.
- Complete the assessment form by indicating the working distance and reading rate with and without prescribed lenses.

Figure 7.2   Visual Access: Regular Print

Section I: Accessing Print

A. Visual Access

1. Regular Print   **Date completed** _____

When accessing print information visually, the student is able to read passages on his or her independent reading level in regular print (12 point)

❑ without prescribed eyeglasses or contact lenses at a distance of

   ____ inches, at approximately   ____ words per minute (wpm).

❑ with prescribed eyeglasses or contact lenses at a distance of

   ____ inches, at approximately   ____ wpm.

❑ When reading this size print with or without prescribed eyeglasses or contact lenses the student experiences visual or physical fatigue after ____ minutes (as reported by student or teacher).

Comments: _____

_____

_____

Enlarged Print Produced on a Photocopier

Materials Needed

- Reading passages on the student's independent reading level enlarged to varying percentages of enlargement on a photocopying machine on 8½ × 11, 8½ × 14, and 11 × 17 inch paper
- Retractable tape measure or a sewing tape measure
- Stopwatch

An important first adaptation to assess for students who may be able to access printed information visually is the use of materials enlarged on a photocopying machine (see Figure 7.3). This adaptation is

Figure 7.3   Visual Access: Enlarged Print Produced on a Photocopier

Section I: Accessing Print

A. Visual Access

From this point forward all items should be attempted with student's prescribed spectacles or contact lens in use.

2. Enlarged Print Produced on a Photocopier   Date completed _____

When accessing print information visually the student is able to read

- ❑ materials enlarged to ___% on

- ❑ 8 ½ × 11 inch paper   ❑ 8 ½ × 14 inch paper   ❑ 11 × 17 inch paper

    at approximately _____ inches and at approximately _____ words per minute (wpm).

When reading this size print with or without prescribed eyeglasses or contact lenses the student experiences visual or physical fatigue after _____ minutes (as reported by student or teacher).

- ❑ The student is willing to use materials enlarged by a photocopying machine on

- ❑ 8 ½ × 11 inch paper   ❑ 8 ½ × 14 inch paper   ❑ 11 × 17 inch paper

- ❑ to complete assignments in the regular classroom.

- ❑ at home to complete school assignments.

- ❑ while working with the teacher of students with visual impairments.

Comments: _____
_____
_____

readily available, and the student may already be using materials enlarged in this way. If so, the examiner may be able to obtain the information to complete the questions about this method of enlarging print, such as the percentages of enlargement typically required by the student, from the teacher of students with visual impairments. If not, the examiner will need to prepare appropriate materials enlarged on a photocopying machine on various sizes of paper (8½ × 11 inch, 8½ × 14 inch, 11 × 17 inch) and at various degrees of enlargement, depending on the size of the original and the capabilities of the photocopying machine. Some machines allow enlargements in single-digit increments between 100 percent and 200 percent. Typical enlargements are 130 percent, 145 percent, 150 percent, and so forth. The examiner will want to assess the student's ability to work with several different levels of enlargement. Additional sizes can be assessed if desired and the form modified accordingly to record the results.

It is important to record the percentage of enlargement setting on the copying machine, the size of paper being used, and the number of times that a document is enlarged to produce the material used for the assessment. The examiner will also want to determine the student's willingness to use these types of materials in various settings. This information will be important when formulating the recommendations for the use of this adaptation for certain types of materials and tasks. It will also be essential data in determining the efficiency and effectiveness of photocopier enlargement as a tool for assisting the student to access printed information for short reading tasks and in determining the usability of regular print and enlarged materials. Enlarging

text on a photocopier may not be an adequate adaptation to permit a student to complete most tasks, but it will be important to determine if it can be used to allow the student to read some classroom materials and perform certain tasks.

From this point on, the student should be assessed wearing any spectacles (eyeglasses) or contact lens that have been prescribed. The procedure used to get a basic understanding of the student's ability to read information enlarged on a photocopier is similar to that used with regular print materials.

Procedure
- Ask the student to read the text produced at the first level of enlargement. Measure the working distance.
- Have the student read aloud for three minutes to measure his or her reading rate.
- Repeat these steps with the text samples at other levels of enlargement and record the level that the student prefers.
- Ask the student or his or her teacher to estimate how long the student can read materials enlarged in this format before experiencing visual or physical fatigue.
- Determine how comfortable the student would be using these materials in various settings.

Large Print

Materials Needed
- Copy of the sample text shown in Appendixes 7B, 7C, and 7D, or similar documents
- Color photographs of various sizes
- One-page sample of 1-inch-high line drawings (picture symbols)

- One-page sample of 2-inch-high line drawings (picture symbols)
- One-page sample of 3-inch-high line drawings (picture symbols)
- Retractable tape measure or a sewing tape measure
- Reading stand
- Stopwatch

A critical part of the assessment is to determine the distances at which the student can see a visual target or read print in various point sizes and fonts (see Figure 7.4.). This information will assist the assessment team in recommending appropriate large-print materials to be used in the student's education program. It may be available from the clinical low vision evaluation and the learning media assessment that the assessment team should have reviewed previously (see Chapter 6). If not, then this aspect of the student's visual performance will need to be examined. This section of the assessment should be completed with the student wearing prescribed eyeglasses or contact lenses.

Although information about a student's clinical visual acuity in Snellen notation (such as 20/200 OD, 20/100 OS) is often given to teachers of students with visual impairments, it is of little practical value in helping the general classroom teacher evaluate and produce instructional materials for a student. Instead, providing the teacher with examples of simple photographs, simple black-and-white line drawings, and print sizes that the student can see at various distances will be more helpful to the teacher in selecting appropriate materials for the student to use. For example, a student might be able to see and identify a 1-inch-high black-and-white line drawing of a house at a working distance of approximately 6 inches and a 3-inch drawing of a school bus at approximately 12 inches. This type of information can help a general classroom teacher better understand how well the student will be able to see various materials presented to the class.

The use of photographs and drawings is evaluated as well as that of text because students are expected to view graphical information to complete many educational activities (such as completing worksheets that include pictures), whether or not they know how to read. To produce the 1-inch, 2-inch, and 3-inch black-and-white drawings of common objects needed to conduct this section of the assessment, the examiner can consult the school's speech therapist about using a computer program that prints picture symbols used for communication boards. It is helpful to print out larger, full-page versions of the drawings that will be used in the assessment and show them to the student before proceeding to make sure that the student is familiar with the objects depicted and can identify them. The student can then be asked to identify the objects in the smaller drawings. The examiner will need to measure the student's working distances and record them.

The ideal arrangement of large print is to display as much text as possible on a given page in a size that the reader can view at a comfortable working distance. The size of text that is comfortable for the student to read may vary from task to task; therefore it is necessary to measure the working distance used by the student with several point sizes and fonts.

To determine the point size that will be comfortable for the student to read to accomplish different tasks, the examiner will need to create simple text samples in various point sizes and fonts, similar to

Figure 7.4   Visual Access: Large Print

Section I: Accessing Print

A. Visual Access

3. Large Print   **Date completed** _____

The student is able to identify the following pictures of common objects:

_____ -inch high color photograph at a distance of approximately _____ inches.
❑ 3-inch high black-and-white line drawing at a distance of approximately _____ inches.
❑ 2-inch high black-and-white line drawing at a distance of approximately _____ inches.
❑ 1-inch high black-and-white line drawing at a distance of approximately _____ inches.

When accessing large print with prescribed eyeglasses or contact lenses (if appropriate), the student is able to read
❑ 72-point print at a distance of approximately _____ inches.
❑ 60-point print at a distance of approximately _____ inches.
❑ 48-point print at a distance of approximately _____ inches.
❑ 36-point print at a distance of approximately _____ inches.
❑ 30-point print at a distance of approximately _____ inches.
❑ 24-point print at a distance of approximately _____ inches.
❑ 18-point print at a distance of approximately _____ inches.
❑ 14-point print at a distance of approximately _____ inches.
❑ 12-point print at a distance of approximately _____ inches.

The student's preferred font is ❑ Arial ❑ APHont ❑ Tahoma ❑ Verdana
    ❑ other (specify): _____

The student's preferred point size with prescribed eyeglasses or contact lenses is
    ❑ 14 ❑ 18 ❑ 24 ❑ 30 ❑ 36 ❑ 48 ❑ 60 ❑ 72

The student prefers text in
    ❑ regular style
    ❑ bold style

The student is able to read continuous text in preferred font and point size at approximately
    ___ words per minute.

When reading this size print with or without prescribed eyeglasses or contact lenses the student experiences visual or physical fatigue after ___ minutes (as reported by student or teacher).

The student is willing to use materials printed in the preferred font and point size on 8 ½ × 11 inch paper

___ to complete assignments in the regular classroom.

___ at home to complete school assignments.

___ while working with the teacher of students with visual impairments.

Comments: _____

_____

_____

those in Appendixes 7B, 7C, and 7D. If the student is just learning letters and numbers, materials using individual letters and numbers should be created in the same range of point sizes. The examiner might need to consider how to place materials so that the student can view them best. The optimum viewing position allows the student to view materials while sitting in an ergonomically correct position, taking into consideration the student's preferred viewing angle if he or she has any visual field loss. Issues associated with positioning should be discussed with an occupational therapist or another team member with experience in this area.

Procedure

- If the student is a nonreader, place the photograph in the optimum viewing position for the student, on a reading stand, if possible. Ask the student to identify the photograph and measure the operative working distance.
- Repeat the previous step with the 1-inch-, 2-inch-, and 3-inch-high black-and-white line drawings.

- Place a sample showing different type sizes, similar to the one in Appendix 7B, on a reading stand, if possible, in the optimum viewing position for the student.
- Seat the student in a chair with the reading material approximately 13 to 16 inches from the student's eyes.
- Ask the student to read the 72-point print. If the student cannot read the 72-point print at this distance, ask the student to pick up the page and gradually bring it closer to his or her eyes until he or she *can* read the 72-point line. Many students will automatically bring the text to their usual reading distance, which might be closer than necessary, so the examiner may need to assist the student in determining the greatest distance at which he or she can read the 72-point print.
- Measure the distance at which the student can read the 72-point print and record that distance.
- Follow the same procedure with the other point sizes until you reach the smallest print that the student can read.

- To refine these measurements, repeat the procedure with materials like those provided in Appendix 7C, which shows text in an Arial font starting at 72 points and descending to 12 points, or other simple text.
- Measure the student's reading rate on passages at the student's independent reading level that are printed in the student's preferred font and point size.

To determine the student's preferred type font, the examiner will need to prepare reading samples in various fonts such as Arial, APHont, Tahoma, and Verdana in both regular type and bold style (see the examples in Appendix 7D). These materials can be created using a word processor on a computer and printed out on a laser or inkjet printer. Since the purpose of this part of the assessment is to see how clearly and easily the student can access the text, not to assess reading skills, these materials should be on or below the student's independent reading level in the point size that the student can read at a comfortable working distance.

- Ask the student to select the sample that he or she thinks is easiest to read. If at this point in the assessment the examiner has not yet created appropriate materials in the student's preferred point size, the assessment team may revisit this task at another time, or they may wish to have the teacher of students with visual impairments determine the student's font preference once appropriate samples have been created.
- Once the examiner has determined the student's preferred font, style, and point size, he or she will need to produce a reading passage within those parameters to assess the student's reading rate.
- The examiner should also note the student's willingness to use large-print materials in various settings and can record any notes or comments about the student's performance or preferences.

Nonoptical Devices

After determining the student's ability to read print without the aid of devices (other than prescribed eyeglasses or contact lenses), the assessment team needs to explore how environmental modifications and nonoptical devices may enhance the student's performance. Three items will be explored in this section of the assessment: the student's ability to read handwritten material, the effects of natural and artificial lighting, and the use of reading stands (see Figure 7.5).

Materials Needed

- Samples of the classroom teacher's manuscript (hand-printed) and cursive writing on standard lined notebook paper, bold-lined notebook paper, and unlined paper
- Graphical information of interest to the student
- Reading passages on the student's independent reading level in the student's preferred font and point size
- Incandescent and fluorescent overhead lighting
- Incandescent, fluorescent, and halogen floor lamps and desk lamps
- Blinds, shades, and other controls for natural light from windows
- Desktop reading stand
- Floor reading stand

Figure 7.5   Visual Access: Nonoptical Devices

Section I: Accessing Print

A. Visual Access

4. Nonoptical Devices   **Date completed** _____

When reading print information, the student prefers
- ❏ text written with a pen or pencil on standard lined notebook paper.
- ❏ text written with felt-tip pen on standard lined notebook paper.
- ❏ text written with felt-tip pen on bold-lined notebook paper.
- ❏ text written with felt-tip pen on unlined paper.
- ❏ other (specify): _____.

When reading handwritten information the student prefers
- ❏ manuscript (printed) writing.
- ❏ cursive writing.

When reading, the student
- ❏ prefers overhead lighting
  - ❏ from an incandescent bulb.
  - ❏ from a fluorescent bulb.
  - ❏ from a halogen bulb.
  - ❏ adjusted with a dimmer switch.
- ❏ prefers window lighting adjusted with
  - ❏ blinds.
  - ❏ shades.
  - ❏ other (specify): _____.
- ❏ experiences glare problems on
  - ❏ paper.
  - ❏ desktop.
  - ❏ computer or video magnifier monitor.
  - ❏ whiteboard.
  - ❏ chalkboard.
  - resulting from
    - ❏ overhead lighting.
    - ❏ window lighting (natural light, sunlight).
- ❏ prefers less lighting than currently available.
- ❏ prefers additional lighting from a
  - ❏ desk lamp with a/an
    - ❏ incandescent bulb.

(continued on next page)

Figure 7.5 *(continued)*

- ❑ fluorescent bulb.
- ❑ halogen bulb.
- ❑ LED bulb.
- ❑ floor lamp with a/an
  - ❑ incandescent bulb.
  - ❑ fluorescent bulb.
  - ❑ halogen bulb.
  - ❑ LED bulb.
- ❑ prefers the location of the lighting source to be
  - ❑ over the left shoulder.
  - ❑ over the right shoulder.
- ❑ prefers to have materials placed on a
  - ❑ desktop reading stand.
  - ❑ portable reading stand.
  - ❑ floor-standing reading stand.

The student is willing to use these devices and accommodations (the examiner may wish to list them individually)
- ❑ to complete assignments in the regular classroom.
- ❑ at home to complete school assignments.
- ❑ while working with the teacher of students with visual impairments.

Comments: _____
_____
_____
_____
_____

Handwritten Materials

Students are often given educational materials prepared by their teacher in their own handwriting, so it is important to assess whether a student can read materials in this format. The teacher of students with visual impairments or the classroom teacher may be able to provide this information, but if not, the examiner will need to obtain writing samples, preferably of the classroom teacher's manuscript (printed) and cursive writing on various types of paper.

Procedure

- If the student is able to read some of these materials, the examiner will need to determine how effective this format is for conveying information to the student. This determination can be based on feedback from the classroom teacher and the teacher of students with visual impairments, as well as on the examiner's observation of the student's ability to read the information.

- If the student is unable to read any of the handwritten samples, the examiner will need to determine in what alternate way these types of materials are typically provided to the student in the classroom and note it in the space reserved for comments.

Lighting

Conducting this section of the assessment effectively requires a good deal of planning because of the number of lighting conditions that need to be assessed and the difficulty of acquiring the different types of artificial and natural lighting needed. Lighting is a critical factor in students' successful use of technology tools for accessing both printed and electronic information visually, and assessment of a student's lightning needs encompasses such considerations as including type of lighting, location of lighting source, and lighting sources associated with glare. Improper placement of the lighting source will result in excessive amounts of glare reflecting off the viewing surface. Control of these factors is essential. If the student has never tried using additional light sources, the examiner will want to evaluate the student's performance with various desk and floor lamps that use incandescent, fluorescent, halogen, and LED (light emitting diodes) bulbs. Dimmer switches to control artificial lighting more precisely may also prove valuable. Talking to both the teacher of students with visual impairments and the student about lighting preferences will help the examiner determine which conditions are most helpful to the student.

The examiner may not be able to investigate all the items related to lighting suggested on the assessment checklist form, but it is nevertheless important to begin to examine the effects of lighting on the student's ability to access printed materials. The teacher of students with visual impairments may already have this information or may be able to conduct this section of the assessment at another time.

Procedure

- Ask the student to view graphical and textual information under artificial lighting.
- Ask the student to view and read some of the materials to determine if the student sees better with, or prefers, specific types of artificial lighting placed in particular positions in relationship to the information being viewed and the student's body.
- Have the student view materials using natural or window lighting.
- Investigate the impact of adjusting shades, blinds, or curtains on the student's ability to comfortably view various objects, graphical materials, and text.

Some environments may have too much light, especially for individuals who are extremely sensitive to light, while others may not have sufficient illumination. Selecting the best lighting source and placement for the student by assessing the effects of various types of lighting will help the examiner determine the lighting conditions that will improve the student's ability to access information visually and complete tasks.

Reading Stands

Students with low vision frequently need to hold print materials at a distance of 6 inches or closer to be able to read them. Some students choose to hold the material close to their eyes, while others place the material on a tabletop or desk and bend over to look at it. Both these options can soon result in physical fatigue. A nonoptical device that can be useful to students when viewing or reading printed information is a reading stand. It is therefore important to provide the student with the opportunity to view materials placed on a reading stand and note the student's reaction.

Procedure

- Determine if the use of a reading stand can place the materials to be viewed in a location that will allow the student to sit up straight with feet on the floor and view the material efficiently enough to complete tasks.
- Determine if a desktop reading stand provides adequate placement or whether an adjustable floor stand with a swing arm is needed to place the materials in the optimum viewing position. This determination will be affected by the size and weight of the material to be viewed, the setting in which it will be used, and the task to be performed with the material. For example, if the student needs to read information in a heavy textbook while typing text into a computer, then the desktop stand may not bring the material close enough for the student to see it. In this case, a floor stand will be needed to hold the heavier material at the appropriate height and viewing distance.

- Note any physical behaviors that might indicate fatigue (see the section on "Visual and Physical Fatigue"). Determine if the reading stands will allow the student to view materials for longer periods of time before experiencing fatigue.
- Note the student's willingness to use the various devices and accommodations in different situations. (The comments section of the assessment checklist form can be used to list specific devices.)
- Note specific information about the adaptations and modifications that were investigated, along with the student's reactions to these adaptations and modifications and any additional information from the teacher of students with visual impairments and classroom teacher.

It is important to note that information obtained from the student's use of nonoptical devices should be applied throughout the rest of the assessment. If a student finds that an additional lighting source is helpful, if a certain combination of natural and artificial light makes it easier to see, or if using a reading stand makes completing a task easier, these tools should be made available for the remainder of the assistive technology assessment.

Optical Devices

A critical part of the assessment process is determining how the student is using any prescribed optical devices for spot and continuous text reading (see Figure 7.6).

Materials Needed

- List of vocabulary words on the student's independent reading level

Figure 7.6   Visual Access: Optical Devices

Section I: Accessing Print

A. Visual Access

5. Optical Devices   **Date completed** _____

When accessing print materials with the use of a prescribed optical device, the student uses

❑ eyeglasses.

❑ contact lenses.

❑ handheld magnifier.

    type _____

    power _____

    ❑ illuminated   ❑ nonilluminated

❑ stand magnifier.

    type _____

    power _____

    ❑ illuminated   ❑ nonilluminated

❑ telescope.

    type _____

    power _____

❑ video magnifier (specify type):

    ❑ desktop video magnifier.

    ❑ flex-arm camera model.

    ❑ portable model with handheld camera.

    ❑ head-mounted display model.

    ❑ electronic pocket magnifier.

    ❑ digital imaging system.

    ❑ other (specify): _____.

The student is able to read continuous text using the prescribed optical device at approximately

    ___ words per minute without a reading stand.

    ___ words per minute with a reading stand.

(continued on next page)

Figure 7.6 (continued)

When reading regular-size print with the prescribed optical device the student experiences visual or physical fatigue after ___ minutes (as reported by student or teacher).

The student is willing to use these devices (the examiner may wish to list these separately)

❑ to complete assignments in the regular classroom.

❑ at home to complete school assignments.

❑ while working with the teacher of students with visual impairments.

Comments: _____

_____

_____

- Samples of printed telephone numbers and price tags
- Reading passages in a 12-point sans serif font on the student's independent reading level (It may be easiest to use samples from an informal reading inventory, such as the Johns *Basic Reading Inventory* [2008].)
- The student's prescribed optical device (such as a handheld magnifier or monocular telescope)
- Reading stand

During this section of the assessment process, students should use any prescribed eyeglasses or contact lenses in addition to optical devices such as magnifiers that have been prescribed for reading as a result of a medical eye exam or the clinical low vision evaluation. The examiner should be able to determine which devices a student uses from the background information discussed in Chapter 6. Arrangements should be made beforehand for the student to have his or her prescribed devices present during this part of the assessment. The examiner can use the following procedures to obtain some general information about how the student uses his or her devices.

Procedure

- Present the student with a list of words and ask the student to read them aloud using the magnifier or other device.
- Present the student with telephone numbers and price tags and ask student to read them aloud using the device.
- Present the student with reading passages and ask the student to read them aloud while using the device.
- Note the student's approximate reading rate on the passages.
- Place the reading material on a reading stand and ask the student to read it aloud. Note any differences in reading rate.
- Note any physical behaviors that might indicate fatigue. Determine if the device or devices used will allow the student to view materials for

longer periods of time before experiencing fatigue.

- Note the student's willingness to use the various devices and accommodations in different situations.

Video Magnifiers (CCTVs)

Many students benefit from the use of video magnifiers (also known as closed-circuit television systems or CCTVs). Given the range of these devices that is available (see Chapter 2), assessing the potential helpfulness of video magnifier use for a student involves a number of determinations.

A student's clinical low vision evaluation may or may not have recommended the use of a video magnifier. In some cases where there was no clear recommendation about this technology, the teacher of students with visual impairments may have exposed the student to the device and found that it is of value to the student. In either case, the examiner will want to explore the student's possible use of a variety of video magnifiers.

Materials Needed

- Reading passages in 12-point sans serif font on the student's independent reading level
- One-page sample of 1-inch line drawings (picture symbols)
- One-page sample of 2-inch line drawings (picture symbols)
- One-page sample of 3-inch line drawings (picture symbols)
- Samples of visual tracking exercises (see the Resources section for possible sources)
- Sample of the student's handwriting that is at least 3–5 days old
- Retractable tape measure or a sewing tape measure

- Desktop video magnifier with an X-Y table that has an adjustable friction brake and adjustable margin stops
- Flex-arm camera model video magnifier
- Several target drawings or photographs of high interest mounted on a brightly colored piece of poster board
- Portable video magnifier with a handheld camera
- Sample reading passage on the student's independent reading level containing short, one-line sentences that are double or triple spaced
- Electronic pocket model video magnifier
- Head-mounted display model video magnifier
- Digital imaging system video magnifier
- Stopwatch

Video magnifiers (CCTVs) are one of the more widely used electronic optical devices by individuals with low vision. Many varieties are available, but they all offer the same basic ability to electronically display enlarged images. Users need basic motor and cognitive skills to take advantage of this technology, although they do not necessarily need to be able to read. This section of the assessment will involve procedures to assess the student on several different types of video magnifiers (see Figure 7.7). Since technology changes so rapidly, new models are always being introduced. The assessment team may want to explore newer models than those discussed in this chapter, because they may offer additional features.

The examiner will need a collection of simple monochrome line drawings and appropriate reading selections to conduct this section of the assessment (see Figure 7.7).

Figure 7.7   Visual Access: Video Magnifier

Section I: Accessing Print

A. Visual Access

6. Video Magnifier (CCTV)   **Date completed** _____

Desktop Video Magnifier

When accessing print materials with the use of a desktop video magnifier (closed-circuit television or CCTV), the student is able to view a (insert a number to indicate the size)

___-inch-high graphic and ___-inch-high text on a __-inch-monitor
at a working distance of approximately 10–13 inches.

___-inch-high graphic and ___-inch-high text on a __-inch-monitor
at a working distance of approximately ___ inches.

The student's polarity preference when viewing text on a video magnifier is
___ dark on light.
___ light on dark.

The student's color preference is
_____ text on a _____ background.

The student is able to manipulate the controls of the video magnifier, with instructions from the examiner, to

❑ adjust the size of the image.
❑ focus the image if the unit does not have auto focus.

When using the video magnifier, the student is able to

❑ write a short sentence legibly on regular notebook paper while
   ❑ looking at the screen or monitor.
   ❑ looking at the paper.

❑ write a short sentence legibly on bold-lined paper while
   ❑ looking at the screen or monitor.
   ❑ looking at the paper.

When using the video magnifier, the student is able to read a 3- to 5-day-old sample sentence of his or her handwriting on

❑ blue-lined notebook paper.
❑ bold-lined writing paper.

The student is able to

❑ independently use an X-Y table for viewing materials with friction brake and margin stops are adjusted by examiner.

Comments: _____

❑ independently adjust friction brake and margin stops after demonstration by examiner.

Comments: _____

❑ independently manipulate the controls of the unit (knobs, buttons, switches, etc.).

Comments: _____

The student is able to read approximately ___ words per minute (wpm) when the friction brake and margin stops are adjusted properly by the examiner.

When reading this size print with or without prescribed eyeglasses or contact lenses the student experiences visual or physical fatigue after ___ minutes (as reported by student or teacher).

The student is willing to use these devices (the examiner may wish to list these separately)

❑ to complete assignments in the regular classroom.
❑ at home to complete school assignments.
❑ while working with the teacher of students with visual impairments.

Comments: _____
_____
_____

Flex-Arm Camera Video Magnifier

When accessing print materials with the use of a flex-arm camera model video magnifier, the student is able to

❑ locate and operate the controls.
❑ use the device's X-Y table or manipulate the reading material without a table.
❑ rotate and adjust the camera for distance viewing.
❑ locate the distance target.
❑ identify the distance target.

The student is able to read approximately ___ wpm when the friction brake and margin stops are adjusted properly by the examiner.

(continued on next page)

Figure 7.7 (continued)

When reading this size print with or without prescribed eyeglasses or contact lenses the student experiences visual or physical fatigue after ___ minutes (as reported by student or teacher).

The student is willing to use these devices (the examiner may wish to list these separately)
- ❑ to complete assignments in the regular classroom.
- ❑ at home to complete school assignments.
- ❑ while working with the teacher of students with visual impairments.

Comments: _____
_____
_____

Portable Video Magnifier with Handheld Camera

When accessing print materials through the use of a portable video magnifier with a handheld camera, the student is able to
- ❑ locate and operate the controls.
- ❑ maintain an angle of the camera with the text that is adequate for reading while moving the camera.

The student is able to read approximately ___ wpm when using this device.

When reading this size print with or without prescribed eyeglasses or contact lenses the student experiences visual or physical fatigue after ___ minutes (as reported by student or teacher).

The student is willing to use these devices (the examiner may wish to list these separately)
- ❑ to complete assignments in the regular classroom.
- ❑ at home to complete school assignments.
- ❑ while working with the teacher of students with visual impairments.

Comments: _____
_____
_____

Head-Mounted Video Magnifier

When accessing print materials through the use of a video magnifier with a head-mounted display, the student is able to
- ❑ locate and operate the controls.
- ❑ locate the distance target.
- ❑ identify the distance target.

The student is willing to use these devices (the examiner may wish to list these separately)

- ❑ to complete assignments in the regular classroom.
- ❑ at home to complete school assignments.
- ❑ while working with the teacher of students with visual impairments.

Electronic Pocket Video Magnifier

When accessing print materials through the use of an electronic pocket video magnifier, the student is able to

- ❑ locate and operate the controls.
- ❑ maintain the camera at an adequate angle to the text for reading while moving the device.
- ❑ operate a model with the camera on the side of the unit.
- ❑ operate a model with the camera in the middle of the unit.

The student is able to read approximately ___ wpm when using this type of device.

When reading this size print with or without prescribed eyeglasses or contact lenses the student experiences visual or physical fatigue after ___ minutes (as reported by student or teacher).

The student is willing to use these devices (the examiner may wish to list these separately)

- ❑ to complete assignments in the regular classroom.
- ❑ at home to complete school assignments.
- ❑ while working with the teacher of students with visual impairments.

Comments: _____
_____
_____

Digital Imaging System

When accessing print materials through the use of a digital imaging system video magnifier, the student is able to

- ❑ locate and operate the controls.

The student is able to read approximately ___ wpm when using this type of device.

When reading this size print with or without prescribed eyeglasses or contact lenses the student experiences visual or physical fatigue after ___ minutes (as reported by student or teacher).

The student is willing to use these devices (the examiner may wish to list these separately)

- ❑ to complete assignments in the regular classroom.
- ❑ at home to complete school assignments.
- ❑ while working with the teacher of students with visual impairments.

Comments: _____
_____
_____

Starting with drawings, pictures, and even objects can generate interest for student readers and nonreaders alike. If feasible, the examiner will want to assess the student's ability to use as many types of video magnifiers as possible and to note the student's willingness to use each device in various settings.

Desktop Video Magnifiers

Assessing a student's ability to use a desktop video magnifier requires quite a few steps. There are numerous features, options, and controls that will need to be investigated. Many of these items will need to be repeated for the other types of video magnifiers. The procedure is outlined in Appendix 7E, "Procedure for Completing the Assessment for Desktop Video Magnifiers."

Flex-Arm Camera Models

Assessing the student's potential use of a flex-arm camera model requires the examiner to repeat several of the steps from the desktop assessment. The first is to determine whether the student has the physical ability to manipulate the device's controls. If the device does not have an X-Y table similar to desktop models, then the examiner will need to demonstrate to the student how the material to be viewed needs to be moved under the camera. The examiner should note the student's coordination while performing this task and how this might affect the student's ability to read text continuously for several pages. The final assessment task for this type of video magnifier is to investigate the student's ability to rotate the camera and manipulate it for distance viewing.

Procedure

- To provide an age-appropriate target for the student to locate using the device, mount a drawing or photograph of high interest to the student on a piece of poster board of a color that offers a high degree of contrast to the target image and creates a wide border around the image to aid the student in locating it without using the video magnifier.
- Place the target in the examination room approximately 20 feet away from the student in front of a surface that will also offer good contrast to the color of the poster board. The student should be able to visually identify the location of the poster board without the use of the video magnifier.
- Explain to the student that one of the features of this type of video magnifier is its ability to be used for distance viewing and point out the general location of the target.
- Ask the student to point to the target with his or her finger. If the student does not locate the target with verbal direction, the examiner might need to walk over to the target and point it out to the student.
- Ask the student to decrease the magnification of the unit to its lowest setting, and then rotate and point the camera toward the target. Have the student maneuver the camera and search for the color of the poster board.
- Ask the student to zoom in on the image and identify it.
- Note the student's ability to manipulate the device and add any necessary comments.
- Present a reading passage on the student's independent reading level and measure the student's reading rate.

Portable Video Magnifier with Handheld Camera

A portable video magnifier with a handheld camera can be easily transported to various locations but requires good hand coordination to manipulate the camera. The examiner will be attempting to gather data about the potential use of this type of tool for completing short reading tasks.

Procedure

- Demonstrate the basic controls of the device and then ask the student to make some adjustments, such as in the size, polarity, and color options of the display.
- Once the student has become familiar with the controls, ask him or her to read an appropriate reading sample and observe the way in which the student maneuvers the device. It might be best to start with short, one-line sentences that are double or triple spaced and then proceed to longer samples.
- Present a reading passage on the student's independent reading level and measure the student's reading rate.

Head-Mounted Video Magnifier

Video magnifiers that use a head-mounted display can be used for both distance and near viewing tasks. Although most users prefer to use this kind of device just for distance viewing, with training and practice continuous text reading can also be accomplished.

Procedure

- Demonstrate the controls and ask the student to first locate a distance target similar to the one used in the evaluation of the flex-arm camera model video magnifier.

- Help the student to adjust the device for near viewing.
- Ask the student to read one of the sample reading passages.

Electronic Pocket Video Magnifier

A wide variety of electronic pocket video magnifiers are available, and there is one major difference from all other types of video magnifiers that should be noted for assessment purposes. Some of these devices have the camera mounted in the middle, while others have the camera mounted at one end of the unit. This type of device requires physical coordination similar to that required for portable units using a handheld camera. The user must be able to move the device over the viewing material and maintain an adequate angle for reading. The device can be used with either one or two hands. The examiner will want to determine if the student has adequate coordination to manipulate the device successfully for continuous text reading.

Procedure

- Demonstrate the controls of the device, assist the student in selecting his or her settings and configuration, and then ask the student to read one of the word lists or reading passages.
- Determine the usefulness of the device for short reading tasks and longer reading assignments by observing and noting the student's performance.
- Present a reading passage on the student's independent reading level and measure the student's reading rate.

Digital Imaging System

The student's use of a video magnifier that uses a digital-imaging process to enlarge printed text will also need to be evaluated.

Procedure

- Demonstrate the basic controls of the device and then ask the student to use them, providing verbal assistance if needed.
- Record whether the student has the physical and cognitive ability to use this technology.
- Present a reading passage on the student's independent reading level and measure the student's reading rate.

Specialized Scanning Systems for Accessing Print Information Visually

Materials Needed

- Computer
- Flatbed scanner
- Optical character recognition software (such as Kurzweil 1000 and 3000, OpenBook, and WYNN)
- Reading samples on the student's independent reading level

As explained in Chapter 2, computer-based systems can provide visual access to printed information for individuals with low vision. Text and images can be scanned into the computer with an optical scanner and accessed with software that will enlarge the scanned image. The Microsoft Imaging program provided with the Windows operating system provides the basic features to scan information and display an enlarged version of it. This program is not designed specifically for this purpose but it can be a useful tool for some individuals. Specialized optical character recognition (OCR) programs of this nature, such as Kurzweil 1000 and OpenBook for text, and Kurzweil 3000 and WYNN for text and graphics, which are designed to be used by individuals with visual impairments or reading difficulties, offer features that make them much easier to use than the basic imaging programs.

The objective of this section of the assessment (see Figure 7.8) is to determine if the student has the cognitive and physical abilities to use these tools. Navigating through the enlarged image while using the imaging program is difficult for many students. To prepare for this section of the assessment, the examiner will need to scan some appropriate text and graphical materials and save them as electronic files on the computer.

Procedure

- Demonstrate the magnification and navigation controls of the programs being assessed and ask the student to execute these controls with the keyboard and the mouse.
- Provide verbal prompts and general assistance when needed.
- Note whether the student is able to use the navigation features of the imaging program and whether he or she can access the printed information more efficiently with the added features provided by the specialized programs.

Visual and Physical Fatigue

Regardless of what devices and adaptations a student with low vision might use, accessing printed information visually often results in both visual and physical fatigue. Visual fatigue results from excessive stress on the eyes, manifested in painful irritation or burning, often accompanied by tearing, watering, or redness of the eyes. Additional symptoms of visual fatigue can include double vision, headaches, reduced visual clarity

Figure 7.8   Visual Access: Scanning Systems for Accessing Print Information Visually

Section I: Accessing Print

A. Visual Access

7. Scanning Systems for Accessing   Date completed _____
   Print Information Visually

When viewing print materials scanned into the computer using a standard imaging program (Microsoft Imaging, PaperPort, etc.), the student is able to

- ❑ operate the scanner.
- ❑ navigate the enlarged screen with the
    - ❑ keyboard.
    - ❑ mouse.

When viewing printed materials scanned into the computer with a specialized scanning system (such as Kurzweil 1000 or 3000, OpenBook, or WYNN), the student is able to

- ❑ operate the scanner.
- ❑ adjust the magnification to the desired size using the
    - ❑ keyboard.
    - ❑ mouse.
- ❑ adjust the rate and other speech parameters.
- ❑ navigate the image horizontally and vertically using the
    - ❑ keyboard.
    - ❑ mouse.
- ❑ select items from the menus and tools from the toolbar with the
    - ❑ keyboard.
    - ❑ mouse.

The student is willing to use these devices (the examiner may wish to list these separately)

- ❑ to complete assignments in the regular classroom.
- ❑ at home to complete school assignments.
- ❑ while working with the teacher of students with visual impairments.

Comments: _____

_____

_____

or acuity, and reduced sensitivity to contrast. Signs of physical fatigue for students with low vision include headaches, back and shoulder pain from bending over to read, and sore arm muscles from holding books up close for viewing.

The examiner may not have an opportunity in the course of the assessment to observe the student reading for an extended period of time in order to find out whether he or she is becoming fatigued. The teacher of students with visual impairments may be able to provide some information about whether the student typically develops fatigue when completing tasks that require the use of vision. If not, the examiner may want to question the student, the student's parents, classroom teachers, and other service providers who work with the student.

If fatigue is a major factor affecting the student's ability to complete educational tasks, the examiner will need to schedule assessment sessions at which he or she can observe the student using various devices for extended periods to determine how each affects the onset of fatigue (see Figure 7.9). These observations may indicate that the student will benefit from using different tools at different times during the day, depending on the reading and writing requirements of the task to be completed and the degree of fatigue experienced by the student. Data may need to be gathered on the student's tendency to tire when using regular print, enlarged print, and large print with or without the use of optical devices or other adaptations. Another factor that affects fatigue is the fluctuating vision experienced by many individuals with low vision. Some students may be able to use their vision quite well early in the day, but then find that it is not very useful in the late afternoon or evening. Information about whether the student experiences this

Figure 7.9   Visual Access: Visual and Physical Fatigue

Section I: Accessing Print

A. Visual Access

8. Visual and Physical Fatigue   **Date completed** _____

The student experiences visual/physical fatigue after reading

    ❑ for ___ minutes **without** adaptations.
    ❑ for ___ minutes **with** adaptations.

Comments:
(Please indicate fatigue factors for each visual access tool used by the student.)

_____

_____

_____

type of fluctuating vision should be available from the teacher of students with visual impairments, the regular classroom teacher, or the student's parents. It is important to note this information, because it will greatly affect the usefulness of various tools when the student is experiencing visual or physical fatigue.

It is extremely important to determine how long the student can work with each device or adaptation before experiencing fatigue in order to determine a particular tool's effectiveness and efficiency for the student. The examiner will want to note these factors, perhaps by simply noting the name of the device followed by the number of minutes the student can use the device before experiencing fatigue. More detailed information can be incorporated into the recommendations and final report of the assessment (see Chapter 8).

TACTILE ACCESS AND BRAILLE

Some students may find that the tools for accessing print information visually are not adequate for all tasks, and that they experience visual fatigue to the extent that at times they are not able to use their vision effectively. These students and those who already use braille will want to investigate tools that allow them to access information tactilely. This section of the assistive technology assessment process is *not* intended to be used to determine if braille should be the student's primary reading medium. The information from the student's learning media assessment described in Chapter 6 will guide the assessment team in identifying the student's reading media and exploring his or her potential for using tools that provide tactile access to information. The

examiner will want to be sure to explore the option of tactilely accessing both graphical and print information. Therefore, in this section of the assessment (see Figure 7.10) only the student's ability to use tactile graphics and a refreshable braille display to access print information will be explored. (For more information on these tools see Chapter 2.) In general, information about the student's ability to read braille should be available from the teacher of students with visual impairments as part of regular progress monitoring of the student's work in language arts and may be helpful in judging a student's performance during assessment. (Other tools for working with tactile information are assessed in the succeeding sections of the assessment form, "Accessing Electronic Information," and "Communicating through Writing.")

Tactile Graphics

Materials Needed

- Samples of various types of tactile graphics that include these tactile features:

  ▶ solid lines of various thickness;
  ▶ dashed lines;
  ▶ dotted lines;
  ▶ two, three, and four tactile fill patterns (texture added within the outline of an area) separated into clearly defined sections;
  ▶ a map or drawing where the boundaries of the textual changes are less well defined.

- Samples of various types of tactile graphics, including those

  ▶ tooled onto braille paper;

Figure 7.10 Tactile Access and Braille

Section I: Accessing Print

B. Tactile Access and Braille   **Date completed** _____

When accessing graphical information the student is able to discriminate tactilely
- ❑ solid lines of various thickness.
- ❑ dashed lines.
- ❑ dotted lines.
- ❑ raised-line drawings of simple shapes.
- ❑ the boundary between two clearly defined textured fill patterns.
- ❑ the boundary between three clearly defined textured fill patterns.
- ❑ the boundary between four clearly defined textured fill patterns.

The student is able to identify tactile information most accurately when it is presented as a simple tactile graphic
- ❑ tooled onto braille paper.
- ❑ produced as a collage of varying textures.
- ❑ thermoformed onto plastic.
- ❑ embossed as dots and lines onto braille paper by a computer-controlled braille embosser.
- ❑ produced as raised lines and patterns on capsule paper.

The student is able to read materials in
- ❑ uncontracted braille.
- ❑ contracted braille.

Results of formal or informal braille assessments conducted by the teacher of students with visual impairments are attached.
   Student's oral braille reading rate is _____ words per minute (wpm).
   Student's silent braille reading rate is _____ wpm.

When accessing print information with a refreshable braille display, the student is able to
- ❑ read instructional-level text.
- ❑ press correct key combination to issue forward and reverse navigation commands
   - ❑ with verbal prompt.
   - ❑ without verbal prompt.
- ❑ read ____ wpm orally and ____ wpm silently.

The student is willing to use these devices (the examiner may wish to list these separately)
- ❑ to complete assignments in the regular classroom.
- ❑ at home to complete school assignments.
- ❑ while working with the teacher of students with visual impairments.

Comments: _____

_____

_____

- produced as a collage of varying textures;
- thermoformed onto plastic;
- embossed as dots and lines onto braille paper by a computer controlled braille embosser;
- produced as raised lines and patterns on capsule paper.
- Braille samples of text on the student's independent reading level

This section of the assessment begins with an evaluation of the student's ability to work with tactile materials. Teacher-made tactile graphics or commercial products can be used to determine the student's ability to obtain information tactilely. Because tactile graphics produced through different production methods vary in their ability to convey information, students should be assessed using samples of tactile graphics produced using the various methods discussed in Chapter 4—tooling, collage, thermoform, embossing on paper by a computer-controlled braille embosser, and raised drawings on encapsulated paper—and that vary from simple to complex.

Procedure

- Determine if the student can identify raised-line drawings of simple shapes and objects. Ask the student to identify these simple graphics rendered by the various production methods available and to indicate which format is easiest to feel.
- Show the student a graphic with four or five straight lines of the same height about 1 inch apart. Ask the student to identify the number of lines.
- Show the student a graphic with four lines of one height and a single

higher line and ask the student if there is anything different about these lines. Ask the student to identify what is different.
- Repeat this approach to determine if the student is able to distinguish and identify graphics using solid, dashed, and dotted lines and lines made up of a pattern of dots and dashes.
- Ask the student to distinguish between different types of textured fill patterns, including those where the boundaries of the textual changes are less well defined.
- Show the student graphics produced by a variety of tactile graphic production methods and note the methods that the student is best able to use for interpreting simple, intermediate, and complex graphics.

Braille Reading Rate

Before evaluating a student's use of tactile information and the materials and equipment that best support it, such as a refreshable braille display, it would be wise for the examiner to acquire the results of any braille assessments that have been conducted with a student who reads braille to determine the effects of the different devices tried during the assessment on his or her braille reading ability. If none have been administered, then the evaluation team will want to have the teacher of students with visual impairments administer some braille assessments in addition to the assistive technology assessment. (Some braille assessment instruments are available from the web site of the Texas School for the Blind and Visually Impaired; see the Resources section.) Particular attention should be paid to the student's mastery of the mechanics of braille reading, word attack skills, reading fluency, comprehension, and writing rate to help the examiner and the assistive technology specialist determine whether to recommend an electronic refreshable braille display for the student.

If the student's braille reading rate is not available at the time of the assessment, the examiner will need to make an informal assessment, or be sure to include any additional information gathered by the teacher of students with visual impairments in doing an assessment of the student's braille reading skills.

Materials Needed

- Sufficient correctly formatted braille materials at the student's independent reading level so that he or she can practice oral and silent reading before the timed assessment. (It may be easiest to use an informal reading inventory, such as the Johns *Basic Reading Inventory*, which is available in braille from the Texas School for the Blind and Visually Impaired in its *Assessment Kit* [Sewell, 1997].)

Procedure

- Have the student practice reading a braille passage to become comfortable with reading the material aloud.
- Time the student reading an additional passage on his or her independent reading level
- Calculate the rate and record it.
- Repeat this procedure with the student reading silently to determine an informal silent reading rate.

Refreshable Braille Display

The final area of tactile access to print to assess is the student's ability to use a refreshable braille display. If the school does not have access to a refreshable braille display, the assessment team will need to investigate alternative sources to borrow one for the assessment. (Sidebar 6.4, "Wait! I Don't Have One of Those!" in Chapter 6 gives suggestions on how to explore these resources.) The student's tactile sensitivity to the pins used to display the dots should be noted, along with his or her ability to manipulate the control keys and understanding of the concept of changing the display to read forward and backward along the braille line.

Procedure

- Demonstrate the braille display and allow the student to read the display with the examiner controlling the unit.
- Ask the student to read the text on the display.
- Show the student how to advance the display to the next segment of text and allow the student to manipulate the control.
- Ask the student to read aloud the text on the display and advance the display when needed.
- Practice doing this with the student for several minutes and determine if the student is physically able to operate the device.
- Note how many repetitions of the command were required before the student performed the advance command without a verbal prompt.
- After the student becomes comfortable reading with the display, ask the student to read a passage aloud and time the student to get a rough reading rate.

AUDITORY ACCESS

Before administering the auditory access section of the assessment, it is helpful for the examiner to consult the student's psychological evaluation (if one is available) and note his or her performance on tasks that require the use of auditory skills. The examiner should be aware of any auditory discrimination or auditory memory deficits, and if the student has any auditory processing issues. If these exist, the examiner may wish to consult with the school psychologist to discuss how these characteristics might affect the student's abilities to access information auditorily. During this part of the assessment, the examiner will want to determine if the student has the auditory skills to discriminate various sounds, understand recorded and synthesized speech, comprehend information presented in this format, and remember what is heard. If the student has undergone assessments such as the Listening Assessment of the *Brigance Comprehensive Inventory of Basic Skills—Revised* (Brigance, 1999) or the Listening Skills component of the *Assessment Kit* from the Texas School for the Blind and Visually Impaired (Sewell, 1997), these tests will also supply information about the student's auditory discrimination (such as the ability to discriminate beginning and ending consonants, medial vowels, and blends), auditory memory (ability to repeat sentences or follow multistage directions), and listening comprehension.

Live Readers and Recorded Information

This section of the assessment seeks to gather data about the student's ability to understand and retain information presented aloud by a live reader (the examiner) or different types of audio players (see Figure 7.11). Does the student remember and understand what he or she hears? Can the student understand recorded or synthesized speech, and can the student comprehend the information presented? Is the student physically able to manipulate an audio player and its controls?

Although some recorded information and books are still available on cassette tapes, most are currently available on CDs (compact discs) or in MP3 or other audio file formats. This technology is changing rapidly, and in the near future most recorded books will be available on CDs or simply as electronic files. They will either be recorded or scanned into a computer and reproduced through synthesized speech, and then saved on some type of easily portable memory storage device, such as a flash drive, SD (secure data) card, or memory stick. Regardless of the storage medium, however, some type of device will be needed to play or listen to the information. These new devices will have controls similar to those found on cassette players, which must be understood and physically manipulated by the user. Therefore, most of the items to be explored in this part of the assessment can be completed even if the examiner has access only to a modified tape player or recorder with the features discussed in Chapter 2. Preferably, the examiner will be able to explore the various media available at the time of the assessment (cassettes, CDs, memory storage devices, MP3 files, digital books, and so forth), paying particular attention to the recording medium used for textbooks and other educational materials that will be needed by the student.

Materials Needed

- APH Handicassette II or other modified tape player or recorder

Figure 7.11   Auditory Access: Live Readers and Recorded Information

Section I: Accessing Print

C. Auditory Access

1. Live Readers and Recorded Information   Date completed _____

When listening to instructional level information read aloud by the evaluator, the student is able to
- ❑ repeat words and simple phrases without having them repeated more than twice.
- ❑ paraphrase the information (a sentence or story).
- ❑ answer simple comprehension questions.

When listening to an analog or digital recording of a story, the student is able to
- ❑ repeat words and simple phrases without having them repeated more than twice.
- ❑ paraphrase the information (a sentence or story).
- ❑ accurately answer simple comprehension questions.

When using an analog or digital player-recorder, the student is able to
- ❑ insert and remove a tape or CD from the player-recorder.
- ❑ activate play, pause, stop, fast forward, and rewind functions (underline those demonstrated).
- ❑ understand and comprehend compressed or "fast" speech.
- ❑ manipulate variable speed and pitch controls.
- ❑ identify index tones, bookmarks, and page locators.

The student is able to
- ❑ listen to recorded speech and follow along with a print copy of the text.
- ❑ listen to recorded speech and follow along with a braille copy of the text.
- ❑ listen to synthesized speech and follow along with a print copy of the text.
- ❑ listen to synthesized speech and follow along with a braille copy of the text.

The student is able to read approximately
____ words per minute (wpm) when listening and reading print or braille.

The student is willing to use these devices (the examiner may wish to list these separately)
- ❑ to complete assignments in the regular classroom.
- ❑ at home to complete school assignments.
- ❑ while working with the teacher of students with visual impairments.

Comments: _____
_____
_____

- Digital Talking Book player
- Digital recorder
- Digital book player
- Sample recordings on topics of high interest to the student
- Reading passage containing a few paragraphs on a topic of high interest to the student that can be read aloud by the examiner
- Reading passages on the student's independent reading level in print, braille, audio recording, and produced by synthesized speech

Procedure

- Read an appropriate grade-level passage to the student. (It may be easiest to use samples from an informal reading inventory, such as the Johns [2008] *Basic Reading Inventory*.)
- Ask the student to relate some details of the story and to answer some simple factual questions.
- Note if the student is able to paraphrase the information presented in the story.
- Dictate some simple sentences and ask the student to braille, write, type, or speak the sentences. Note the student's ability to remember the dictation and how many times the information must be repeated.
- Demonstrate the features of the player or recorder being used, including start, stop, pause, review, and fast-forward.
- Direct the student to perform different tasks that will demonstrate his or her ability to manipulate the controls and understand their functions, such as the following:

  ▶ Press the fast-forward button.
  ▶ Press the play button.
  ▶ Press the stop button.
  ▶ Press the rewind button.
  ▶ Press the stop button.
  ▶ Press the play button.
  ▶ Press the pause button.
  ▶ Press the stop button.

- Demonstrate the player or recorder's variable speed and pitch controls by playing an audio recording or an age-appropriate passage.
- Gradually increase the rate at which the audio information is being played, and adjust the pitch control until the reader's speech is at its normal-sounding pitch.
- Ask the student if he or she can understand the reader.
- Stop the recorder and ask the student to repeat or paraphrase what he or she just heard.
- Repeat this step several times.
- Increase the rate once again, adjust the pitch of the speech, and ask the student to repeat or paraphrase what he or she hears.
- Ask the student to increase the rate slightly and then adjust the pitch until it sounds like a normal pitched voice.
- Repeat the steps involving the player or recorder for any different type of device.
- Note the results, along with any comments or observations.

Audio-assisted reading, discussed in Chapters 2 and 3, pairs the use of audio information with either print or braille. Many individuals find accessing information in two modalities to be very helpful. The examiner will want to provide the student with an opportunity to explore this option and note the student's relative success using this methodology. After providing the student with an opportunity to practice using this reading technique, the examiner should conduct an informal measurement of the student's reading rate when listening to and reading in print or braille a selection on his or her independent reading level.

Specialized Scanning Systems for Accessing Print Information Auditorily

Materials Needed

- Computer system with a flat bed scanner
- Optical character recognition software (such as Kurzweil 1000 and 3000, OpenBook, and WYNN)
- Reading samples at the student's independent reading level

As noted earlier and in Chapter 2, specialized computer-based scanning systems such as Kurzweil 1000 and 3000, WYNN, and OpenBook are designed to be used by individuals with visual impairments or reading difficulties and offer numerous features that make them much easier to use than mainstream optical character recognition (OCR) programs. Text that is scanned into the computer with an optical scanner can be accessed auditorily with software that will verbalize the text using synthesized speech. The objective of this section of the assessment (see Figure 7.12) is to determine if the student has the cognitive and physical ability to use these tools. The examiner will need to scan some appropriate text into the computer and save it as an electronic file.

Procedure

- Demonstrate the speech and navigation controls of the programs.
- Ask the student to execute these controls with the keyboard or mouse.
- Note if the student is able to use the navigation features of the program and understand the basic functions of the menu system, submenus, dialog boxes, and their controls.

READING RATES

The section of the assessment checklist on reading rates (see Figure 7.13) is not a separate part of the assessment, but rather an optional section to organize information that can be used when needed to demonstrate to a student, parents, teachers, or administrators the benefits of using particular adaptations and assistive technology for accessing print information and reading. Most of the information to complete this section will already have been gathered and available in previous sections of the form.

Often students do not want to use technologies or adaptations that might make them look "different," but it is sometimes difficult to know which adaptations will be acceptable to a student and which will not. Students may not always need to use the adaptation that provides the greatest reading efficiency for every reading task or in every environment, but the data in this section might help a student understand the efficiency of using a particular adaptation to accomplish certain tasks in certain settings. Some adaptations or devices require more practice than the time spent during the assessment will offer before the efficiency they provide is evident. In general, it may be best not to reveal to the student the exact intent of the procedures carried out with the different reading approaches and technologies. If the student is aware of the examiner's efforts to determine the approach that yields the best reading rate, he or she may choose to read more slowly with a device that is disliked. Therefore, it is important to measure the reading rates with each device separately and before the discussion about the student's willingness to use the tools in various settings. The ultimate goal is to help the student and all parties involved understand that better results may be obtained by using different adaptations for different tasks.

ACCESSING INFORMATION PRESENTED AT A DISTANCE

The final area to examine related to accessing print involves ascertaining how the student typically accesses print information

Figure 7.12   Specialized Scanning Systems for Accessing Print Information

Section I: Accessing Print

C. Auditory Access

2. Specialized Scanning Systems for Accessing Print Information Auditorily   Date completed _____

When accessing printed materials scanned into the computer with a specialized scanning system (such as Kurzweil 1000 and 3000, OpenBook, and WYNN), the student is able to
- ❏ adjust the rate and other speech parameters.
- ❏ navigate through the document when provided instruction by the evaluator.
- ❏ select items from the menus or tools from the toolbar when provided instruction by the evaluator.

When listening to text read by the program, the student is able to
- ❏ repeat words and simple phrases without having them repeated more than twice.
- ❏ paraphrase the information (sentence or story).
- ❏ accurately answer simple comprehension questions.

The student is willing to use these devices (the examiner may wish to list these separately)
- ❏ to complete assignments in the regular classroom.
- ❏ at home to complete school assignments.
- ❏ while working with the teacher of students with visual impairments.

When accessing print materials using audio-assisted reading the student is able to read ____ words per minute (wpm).

Comments: _____
_____
_____

displayed in the classroom at a distance—for example, information on a chalkboard or whiteboard, on an overhead or computer projector, on a video monitor, or on other electronic display devices. This information can be obtained from the teacher of students with visual impairments, the classroom teacher, and the student.

Print information is displayed in classrooms for two basic purposes: Some information is intended simply to be read, whereas other information is meant to be copied or recorded by the students. As explained in Chapter 2, there are a wide variety of adaptations and devices that can help students access information at a distance, depending on both what they need to do with the information and their individual needs (see Figure 7.14). Some students are able to sit close enough to information to read it, others may choose to walk up and read the information, and still others may use an optical or electronic device. Another option is to provide the student an accessible copy of the information. For some students, having someone read or dictate information while he or she brailles, writes, types, or records it is a workable option.

Probably the most critical information to obtain about the methods a student uses for accessing information displayed at a distance is how effective these tools are for the student. Do they allow the student to access the information in a reasonable amount of time? Has the student tried other options? The examiner should note this information and be ready to discuss the need for any changes in the final report presented to the IEP team.

Figure 7.13   Reading Rates

Section I: Accessing Print

D. Reading Rates   **Date completed** _____

Optional; may be used to support use of various adaptations.

When accessing print information, the student is able to read

____ words per minute (wpm) orally when reading materials in 12-point type using prescribed spectacles or contact lenses.

____ wpm orally when reading materials in the optimum point size and font:

____ -point print and _____ font.

____ wpm orally when reading with a prescribed optical device.

____ wpm orally when reading with a video magnifier (CCTV).

____ wpm orally when reading braille.

____ wpm when using audio-assisted reading.

Comments: _____

_____

_____

Figure 7.14   Accessing Information Presented at a Distance

Section I: Accessing Print

E. Accessing Information Presented at a Distance

Date completed _____

When accessing information presented at a distance on a chalkboard or whiteboard or by an overhead or computer projector or TV/VCR/DVD, the student reported that he or she

- ❑ sits close enough to view the information, at a working distance of approximately _____ feet.
- ❑ uses a handheld or spectacle-mounted telescope.
- ❑ uses a video magnifier with distance-viewing capabilities.
- ❑ gets an accessible copy from the teacher.
- ❑ uses a peer notetaker.
- ❑ uses an electronic whiteboard connected to an accessible computer.
- ❑ has information read aloud by a peer or paraeducator and
  - ❑ brailles information on a braillewriter.
  - ❑ writes information on paper.
  - ❑ inputs information into computer or accessible personal digital assistant.
  - ❑ records information on tape recorder or digital recorder.
- ❑ other (specify): _____.

Are these options working adequately?

- ❑ Yes
- ❑ No

Explain briefly:

_____

_____

The student is willing to use these devices and accommodations (the examiner may wish to list them individually)

- ❑ to complete assignments in the regular classroom.

Comments: _____

_____

_____

The examiner will also need to investigate how information is presented in the student's classes to see whether other technology tools might be useful. For example, if the classes use whiteboards, the examiner will want to expose the student to technology that offers the option of displaying the information written on the whiteboard on a computer to determine the potential of this tool for use in accessing information presented at a distance.

SECTION II: ACCESSING ELECTRONIC INFORMATION

Computer Access: Output Devices

- Visual Access
- Tactile Access
- Auditory Access

Computer Access: Input Devices

- Keyboard Input
- Pointing Device Input

Accessing Electronic Information Using a Personal Digital Assistant (PDA)

Electronic Calculators and Dictionaries

- Electronic Calculators
- Talking Dictionaries

As more and more information becomes available electronically, the need for tools to help students who are blind or visually impaired to access this information also increases. Chapter 3 provides information about the various ways students can obtain information from computers, the Internet, or other electronic devices and tools. Generally, a computer system with the appropriate adaptations will provide a student with visual impairments with an ideal tool for accessing electronic information as well as producing written communication. In assessing the types of technology that will provide the greatest benefit for a student, the examiner needs to look at the most efficient methods the student can use to both input electronic information and to retrieve—output—it visually, tactilely, or auditorily.

COMPUTER ACCESS: OUTPUT DEVICES

Accessing a computer's output generally refers to the information on its monitor or visual display. As with other information discussed in this book, students may use vision, hearing, or touch, or some combination of these senses, to obtain this information.

Visual Access

Materials Needed

- Windows-based computer system (The assessment can be conducted with a Macintosh computer, but the examiner will need to modify the assessment checklist, if used, and make sure that the basic intent of all the items is covered.)
- Appropriate reading samples saved as documents on the computer in 14, 18, 24, 30, and 36 points in each of the following fonts: Arial, APHont, Tahoma, Verdana
- Hardware screen magnifier (such as a Fresnel lens that attaches to the monitor)

- Fully adjustable articulating monitor arm and an LCD (liquid crystal display) monitor
- Full-featured screen magnification program

There are a number of options that students with low vision can use to access the information on a computer (see Figure 7.15). When beginning to assess a student with low vision on a computer, the examiner should make sure that any eyeglasses or contact lenses the student uses are in place. The examiner should also take the opportunity to observe the student's position at the computer itself. Students with low vision may bend over to get close to the monitor to see the display, which usually causes their abdomen to push against their wrists and hands, resulting in inefficient keyboarding. Although this posture may not be a problem for short reading and writing activities, it will not be efficient for most educational tasks. In reviewing the adaptations available for accessing the computer, the examiner should keep in mind which options will best allow the student to work from a good ergonomic position.

Most students will require some type of adaptation or modification to work efficiently with a computer system, but some will not use any. The examiner should first assess the student's functioning on the computer without adaptations, by asking the student to read and identify screen elements such as menus, icon titles, and dialog boxes, and then repeat the same steps with various types of adaptations.

Procedure

- Ask the student to read the names of some of the icons on the computer screen when it is displaying the standard Windows Desktop, and measure his or her working distance.
- Open the Windows Start Menu (by left clicking on the Start button one time, pressing Control + Escape, or by pressing the Windows key if one is available on the keyboard being used). Ask the student to read items on this menu.
- Measure the working distance at which the student can read this menu.
- Press the Escape key to retract or hide the Start Menu.
- Right click on any icon. Select the Properties item from the menu that will appear. A dialog box will be displayed.
- Ask the student to read text in the dialog box.
- Measure the working distance at which the student can identify these items.
- Note the working distance and the monitor size being used.

If the student is able to identify the various screen elements and read the text, even with a short working distance, the examiner may want to repeat these steps with larger monitors and an adjustable monitor stand, as described in the following section on screen-enlarging hardware.

To ascertain the best type sizes and font for the student, the examiner can use the prepared word-processing file containing appropriate words and sentences in various fonts and point sizes, from 14 to 36:

- Open the prepared word-processing file.
- Open the View Menu and select Normal.

Figure 7.15 Computer Access: Visual Output Devices

Section II: Accessing Electronic Information

A. Computer Access: Output Devices

1. Visual Access   **Date completed** _____

The student is able to view electronic information on a desktop computer or in the computer lab without additional adaptations and identify or read

    ❏ text   ❏ icon titles   ❏ menus   ❏ dialog boxes   ❏ other system items on a

        ❏ 17-inch monitor at approximately ___ inches.
        ❏ 19-inch monitor at approximately ___ inches.
        ❏ 21-inch monitor at approximately ___ inches.
        ❏ other (specify): _____

The student prefers viewing text in a word-processing program on the computer in
    ___-point type in   ❏ regular   ❏ bold print
    ❏ Arial
    ❏ APHont
    ❏ Tahoma
    ❏ Verdana
    ❏ other (specify): _____
    displayed on a ___ -inch monitor at approximately ___ inches.

The student is able to view electronic information on a
    ___ -inch computer monitor with the use of
        ❏ screen magnification hardware at approximately ____ inches.
        ❏ an articulated flexible monitor stand at approximately ___ inches.

The student is able to view electronic information using the computer operating system's screen enhancements such as
    ❏ screen resolution (specify): _____.
    ❏ Windows Display Appearance Scheme (specify): _____.
    ❏ Windows Display Appearance Settings. (*Record specific settings selected on the Windows Display Properties Appearance Checklist appendix to this form.*)

    ❏ Microsoft Magnifier
        ❏ magnification level: _____
        ❏ other setting (specify): _____

The student is able to use the Microsoft Magnifier to
- ❑ identify screen elements.
- ❑ read text in menus, dialog boxes, and text documents.
- ❑ navigate around the screen.
- ❑ locate the file names listed in the Open file dialog box.
- ❑ select a requested file to open.

(If the school district uses Macintosh computers, complete the previous sections for the accessibility features provided in the computer's operating system.)

When using a dedicated screen magnification program, the student is able to
- ❑ read 12-point print enlarged to _____× magnification at a working distance of approximately 13 inches.
- ❑ locate and select menu items, buttons, and other screen elements with the mouse or other pointing device.
- ❑ locate and select menu items, buttons, and other screen elements using keyboard commands.
- ❑ navigate around the screen and maintain orientation.
- ❑ use an automatic reading feature at a speed setting of _____.

The student's color preference is _____ text on a _____ background.

❑ The student is unable to access the computer visually.

The student is willing to use these devices (the examiner may wish to list these separately)
- ❑ to complete assignments in the regular classroom.
- ❑ at home to complete school assignments.
- ❑ while working with the teacher of students with visual impairments.

Comments: _____
_____
_____

- Open the View Menu again and select Zoom.
- From the Zoom dialog box, select the Page Width radio button to display the text at the full width of the monitor. In most cases this will have the effect of enlarging the image of the text.
- Ask the student to read the text. Some students may need text at a point size larger than 36 points. Be prepared to present appropriate text at larger sizes if necessary.
- Measure the working distance and identify the point size and font that the student can read at approximately 10–13 inches distance and record this information.

Screen-Enlarging Hardware

Adaptations that enlarge the image on a computer monitor are available as either hardware attachments or software applications, and a student's use of these options need to be explored.

Large Monitor. The simplest hardware adaptation is a larger monitor. At the time of this writing, most stand-alone computers are equipped with a 17-inch CRT (cathode ray tube) monitor or an LCD (liquid crystal display) monitor. If different monitors are available, try the same procedure as in the previous section with a 19-inch, 21-inch, or even larger monitor. When using a larger monitor, the examiner will need to be aware that the distance between the student's eyes and the edges of the monitor dramatically increase with monitors 25 inches and larger. With large monitors like these, the text that is farther away may be as hard to see as smaller text that is closer—possibly negating the effects of the increased text and object size. Therefore, the student's ability

to view information presented at different locations on the monitor needs to be carefully assessed before recommending the use of a very large monitor. The objective is to determine the combinations of font, point size, and monitor size that will allow the student to access the computer at a comfortable distance. Knowing these combinations will enable the assessment team to recommend appropriate tools for various tasks performed on the computer.

Hardware Screen Magnifiers. Several hardware screen magnifiers are available that attach to the front of the monitor and magnify the screen's image approximately 1.25×–2×.

- Place one of these devices on the monitor, if available, and ask the student to read or identify the various Windows screen elements, as done earlier without adaptations.
- Measure and note the working distance.

Many students will experience only a very slight improvement in their ability to read the screen using this type of device. Careful measurement is required, therefore, because the student may be reading the screen at the same working distance he or she does without the device or at only one or two inches further away and thus this type of device may not be of sufficient benefit.

Flexible Monitor Stand. Another hardware option that the examiner will need to investigate is a monitor stand with an articulated flexible arm. This standard office accessory allows the monitor to be placed on a platform that is suspended above the table. Its height and the distance from the viewer's eyes can be easily adjusted for maximum viewing. The objective here is to determine if the monitor stand can place the monitor screen at the appropriate height and distance from the user to allow the student to comfortably view the screen while maintaining an ergonomically correct posture. Monitor arms for LCD monitors are more flexible than those for CRT monitors, but the stands for CRTs will provide adequate positioning for some students. The flexible monitor stand can be a very good solution for some students because it requires little adaptation to the computer system and is a typical piece of office furniture—a point that may be important to some students who are uncomfortable using adaptive devices. Although many examiners may not have access to this type of equipment, if the student can read visually the basic screen elements (menus, dialog boxes, and so forth) at a distance of 6 inches or more, then a flexible monitor arm may be a viable solution.

Software Options

Most computer operating systems offer accessibility options that allow the user to adjust the display of information on the screen. The user can adjust the screen resolution; the text font, size and color; the background color; and the size of other screen elements.

Accessibility Wizard and Display Preferences. Microsoft Windows 98 and higher operating systems also offer an Accessibility Wizard that can be used to guide the examiner through a series of settings designed to make the screen display accessible for users with low vision. (See Appendix 7F, "Assessing Display Settings Using the Accessibility Wizard.") If these settings are not sufficient, additional adjustments can be made in the Display Properties menu to improve the visibility of the display for individual users. (See Appendix 7G, "Procedure for Assessing

Student Display Preferences," for instructions on how to adjust these options to produce the best display setting for the user and record your findings on the Windows Display Properties Appearance Checklist [Figure 7.16], which is an appendix to the assessment checklist form.) The examiner will need to develop a good working knowledge of these features before presenting them to the student.

Although the adjustments that can be made using the options built into the Windows operating system may be sufficient for some students to work in a word-processing program, they do not magnify all items displayed on the screen by applications, such as an encyclopedia or educational program. The advantage of these accessories, however, is that they are provided with the computer at no additional expense. If a student is able to work efficiently with this level of adaptation, along with using a word processor's ability to enlarge fonts, this combination can provide an effective and affordable tool for accessing some electronic information and for producing written communication.

Microsoft Magnifier. Another accessibility feature offered by the Windows operating system is a program called Microsoft Magnifier. It is accessed through the Accessibility Wizard (as described in Appendix 7F) or through the Accessibility menu. (See Appendix 7H, "Assessing the Student's Ability to Use Microsoft Magnifier," for instructions on assessing the student's use of this feature.) The Microsoft Magnifier and the other accessibility options may offer adequate access for some individuals with low vision, but many students will need the power of a full-featured screen magnification program.

Screen Magnification Software. Dedicated screen magnification software programs

Figure 7.16   Windows Display Properties Appearance Checklist

Appendix: Windows Display Properties Appearance Checklist

Items Adjusted

❑ 3D Objects
    Color _____

❑ Active Title Bar
    Size _____   Color _____
    Font _____
            ____ Size ____ Color ____ Bold ____ Italic

❑ Active Window Border
    Size _____   Color _____

❑ Application Background
    Color _____

❑ Caption Buttons
    Size _____

❑ Desktop
    Color _____

❑ Icons
    Size _____
    Font _____
            ____ Size ____ Bold ____ Italic

❑ Icon Spacing (Vertical)
    Size _____

❑ Icon Spacing (Horizontal)
    Size _____

❑ Inactive Title Bar
    Size _____   Color _____
    Font _____
            ____ Size ____ Color ____ Bold ____ Italic

❑ Inactive Window Border
    Size _____   Color _____

❏ Menu
  Size _____   Color _____
  Font _____
          ____ Size ____ Color ____ Bold ____ Italic

❏ Message Box
  Font _____
          ____ Size ____ Color ____ Bold ____ Italic

❏ Palette Title
  Size _____
  Font _____
          ____ Size ____ Bold ____ Italic

❏ Scrollbar
  Size _____

❏ Selected Items
  Size _____   Color _____
  Font _____
          ____ Size ____ Color ____ Bold ____ Italic

❏ ToolTip
  Color _____
  Font _____
          ____ Size ____ Color ____ Bold ____ Italic

❏ Window
  Color _____

provide the additional features and greater magnification needed by many users. In addition, they offer features to customize the way that information is displayed on the screen. Some programs offer an automatic reading or review mode, and others even offer paired synthesized speech with the review mode and other speech features. Appendix 7I, "Completing the Screen Magnification Software Assessment," provides step-by-step directions for assessing the student's potential for using screen magnification software.

Some students may require a high degree of magnification (5× or more) to view the screen at a comfortable working distance. When using a high degree of magnification, only a small amount of information can be displayed on the screen at any one time, which can decrease the user's speed and efficiency. In such cases, the examiner should also investigate the user's potential for accessing electronic information both visually and auditorily, auditorily alone, or tactilely.

Tactile Access

Materials Needed

- Computer with screen-reading software and a dedicated refreshable braille display or an accessible personal digital assistant (PDA) with a braille display
- Appropriate reading passages saved as a document on the computer or accessible PDA

Accessing electronic information tactilely entails the use of an electronic refreshable braille display in one of two forms: a dedicated device that connects directly to the computer, or a display that is part of an accessible personal digital assistant (PDA), which can be connected to a computer. For many braille readers this technology offers the ideal access to computers and electronic information, and it is becoming more affordable. However, the use of electronic refreshable braille displays is not widespread in the schools, and many teachers of students with visual impairments may not have access to one to complete this section of an assistive technology assessment. If the student is a braille reader, it is very important that the examiner acquire a braille display for the assessment process. Many students will be much more efficient at accessing information through the use of braille than with synthesized speech. A braille display can also be a valuable tool for less experienced braille readers to improve their braille-reading skills. If a braille display is not available, the examiner may need to contact a vendor to assist with this section of the assessment, as discussed in Chapter 6.

The objective of the assessment done with a braille display (see Figure 7.17) is to determine whether the student has the tactile sensitivity to read the refreshable braille and the cognitive ability to execute the necessary commands and to understand the concepts involved in navigating around the text being displayed.

Procedure

- Ask the student to read some prepared sentences on the braille display and note the results.
- Demonstrate the commands required to navigates by line, sentence, word, and character, and then ask the student to execute some of these commands.
- Ask the student to enter a few sentences and then read them back.
- Note the student's performance and add any necessary comments.

Auditory Access

Materials Needed

- Computer system with screen-reading software
- A variety of speech synthesizers, both software and hardware
- Documents or files containing appropriate statements, questions, and reading passages prepared for all synthesizers
- Talking word processor program

All modern computers can produce synthesized speech through the use of a dedicated speech synthesizer, or the computer's sound card, speakers, and the appropriate software (see Chapter 3 for more details). For many individuals who use their sense of hearing to obtain information, the use of synthesized speech is an effective way to access electronic information.

Figure 7.17   Computer Access: Tactile Output Devices

Section II: Accessing Electronic Information

A. Computer Access: Output Devices

1. Tactile Access   Date completed _____

When accessing electronic or computer-based information tactilely, the student is able to
- ❑ read braille text displayed on a dedicated braille display connected to a computer.
- ❑ read braille text displayed on an accessible PDA braille display connected to a computer.
- ❑ execute navigation commands with instruction.
- ❑ enter text through the braille keyboard, if available.

The student is willing to use these devices (the examiner may wish to list these separately)
- ❑ to complete assignments in the regular classroom.
- ❑ at home to complete school assignments.
- ❑ while working with the teacher of students with visual impairments.

Comments: _____
_____
_____

Assessment of a student's potential to use auditory access to a computer must answer two questions:

- Can the student understand and comprehend synthesized speech?
- Does the student have the physical and cognitive ability to execute the commands that control the program?

Most speech synthesizers today are software based, although hardware synthesizers are still available. The examiner will want to have several of each available for the assessment, if possible. Software synthesizers are usually available as part of programs that speak and use the computer's sound card to produce the speech, such as a talking word processor.

Synthesized Speech

In assessing a student's ability to use synthesized speech with computers, the first item to determine is the quality of speech that the student is able to understand and work with efficiently. Several talking word processors are available that can be used to assess the student's ability to understand synthesized speech. The examiner will need to create a variety of speech samples with each software synthesizer available. Some of these may be from talking word processors and some may be from dedicated screen-reading software. The examiner can follow the procedures outlined here with several different synthesizers and a screen-reading program to complete this part of the assessment.

Procedure

- Prepare files with the available software that speak age-appropriate statements and questions, such as, "Hello, _____." "This computer talks funny." "How old are you?" and "What is your favorite food?" Note the student's ability to understand sentences and words.

- Press letters on the computer keyboard and ask the student to identify them. Start with letters that have distinctive sounds (such as *a, f, h, o, s, w*).

- If the student is able to identify the distinctive-sounding letters, try using more confusing letters (*b, c, d, e, p, t, z*).

If no software or hardware synthesizers are available, a talking calculator or talking dictionary can be used to determine the student's ability to understand synthetic speech. If a student is able to understand the often unclear synthetic speech produced by one of these devices, he or she will likely be able to understand the higher quality speech produced by computer-based speech synthesizers.

If the student is able to answer the questions correctly and respond to the statements spoken, he or she will most likely be able to work with the quality of speech produced by the synthesizer being used. Most students who do not have any physical hearing loss or auditory processing deficits will be able to learn to understand synthesized speech and use it efficiently, even if they do not understand it perfectly the first time they hear it. During the assessment the student may need to hear multiple samples of each synthesizer in order to acclimate to its unique sound. This may require the examiner to have multiple files prepared for the assessment or be familiar enough with the equipment and the student to create statements and questions during the assessment.

Other software synthesizers are included as part of screen-reading programs, some screen magnification programs, and specialized scanning programs such as those developed by Kurzweil and OpenBook. The assessment procedure should be repeated with a variety of software speech synthesizers used in talking word processors and screen-reading software. The examiner can evaluate the student's performance with a variety of speech synthesizers by obtaining demonstration copies of these programs (see Chapter 6). The specific software and hardware synthesizers listed on the assessment form provided here (see Figure 7.18) are simply suggestions to make assessment teams aware of some of the common software programs that offer a software synthesizer. Examiners should feel free to use the synthesizers that they can access and note what is used in the "Other" section.

Hardware synthesizers may be a little harder to acquire for an assessment, but the assessment team ought to try to obtain several if at all possible (see Chapter 3 for more information about the advantages and disadvantages of hardware and software synthesizers). These vary in speech quality, and it is important to determine which ones the student can understand. Again, the examiner will need to prepare speech samples prior to the assessment and become familiar with the operation of the synthesizers. Most accessible PDAs contain hardware synthesizers. Hardware synthesizers require the use of a screen-reading program, so the examiner will need to have one installed for this part of the assessment. Many of these programs are able to speak punctuation, but this feature should be turned off for the assessment.

Figure 7.18 Computer Access: Auditory Output Devices

Section II: Accessing Electronic Information
A. Computer Access: Output Device

3. Auditory Access   Date completed _____

When accessing electronic information auditorily, the student is able to understand synthesized speech produced by

software synthesizers:
- ❑ Intellitalk
- ❑ TrueVoice
- ❑ OpenBook
- ❑ Other (specify): _____
- ❑ Write:Outloud
- ❑ DECTalk Access 32
- ❑ Microsoft Speech Engine
- ❑ Kurzweil
- ❑ Eloquence (JAWS)

hardware synthesizers:
- ❑ Type 'n Speak, Braille 'n Speak, Braille Lite
- ❑ Double Talk LT
- ❑ DECTalk Express
- ❑ Other (specify): _____

When accessing electronic information auditorily through synthesized speech and a screen reader the student is able to understand and identify
- ❑ sentences and lines.
- ❑ words.
- ❑ distinctive sounding letters (such as *a, f, h, o, s, w*) when spelled in words.
- ❑ similar sounding letters (*b, c, d, e, p, t, z*) when spelled in words.
- ❑ distinctive sounding letters (such as *a, f, h, o, s, w*) when spelled in isolation.
- ❑ similar sounding letters (*b, c, d, e, p, t, z*) when spelled in isolation.

When accessing electronic information auditorily through synthesized speech and a screen reader the student is able to execute navigation commands with instruction to
- ❑ read by characters.
- ❑ read by words.
- ❑ read by sentence and lines.
- ❑ move forward (to the next character, word, line).
- ❑ move backward (to the prior character, word, line).

❑ When accessing electronic information auditorily, the student was **not** able to grasp the concept of navigation.

The student is willing to use these devices (the examiner may wish to list these separately)
- ❑ to complete assignments in the regular classroom.
- ❑ at home to complete school assignments.
- ❑ while working with the teacher of students with visual impairments.

Comments: _____
_____
_____

Some students may have difficulty understanding the speech produced by some synthesizers but not by others. If this occurs, the examiner will want to further investigate the synthesizers the student can understand. To do this, the student should be asked to identify words and letters spoken individually. The examiner may find that the student is able to use context clues to understand statements and questions spoken by some synthesizers, but not understand individual words and letters. It will therefore be necessary to evaluate other synthesizers and determine which ones provide comprehensible speech for distinguishing words and letters. The student will need this level of understanding to use this tool effectively.

Navigation Using Screen-Reading Software

Once it has been determined whether the student can understand synthesized speech, it will be necessary to assess his or her ability to comprehend how a system conveys information and the concept of moving or navigating through a document using the screen reading program's keyboard commands.

Procedure

- Demonstrate the navigation commands used to read through a document by sentences, words, and characters
- Tell the student the commands to make the screen-reading program speak the current line or sentence and ask the student to execute that command.
- Repeat this step for the commands to read forward and backward through the text by words and characters.
- After the student has had several opportunities to execute these commands, ask him or her to read forward

and backward by several lines, sentences, words, or characters. Remind the student of the keystrokes used to execute the commands, if necessary.
- Record the student's responses and any appropriate comments.

As with most of the other devices and adaptations investigated in the assessment, the examiner will want to ask the student if he or she will be willing to use the technology to complete work at home, with the teacher of students with visual impairments, and in the regular classroom.

COMPUTER ACCESS: INPUT DEVICES

Once the examiner has gathered data about how the student will access the output of the computer—that is, its display—the next step is to determine what tools the student will use to input information or interact with the computer. Entering information into the computer can be accomplished in several ways, but the two most widely used input devices are still the traditional QWERTY (typewriter style) keyboard and the mouse or some other type of pointing device. Most students with visual impairments will be able to use one or both of these methods. If other input devices are needed, such as alternative keyboards—including six-key braille keyboards, switches, and voice recognition—the student's performance with these devices should be assessed by someone who is experienced in their use.

Keyboard Input

Keyboarding is an essential skill for students who are blind or visually impaired. Some students will already have some keyboarding skills, and others will have little or none. These skills may or may not include "touch typing," in which the keys are pressed while the individual is not looking at them. The procedures outlined in this section will help the examiner determine the student's basic knowledge of the keyboard and whether he or she is able to make use of it (see Figure 7.19). Because of the importance of keyboarding skills, the focus of the assessment is to provide the examiner with the data needed to make recommendations about the student's needs for keyboarding instruction and practice.

Materials Needed
- Accessible computer with word processing software and a standard QWERTY keyboard (preferably not a laptop)
- Flexible arm copy holder
- Prepared text samples in the student's preferred format (print or braille)

Procedure
- Open a blank word-processor file and the student's preferred method of screen access, as determined earlier in the assessment (such as a screen reader or screen magnifier).
- Ask the student to enter some simple text, such as his or her name, a few short sentences, and the alphabet.
- Note the student's ability to locate the alphanumeric keys and hold down the shift key to make a capital letter and how many fingers of each hand he or she uses when entering text.
- While the student is typing, observe his or her posture (the student should be sitting up straight with feet on the floor), the angle of the wrists and hands in relation to the keyboard, and the curvature of the fingers. Are

these mechanics of keyboarding consistent with best practices?
- Survey the student's ability to strike the intended key or its neighbor (a "miss-hit"), and his or her ability to lift the fingers before a letter is repeated ("key repeat").
- If the student has vision, determine whether the student is looking at the keys while typing or if he or she can enter text without looking at the keys.
- If the student has sufficient vision, set up a flexible arm copy holder that clamps onto the edge of a table. Place appropriate text samples in the student's preferred type size and font on the copy holder, or give the student the text samples in braille, and ask the student to enter the text into the computer.
- Read a text sample to the student and have him or her input the text into the computer.
- Obtain an estimate of the student's keyboarding speed when typing from dictation or from copy in print or braille.

If the student demonstrates physical difficulties while using the standard keyboard, there are various hardware and software adaptations that can help. Students with low vision and a physical deficit that will prevent them from becoming touch typists may benefit from enlarged identifying letters on the keys, referred to as "zoom caps." There are also enlarged keyboards that the examiner might wish to investigate. The examiner may also wish to seek assistance from an occupational or physical therapist to assess the student's ability to use some of the adaptations listed on the assessment form. Many of the keyboard utilities listed,

Figure 7.19   Computer Access: Keyboard Input

Section II: Accessing Electronic Information
B. Computer Access: Input Devices

1. Keyboard Use   Date completed _____

❑ The student is able to use a standard keyboard without adaptation.

The student

❑ demonstrates keyboard awareness (has a general knowledge of the key locations).
❑ is able to search for keys and type individual letters.
❑ is able to locate and identify alphanumeric keys.
❑ is able to locate and identify function keys.
❑ is able to activate two keys simultaneously.
❑ is able to touch type while looking at his or her hands
  ❑ from dictation.
  ❑ from braille copy.
  ❑ from copy that is presented in the student's preferred font and point size and positioned on a flexible-arm copy holder.
❑ is able to touch type without looking at his or her hands
  ❑ from dictation.
  ❑ from braille copy.
  ❑ from copy that is presented in the student's preferred font and point size and positioned on a flexible-arm copy holder.
❑ does not demonstrate excessive miss-hits or key repeats.
❑ uses good mechanics when typing (posture, wrist elevation, etc.).
❑ types with ___ fingers of right hand and ___ fingers of left hand.
❑ is able to type approximately ___ words per minute (wpm)
  ❑ from dictation.
  ❑ from braille copy.
  ❑ from copy that is presented in the student's preferred font and point size and positioned on a flexible-arm copy holder.

❑ The student is able to utilize a standard computer keyboard with the following adaptations: *(Seek assistance from an occupational or physical therapist as needed.)*
  ❑ zoom caps   ❑ keyguard   ❑ tactile locator dots
  ❑ other (specify): _____

❑ The student is able to utilize a standard computer keyboard with the following keyboard utilities: (*Seek assistance from an assistive technology specialist, occupational therapist, or physical therapist to complete this section.*)

    ❑ sticky keys   ❑ repeat keys   ❑ slow keys

    ❑ mouse keys   ❑ toggle keys

❑ The student is **not** able to utilize a standard keyboard with or without adaptations. *(If checked, refer student for a computer access evaluation.)*

Comments: _____

_____

_____

such as sticky keys, repeat keys, slow keys, mouse keys, and toggle keys (which, for example, make it easier for an individual to use keyboard combinations with one hand, ignore brief or repeated keystrokes, or control the mouse through the keyboard), can be accessed through the Accessibility Wizard discussed earlier in regard to visual access to computer output. If the student is unable to input text successfully using a standard keyboard with or without adaptations, the student should be referred to an assistive technology specialist, a rehabilitation engineer, or occupational and physical therapists for a computer access evaluation to determine the most effective method and tools for the student to use to input information into the computer.

Pointing Device Input

For most students with typical vision or low vision, the most commonly used pointing device is the mouse. However, some individuals prefer a trackball or a touch pad for their pointing device. Some people with low vision and most people who have no usable vision choose not to interact with the computer through a pointing device but prefer to use the keyboard. This section of the assessment evaluates the ability of students to make use of different types of pointing devices for computer input (see Figure 7.20).

Materials Needed

- Accessible computer system with mouse, trackball, and other pointing devices
- Cursor enhancement software

Procedure

- Ask the student to visually locate the Windows standard pointer on the screen. If the student is unable to locate this pointer, then follow the steps below to try larger, darker, or differently shaped pointers:
- Open the Start Menu.
- Select Control Panel.

Figure 7.20   Computer Access: Pointing Device (Mouse) Input

Section II: Accessing Electronic Information

B. Computer Access: Input Devices

2. Pointing Device (Mouse)   **Date completed** _____

The student is able to visually locate the pointer on the screen when it is set to
- ❑ standard size
- ❑ standard large
- ❑ standard extra large

at approximately ___ inches on a ___-inch monitor.

The student is able to visually locate the pointer on the screen when it is set to
- ❑ black
- ❑ black large
- ❑ black extra large

at approximately ___ inches on a ___-inch monitor.

The student is able to visually locate the pointer on the screen set to
- ❑ inverted
- ❑ inverted large
- ❑ inverted extra large

at approximately ___ inches on a ___-inch monitor.
- ❑ other enlarged pointer (specify): _____

at approximately ___ inches on a ___-inch monitor.

The student is able to
- ❑ use the mouse to navigate the desktop and place the pointer on the desired screen element.
- ❑ maintain the mouse or pointer position while clicking or double-clicking.
- ❑ maintain eye contact with the mouse or pointer while navigating the desktop.

The student is able to select the following items with the mouse:
- ❑ pull-down menus
- ❑ toolbar buttons
- ❑ scroll bars
- ❑ tabs in multipage dialog boxes
- ❑ radio buttons
- ❑ edit fields
- ❑ edit combo box

❏   combo box
❏   edit spin box
❏   left-right slider
❏   checkbox
❏   other controls

❏   The student is able to perform most mouse functions using keyboard commands.

❏   The student is **not** able to physically use a standard mouse. (*If checked for a student with low vision using an enlarged pointer or screen magnification software, refer student for a computer access evaluation to determine a more accessible pointing device.*)

Comments: _____
_____
_____

- Select Mouse.
- Select Pointer.
- Select the pull down box for Scheme.
- Select the desired pointer and choose OK.
- Ask the student to locate the pointer and measure the working distance.
- If the student is unable to locate any of these Windows pointers at a working distance of approximately 10–13 inches, then try larger pointers obtained from the Internet (see Chapter 3).
- Once the student is able to locate the pointer, ask him or her to move the pointer around the screen and place it over various screen elements such as icons and menus. Note if the student is able to visually track the pointer as it is moved around the screen.
- Ask the student to select an item by double clicking on that item. Notice if he or she is able to keep the pointer on the intended item.
- If difficulties are noted, repeat the procedure with a trackball or other pointing device.

If the student continues to have difficulty in using the mouse or other pointing device, refer the student for a computer access evaluation.

ACCESSING ELECTRONIC INFORMATION USING A PERSONAL DIGITAL ASSISTANT (PDA)

Materials Needed

- Portable dedicated word processor with scalable fonts
- Accessible PDA with QWERTY keyboard, speech output, and braille display

- Accessible PDA with six-key braille keyboard, speech output, and braille display
- Files saved on these devices that contain appropriate sentences, questions, and reading passages

Although the text and graphics displayed on the small screens of mainstream PDAs are usually too small for most students with a visual impairment to view efficiently, many students can access electronic information by using an accessible PDA with visual, tactile, or auditory output. Some students may find the text displayed in a portable dedicated word processor with scalable fonts adequate for reading notes taken in class or for viewing a file that they wish to read with the flexibility of a portable device, so this option should also be assessed. However, most students will require a PDA with tactile or auditory output for these kinds of tasks. As with other devices that access electronic information, the main issues to resolve are whether the student can comprehend the device's output and can physically manipulate the keys and controls on the device (see Figure 7.21).

To find out whether a student can comprehend the synthesized speech, the examiner can repeat the steps described previously to assess the ability to work with synthesized speech produced by a computer. Similarly, determining a student's ability to access a PDA with a refreshable braille display can be accomplished by asking the student to complete tasks similar to as those used previously with regard to tactile output devices. The examiner will need to prepare appropriate materials, such as simple sentences and questions, for the student to use with these devices for this section of the assessment. The following procedure can be used for each of the devices assessed.

Procedure

- Demonstrate the device by having it speak some simple sentences or questions, such as "Hello John/Susan." "How old are you?" "What is your favorite food?" "What did you have for breakfast today?" (Avoid yes-or-no questions.)
- Ask the student to answer the questions or to repeat what the device speaks.
- Have the device speak single words and ask the student what was said.
- Have the device speak individual letters and ask the student to identify them. Start with letters that have distinctive sounds (such as *a, f, h, o, s, w*). If the student is able to identify these, ask the student to identify letters that sound similar (*b, c, d, e, p, t, z*).
- Ask the student to enter characters, words, and sentences into the device using either the six-key braille keyboard or QWERTY keyboard, depending on which device you are using.
- Demonstrate the commands for reading forward and backward in the text.
- Ask the student to read several sentences from the prepared text. Remind the student of how to execute the commands if necessary.
- After several trials, note whether the student is able to use the advance and reverse commands to read sentences and review words that he or she may not have understood on first hearing.
- Ask the student to locate words in the text that will require him or her to use the advance and reverse commands.
- Determine if the student is able to physically manipulate the device and to press the keys appropriately to execute commands.

Figure 7.21   Personal Digital Assistants

Section II: Accessing Electronic Information

C. Personal Digital Assistants (PDAs)   Date completed _____

The student is able to

❑ read the text displayed on a standard PDA.

❑ read the text displayed on a portable word processor with scalable fonts.
Specify font _____ and point size _____.

❑ understand speech produced by a talking PDA, including
   ❑ sentences or lines.
   ❑ words.
   ❑ distinctive sounding letters (such as *a, f, h, o, s, w*).
   ❑ similar sounding letters (*b, c, d, e, p, t, z*).

❑ read the braille produced by a PDA with a refreshable braille display.

❑ execute navigation commands with instruction.

❑ execute navigation commands without instruction.

❑ enter text through the ❑ braille or ❑ QWERTY keyboard.

The student prefers using a/an
   ❑ portable word processor with scalable fonts.
   ❑ accessible PDA with speech output only.
   ❑ accessible PDA with refreshable braille display and speech output.

The student was able to answer simple comprehension questions about information presented on a/an
   ❑ portable word processor with scalable fonts.
   ❑ accessible PDA with speech output only.
   ❑ accessible PDA with refreshable braille display and speech output.

The student was able to read approximately
   _____ words per minute (wpm) when using a portable word processor with scalable fonts.
   _____ wpm when using an accessible PDA with speech output only.
   _____ wpm when using an accessible PDA with refreshable braille display and speech output.

The student is willing to use these devices (the examiner may wish to list these separately)
   ❑ to complete assignments in the regular classroom.
   ❑ at home to complete school assignments.
   ❑ while working with the teacher of students with visual impairments.

Comments: _____

_____

_____

- Note if the student is able to grasp the purposes of the commands and is able to execute them to perform the requested actions.
- If an accessible PDA with a refreshable braille display is available, ask the student to read the characters and words on the display, and repeat the requests above.

If one of the objectives of the assistive technology assessment is to determine whether the student will benefit from an accessible PDA with a braille display or if one with speech output only will be appropriate, the examiner might wish to conduct this segment of the assessment at another time, as it can be somewhat time consuming. To help make this determination and formulate a recommendation, the student's efficiency in using the two types of output needs to be compared, and the student will need some practice time reading additional passages with each device to master the navigation commands. For the assessment, the examiner will need to prepare several appropriate reading samples with comprehension questions and save them on each type of device, and then do the following:

- Ask the student which device he or she thinks is more effective and which one he or she likes better.
- Ask the student to read a different passage with each device and note the time required.
- Ask the student to respond to the comprehension questions and note the accuracy of the answers to the comprehension questions with each device.

This information can then be used in combination with other information about the student's braille-reading skills to assist in making recommendations about accessible PDAs with braille displays.

ELECTRONIC CALCULATORS AND DICTIONARIES

Students who are blind or visually impaired are able to obtain information from other types of electronic devices in addition to computers. Two particularly useful devices for students are electronic calculators and talking dictionaries (see Figure 7.22).

Electronic Calculators

Materials Needed

- Large-print calculators
- Talking calculators

Calculators with enlarged displays, speech output, or both have become widely available. Some students with low vision may be able to read and operate calculators with large displays. The examiner will wish to acquire a variety of large-print calculators to demonstrate to a student with low vision to determine whether any of them are useful for him or her.

Procedure

- Note the size of the numerals displayed on the calculator.
- Explain the layout of the calculator keypad.
- Demonstrate how to enter numbers and perform operations. Ask the student to enter some numbers and perform some simple operations.
- Note the student's physical ability to enter the numbers and perform operations.
- Check the accuracy of the student's entry and ask him or her to read the display.
- Record the observations.

Figure 7.22   Electronic Calculators and Dictionaries

Section II: Accessing Electronic Information

D. Electronic Calculators and Dictionaries   Date completed _____

The student is able to

❏ use a calculator with an enlarged display containing ___-inch numerals.

❏ accurately locate and press the keys on the calculator keypad.

❏ perform basic operations
   ❏ with prompting.
   ❏ without prompting.

❏ use a talking calculator and
   ❏ demonstrate understanding of the synthesized speech by repeating
      ❏ single digits spoken by the calculator.
      ❏ whole numbers spoken by the calculator.
   ❏ accurately locate and press the keys on the calculator keypad.
   ❏ perform basic functions
      ❏ with prompting.
      ❏ without prompting.

When using a talking dictionary, the student is able to
   ❏ understand and identify distinctive sounding letters (such as *a, f, h, o, s, w*).
   ❏ understand and identify similar sounding letters (*b, c, d, e, p, t, z*).
   ❏ understand and identify individual words.
   ❏ understand definitions spoken as continuous speech.
   ❏ accurately locate and press the keys on the dictionary's keyboard.
   ❏ perform basic functions
      ❏ with prompting.
      ❏ without prompting.

The student is willing to use these devices (the examiner may wish to list these separately)
   ❏ to complete assignments in the regular classroom.
   ❏ at home to complete school assignments.
   ❏ while working with the teacher of students with visual impairments.

Comments: _____
_____
_____

Some students will not be able to see a display, and some will prefer to use a talking calculator. The quality of the speech produced by these devices is, in general, not as good as that of dedicated speech synthesizers. Because a calculator has a limited vocabulary, however, most students will be able to learn to understand it with practice, even if they are not able to understand the speech at first hearing. To assess the student's ability to use a talking calculator, both the student's understanding of the speech produced and ability to manipulate the keys and buttons need to be assessed, as follows:

- Press number and operation keys and ask the student to identify what he or she hears.
- Continue asking the student to identify keys and the results of operations to determine if the student is able to adapt to the synthesized speech and acquire an understanding of the speech through repeated exposure.
- Explain the layout of the calculator keypad.
- Ask the student to press specified keys and observe his or her execution to determine if the student is physically able to operate the keys.
- Note if the student is able to perform the operations independently or needs continued prompting.

Asking the student to perform simple operations with the calculator will help the examiner determine if the student understands the basic use of the device. Many students will need prompting to perform the operations on the first few trials, but will begin to do so independently after some practice.

Talking Dictionaries

Materials Needed

- Talking dictionary

Accessing dictionaries has often been a laborious task for many students who are blind or visually impaired. The talking dictionary offers a highly efficient alternative. Some talking dictionaries speak only the target word and its spelling, but do not speak the definition, which is of limited value to a student who cannot read the definition. However, there are devices that are fully speaking and offer many features to their users. At the time of this writing, one such model is available on a high school or college level and one on an elementary school level. Although the high school model is expensive, it offers many worthwhile features. The examiner should use the device that is most appropriate for the student's age and functioning.

As with other electronic devices, the examiner will be assessing the student's ability to comprehend the speech produced by these devices, determining his or her manual dexterity in manipulating the keys, and observing his or her cognitive capacity to perform tasks with the device. The keys on many of these devices are organized in the traditional QWERTY-style arrangement and are quite small, so they may be difficult for the student to locate. Procedures used with dictionaries are similar to those that have been used previously to assess the student's ability to understand synthesized speech and manipulate a keyboard and controls:

Procedure

- Press letters on the talking dictionary and ask the student to identify them. Begin with letters that have distinctive sounds (such as *a, f, h, o, s, w*). If the student is able to identify the distinctive-sounding letters, the examiner can then try using the more confusing letters (*b, c, d, e, p, t, z*).

- Enter words and have the device speak them to determine if the student can understand the letter sounds put together in words.
- Demonstrate the device by reading a definition one word at a time. Ask the student to identify the words he or she hears.
- Continue reading the definition using continuous speech. Stop and ask the student to repeat what he or she heard.
- Continue reading definitions both with continuous speech and one word at a time and ask the student to explain the meaning of the definitions.
- Ask the student to enter a word into the dictionary using the device's keyboard. Some students may need assistance locating individual keys. Point out the raised dots on the *f* and *j* keys. The examiner may need to assist some students by giving verbal instructions to locate specific keys.
- Assist the student in locating the Read key and the Left and Right arrow keys. Have the student place the pointer and middle fingers of his or her right hand on the Left and Right arrow keys respectively.
- Have the student place his or her left pointer finger on the Read key and press it.
- Instruct the student to press the Left arrow key to stop the speech and read back one word.
- Ask the student to press the Right arrow key three times.

Many students will be able to perform simple navigation functions like these, demonstrating their physical and cognitive ability to use this tool to access information in reference materials.

SECTION III: COMMUNICATING THROUGH WRITING

Nonelectronic Tools for Producing Written Communication

- Writing Tools Using Visual Access
- Writing Tools Using Tactile Access

Electronic Tools Used for Producing Written Communication

- Computer with Flatbed Scanner and Imaging Program
- Accessible Computer with Word-Processing Program
- Electronic Braillewriters
- Accessible PDAs

There are a wide variety of tools that students with a visual impairment can use to produce written communication in print, braille, or both (see Chapter 4). Writing tasks can be organized into two broad categories. First, individuals often need to record relatively small amounts of information in a format that they can read or access later—for example, a student might want to record a friend's name and telephone number. The tools and adaptations that the student chooses to record this type of information may not prove effective for tasks in the second category: longer writing tasks such as a letter, report, or term paper. Determining which tools will best meet the student's needs for short writing tasks and for long writing tasks is the purpose of this section of the assessment. Available writing tools include both nonelectronic and electronic tools that can be accessed visually, tactilely, or auditorily, depending on the student's preferences.

NONELECTRONIC TOOLS FOR PRODUCING WRITTEN COMMUNICATION

Writing Tools Using Visual Access

Materials Needed

- A variety of writing instruments including pencils, pens, felt-tip markers, and erasable pens
- Bold-lined paper, 7/16 inch and 9/16 inch ruled
- Raised-lined paper
- Crayons and a screen board
- Dry-erase markers and a personal sized whiteboard (9 × 12-inch)
- Signature guide
- Desktop video magnifier
- Lists of words and short sentences that are appropriate for the student's reading and spelling level in the student's preferred font and point size or larger
- Sample of the student's handwriting from 3 to 5 days earlier

Because of their widespread availability, paper and pencil or pen are often used by individuals with low vision for producing written communications in print. Some students may be able to write legibly with regular paper and pencil, while others will prefer bold- or raised-lined paper and a writing instrument that produces a dark, bold mark. The initial assistive technology assessment can explore the student's abilities to produce handwriting and use different writing tools (see Figure 7.23).

The examiner will need to acquire writing samples from the student while he or she is trying various combinations of writing paper and writing instruments. To do this, the examiner will need to prepare two lists of words and short sentences that are appropriate for the student's reading and spelling level. The writing sample to be copied will need to be provided in the student's preferred font and point size. In this instance, since the aim is to evaluate the student's writing, not his or her reading, it might be better to produce the text in a larger point size than the student normally prefers to allow the student to view the text more easily while copying.

Allow the student to choose either manuscript or cursive writing when producing the writing sample.

Procedure

- Ask the student to copy words and sentences from one of the lists using paper and pencil or the student's preferred adaptations.
- Dictate the words and sentences from the second list for the student to write and note how he or she performs the task.
- Note any physical difficulties that might be exhibited while the student is writing and record the amount of time it takes the student to accomplish the task.
- Review the samples with regard to legibility and spacing.
- Ask the student to read the samples and note his or her response. Ask the student to sign his or her name. Note if the student uses a signature guide or other adaptation.
- Note the difficulty or ease with which the student is able to write.

Figure 7.23   Writing Tools Using Visual Access

Section III: Communicating Through Writing
A. Nonelectronic Tools for Producing Written Communication

1. Writing Tools for Students Using Visual Access   Date completed _____

When using standard writing tools (pencil, pen, etc.), the student is able to

❑ write manuscript (print) legibly at the rate of
   _____ words per minute (wpm) from dictation,
   _____ wpm from copy, and
      ❑ read his or her handwriting.
      ❑ read a sample of his or her handwriting from 3 to 5 days earlier.

❑ write cursive legibly at the rate of
   _____ wpm from dictation,
   _____ wpm from copy, and
      ❑ read his or her handwriting.
      ❑ read a sample of his or her handwriting from 3 to 5 days earlier.

❑ space appropriately between letters and words.

❑ sign his or her name legibly in cursive using
   ❑ a signature guide.
   ❑ the edge of a card, ruler, or some other similar device.

❑ The student produces legible writing **laboriously** and **with great difficulty** when using standard writing tools.

Comments: _____
_____
_____

The student is able to produce legible **manuscript** (print) writing using

❑ bold-lined paper at the rate of
   ___wpm from dictation,
   ___wpm from copy, and:
      ❑ read his or her handwriting.
      ❑ read a sample of his or her handwriting from 3 to 5 days earlier.

(continued on next page)

Figure 7.23 (continued)

❑ raised-lined paper at the rate of
___wpm from dictation,
___wpm from copy, and
    ❑ read his or her handwriting.
    ❑ read a sample of his or her handwriting from 3 to 5 days earlier.

❑ an erasable pen or   ❑ a thick, dark pencil (such as a primary pencil) at the rate of
___wpm from dictation,
___wpm from copy, and
    ❑ read his or her handwriting.
    ❑ read a sample of his or her handwriting from 3 to 5 days earlier.

❑ a felt-tip pen at the rate of
___wpm from dictation,
___wpm from copy, and
    ❑ read his or her handwriting.
    ❑ read a sample of his or her handwriting from 3 to 5 days earlier.

❑ a whiteboard and erasable marker at the rate of
___wpm from dictation,
___wpm from copy, and
    ❑ read his or her handwriting.
    ❑ read a sample of his or her handwriting from 3 to 5 days earlier.

❑ a video magnifier (specify writing tools and adaptations being used)
_____ at the rate of
___wpm from dictation,
___wpm from copy, and
    ❑ read his or her handwriting.
    ❑ read a sample of his or her handwriting from 3 to 5 days earlier.

___other (specify): _____

The student is able to produce legible **cursive** writing using
❑ bold-lined paper at the rate of
___wpm from dictation,
___wpm from copy, and
    ❑ read his or her handwriting.
    ❑ read a sample of his or her handwriting from 3 to 5 days earlier.

- ❏ raised-lined paper at the rate of
  ___ wpm from dictation,
  ___ wpm from copy, and:
    - ❏ read his or her handwriting.
    - ❏ read a sample of his or her handwriting from 3 to 5 days earlier.

- ❏ an erasable pen or ❏ a thick, dark pencil (such as a primary pencil) at the rate of
  ___ wpm from dictation,
  ___ wpm from copy, and
    - ❏ read his or her handwriting.
    - ❏ read a sample of his or her handwriting from 3 to 5 days earlier.

- ❏ a felt-tip pen at the rate of
  ___ wpm from dictation,
  ___ wpm from copy, and
    - ❏ read his or her handwriting.
    - ❏ read a sample of his or her handwriting from 3 to 5 days earlier.

- ❏ a whiteboard and erasable marker at the rate of
  ___ wpm from dictation,
  ___ wpm from copy, and
    - ❏ read his or her handwriting.
    - ❏ read a sample of his or her handwriting from 3 to 5 days earlier.

- ❏ a video magnifier (specify writing tools and adaptations being used)
  _____ at the rate of
  ___ wpm from dictation,
  ___ wpm from copy, and
    - ❏ read his or her handwriting.
    - ❏ read a sample of his or her handwriting from 3 to 5 days earlier.
- ❏ other (specify): _____

The student is willing to use these devices (the examiner may wish to list these separately)
- ❏ to complete assignments in the regular classroom.
- ❏ at home to complete school assignments.
- ❏ while working with the teacher of students with visual impairments.

Comments: _____
_____
_____

If the student's writing is labored, time consuming, and barely legible, it should be noted. This information will be critical when recommending writing tools for the student and will need to be fully explained in the final assessment report.

Some students' handwriting may not be truly legible, but the student will be able to read it because the student can remember what he or she wrote. To determine if this is the case or if the student can actually read his or her own handwriting—and thus use it as an effective communication tool—the examiner should obtain a sample of the student's handwriting from three to five days earlier and ask the student to read it aloud. The ease with which the student reads the sample should be noted. If the student has difficulty reading it or is unable to do so, the examiner will need to explore other writing tools for the student.

There are several low-tech options that may assist the student with handwriting. The following is a method to assess these different options:

- Ask the student to create a short writing sample using each of the following alternatives: a felt-tip pen and an erasable pen with regular paper, bold-lined paper, and raised-lined paper; a crayon and a screen board; and erasable markers and a whiteboard.
- The examiner can dictate text for the student to write or can pose simple questions and ask the student to respond in complete sentences. Remember that the point of this part of the assessment is to determine the effectiveness of various writing tools, not the student's creativity, spelling, or use of grammar, so the text the student is to write will need to be

easy enough for the student to accomplish without difficulty.
- Review the writing samples as before.
- Ask the student to read back the writing.
- Ask the student if he or she prefers any of the alternatives offered.
- Note the ease or difficulty exhibited by the student using each of these tools and the legibility of his or her writing.
- Repeat these steps with a desktop video magnifier system.

If the student's writing with a particular adaptation is legible and not labored, then this may be a tool that he or she can use to accomplish writing tasks. The examiner may need to ask the student, teacher of students with visual impairments, parents, and classroom teacher to determine if the tool or adaptations will be effective for short writing tasks only or might also serve for longer writing tasks. (See Chapter 8 on recommendations and writing the final report for additional discussion of this issue.)

Writing Tools Using Tactile Access

Braillewriting (embossing) can be performed with both low-tech and high-tech tools, and the ability of a student whose primary learning medium is touch needs to be assessed using both. If the student's ability to write braille was not noted as part of the braille assessment described earlier, the examiner will want to ask the student to produce some writing samples with a manual braillewriter and a slate and stylus. As was done with the assessment of print-writing tools, the examiner will need to prepare lists of words and sentences that are appropriate for the student's reading and spelling levels for the student to copy. One of the lists will need to be in braille.

In this section of the assessment (see Figure 7.24), the examiner will evaluate the student on the use of low-tech and mechanical tactile devices—the Perkins Brailler, the slate and stylus, and signature guides. Electronic options for writing braille are included in the next section of the assessment.

Braillewriter

Materials Needed

- Perkins manual Brailler
- Perkins unimanual Brailler (if needed; for students who have the use of only one hand)
- Extension keys for brailler
- Lists of words and short sentences that are appropriate for the student's reading and spelling level in the student's preferred font and point size or larger

Procedure

- Ask the student to braille the words and sentences using each of the tools available.
- Have the student produce the written communication by both copying it from hard copy braille and from dictation.
- Note the ease or difficulty the student exhibits with the tools and the time it takes to accomplish the task.

Students who do not have adequate finger strength to effectively press the keys of a manual braillewriter should have the opportunity to try extension keys for a standard braillewriter, and their ability to write braille with these adaptations should be assessed. Some students with motor impairments may have difficulty operating the manual brailler

with two hands. These students will need to be provided the opportunity to try using a unimanual brailler to determine if it will be an effective writing tool.

Slate and Stylus

Materials Needed

- Slate and stylus (various models)
- Words and sentences for copying

The last manual braille-writing tool to investigate is the slate and stylus. There are many types of slates and styli available, each with their own advantages. If a student has difficulty with a certain type of slate, the examiner may wish to investigate different models. For example, some students may have difficulty keeping the paper straight when using a pocket slate, but could be more efficient using a board slate (which makes it easier to move the slate down the paper) or a Janus slate, which holds a standard index card rather than a piece of paper.

Procedure

- Ask the student to emboss words dictated by the examiner.
- If the student displays proficiency with this tool, dictate a short sentence and have the student write it using the slate and stylus.
- Provide the student with a list of words and some short sentences for the student to write with the slate and stylus.
- Time the student's approximate writing rate with the slate and stylus.

Signature Writing

Materials Needed

- Signature guide
- Card, ruler, or other straight edge

Figure 7.24 Writing Tools Using Tactile Access

Section III: Communicating Through Writing
A. Nonelectronic Tools for Producing Written Communication

2. Writing Tools for Students Using Tactile Access   Date completed _____

When using a manual braille-writing device, the student is able to use

- ❏ a standard Perkins Brailler to emboss characters, words, and sentences at the rate of
  ___ words per minute (wpm) from dictation.
  ___ wpm from copy.

- ❏ a manual brailler with extension keys to emboss characters, words, and sentences at the rate of
  ___ wpm from dictation.
  ___ wpm from copy.

- ❏ a unimanual brailler to emboss characters, words, and sentences at the rate of
  ___ wpm from dictation.
  ___ wpm from copy.

- ❏ a slate and stylus to emboss characters, words, and sentences at the rate of
  ___ wpm from dictation.
  ___ wpm from copy.

❏ The student is able to sign his or her name legibly in cursive using
  - ❏ a signature guide.
  - ❏ the edge of a card, ruler, or some other similar device.

The student is willing to use these devices (the examiner may wish to list these separately)
  - ❏ to complete assignments in the regular classroom.
  - ❏ at home to complete school assignments.
  - ❏ while working with the teacher of students with visual impairments.

Comments: _____
_____
_____

The ability to sign one's name is an important skill for independence for students who do not have visual access to their writing. The student's ability to write his or her signature with a signature guide or by using the edge of a card, ruler, or some other device should be assessed. If this information is available from the teacher of students with visual impairments, it will not be necessary to have the student demonstrate it during the assessment.

ELECTRONIC TOOLS USED FOR PRODUCING WRITTEN COMMUNICATION

Materials Needed

- Appropriate writing samples for dictation and copying
- Electronic braillewriter

Electronic writing tools offer tremendous opportunities for students with visual impairments to produce high-quality written communications. The efficiency of these tools demands that their potential use be evaluated in the assistive technology assessment (see Figure 7.25). Several of the devices explored in this section are also addressed in other sections of the assessment—such as an accessible computer with a word-processing program, an electronic braillewriter, or an accessible PDA—because they are also used for accessing print, electronic information, or both. The examiner may wish to combine the tasks from this section that use a particular device with those from the previous section, or it may be beneficial for the student to have the repeated exposure to the device.

Computer with Flatbed Scanner and Imaging Program

Materials Needed

- Accessible computer system with flatbed scanner and imaging software
- Appropriate worksheet to be completed

The first tool to investigate is designed for writers who wish to access information visually. One writing task that must often be accomplished in school is the completion of worksheets and other forms. This task can be challenging for some students with low vision. One possible solution is the use of a computer with a flatbed scanner and an imaging program. The objective of this section is to determine if the student has the physical and cognitive skills to use this hardware and software solution.

- Demonstrate the use of the scanner and the software, including the zoom and text insertion features.
- Ask the student to perform the task with prompts from the examiner.
- Note any comments about the student's potential use of this technology.

Accessible Computer with Word-Processing Program

Materials Needed

- Accessible computer with word-processing program
- Appropriate writing samples for dictation and copying in the student's preferred format

An accessible computer with a word processing program is probably the most common electronic writing tool available and may offer the most benefit for students who are blind or visually impaired.

Figure 7.25   Electronic Tools for Producing Written Communication

Section III: Communicating Through Writing

B. Electronic Tools for Producing Written Communication

Date completed _____

When using a computer with a scanner and imaging software, the student is able to
- ❑ scan a worksheet or form.
- ❑ use the software text tool to insert text into the worksheet.

When using an accessible computer running a word-processing program, the student is able to enter characters, words, and sentences at the rate of

___words per minute (wpm) from dictation.

___wpm from copy.

When using the Mountbatten Brailler or another electronic braillewriter, the student is able to emboss characters, words, and sentences at the rate of

___wpm from dictation.

___wpm from copy.

When using an accessible PDA with a QWERTY keyboard, the student is able to enter characters, words, and sentences at the rate of

___wpm from dictation.

___wpm from copy.

When using an accessible PDA with a braille keyboard, the student is able to enter characters, words, and sentences at the rate of

___wpm from dictation.

___wpm from copy.

Comments: _____

_____

_____

Additional Assessment Information:

_____

_____

_____

Procedure

- Demonstrate the basic functions of the word processor.
- Ask the student to enter text from dictation and from copy in the student's preferred format.
- Allow the student an opportunity to practice with the system.
- Evaluate the speed at which the student can enter information from dictation and hard copy and record the data.

Electronic Braillewriters

Materials Needed

- Electronic braillewriter
- Appropriate writing samples for dictation and copying

If a student does not have the finger strength to operate the manual braillewriter with extension keys discussed in the previous section, the examiner may wish to investigate the use of an electric brailler, if one is available. If at all possible the examiner will wish to secure a Mountbatten Brailler or some other electric braillewriter for the assessment. (See the discussion about the Mountbatten in Chapter 4.) Preschool and early elementary students who may also have trouble using a manual braillewriter can be assessed on this device to determine if the student has the finger strength to use it as a tool that will allow him or her to write more easily.

Procedure

- Give the student time to explore the electronic braillewriter and satisfy his or her curiosity about it.

- Have the student produce writing samples from both dictated passages and by copying.
- Note the rate at which the student is able to use this device to write words and sentences from copy and from dictation.
- If appropriate assess the student's ability to understand the synthesized speech from the Mountbatten Brailler and note that information.

Accessible PDAs

Materials Needed

- Accessible PDA with six-key braille keyboard
- Accessible PDA with QWERTY keyboard
- Appropriate writing samples for dictation and copying

Accessible PDAs offer the user a portable writing tool that can be used for either short or long writing tasks. Some devices use a QWERTY typewriter-style keyboard for input, while others use a six-key brailler-style keyboard. PDAs are also available with speech output only, or with a refreshable braille display in addition to speech output. A student's ability to make use of an accessible PDA for writing is assessed in the same way as the use of other electronic devices.

Procedure

- Ask the student to enter characters, words, and sentences into the device as dictated by the examiner.
- Repeat this process with text provided in braille or large print for the student to copy.
- Time the student's data entry and note it on the assessment form.

ADDITIONAL INFORMATION

The examiner may have additional information that he or she feels is pertinent or would like to explain in greater detail some of the information noted elsewhere. For example, it may be necessary to explain why a student only partially completed a task or the specific circumstances under which the student is able to complete a particular task. There also may be information not specifically addressed on the assessment form that the examiner feels is important. If the assistive technology checklist supplied here is being used, this can be noted in the space provided at the end of the form. These types of comments can be useful when the assessment team begins to formulate recommendations for the student.

FOLLOW-UP AND NEXT STEPS

The information compiled during the assistive technology assessment will need to be submitted to the entire assessment team for review. The team may decide to request additional assessment by an assistive technology specialist or rehabilitation engineer if necessary to assess the student's potential use of more sophisticated devices and systems that are not available to the initial examiner. In addition, this follow-up can encompass any additional assessments that might need to be conducted by other specialized personnel, like occupational, physical, or speech therapists.

With the completion of the assessment, the team is now ready to proceed to compiling its recommendations. Individual examiners who have participated in the assessment may find it helpful to complete notes on their recommendations as soon as possible after the assessment. For this purpose, a sample recommendations checklist is included in the following chapter. It can serve as a tool for checking off items that may be beneficial in meeting the student's assistive technology needs and to serve as a reminder of the devices and issues that were addressed throughout the assessment process.

REFERENCES

Brigance, A. H. (1999). *Brigance comprehensive inventory of basic skills—revised*. North Billerica, MA: Curriculum Associates.

Johns, J. (2008). *Basic reading inventory*: *Pre-primer through grade twelve and early literacy assessments* (10th ed.). Dubuque, IA: Kendall/Hunt.

Koenig, A., Holbrook, M., Corn, A., DePriest, L., Erin, J., & Presley, I. (2000). Specialized assessments for students with visual impairments. In A. J. Koenig & M. C. Holbrook (Eds.), *Foundations of education* (2nd ed.), Vol. II: *Instructional strategies for teaching children and youths with visual impairments* (pp. 103–153). New York: AFB Press.

Sewell, D. (1997). *Assessment kit*: *Kit of informal tools for academic students with visual impairments*. Austin: Texas School for the Blind and Visually Impaired.

ASSISTIVE TECHNOLOGY ASSESSMENT CHECKLIST
FOR STUDENTS WITH VISUAL IMPAIRMENTS

Student's Name _Bill Alonso_   Person Completing Checklist _Samantha Higgins_

Student's Grade _10th_   Position _Teacher of Visually Impaired Students_

Student's Date of Birth _3/18/1993_   Date(s) of assessment _10/1, 10/8, & 10/15/08_

This document is a summary of information collected during the above-named student's assistive technology evaluation. Information for this assessment was obtained from the student's learning media assessment, the clinical low vision evaluation, the functional low vision evaluation, and from observation and assessment of the student's use of specific devices, as outlined below.
The assessment covers three main areas:

- **Section I: Accessing Print,** which covers how the student uses visual, tactile, and/or auditory tools to access textbooks, workbooks, assigned novels, and other printed information generally used in the classroom, including information presented on chalkboards or whiteboards
- **Section II: Accessing Electronic Information,** which covers how the student uses visual, tactile, and/or auditory tools to obtain information from electronic means, such as computers, electronic dictionaries and similar devices, digital books, and electronic braille devices
- **Section III: Communication through Writing,** which includes manuscript (print) and cursive writing, braille writing, and the use of electronic writing tools

The assessment sections of this document are followed by a recommendations section. The notations made will become part of the final written report detailing the rationale for each recommendation submitted to the student's Individualized Education Program team.

Directions: Indicate in the space provided the date each section is completed. All items not assessed should be marked NA.

(continued on next page)

Source: Adapted with permission from the "Assistive Technology Vision Aids Assessment," from the Georgia Project for Assistive Technology, Georgia Department of Education, Atlanta.

Section I: Accessing Print

A. Visual Access

1. Regular Print   Date completed   10/1/08

When accessing print information visually, the student is able to read passages on his or her independent reading level in regular print (12 point)

❑ without prescribed eyeglasses or contact lenses at a distance of   NA

____ inches, at approximately   ____ words per minute (wpm).

❑ with prescribed eyeglasses or contact lenses at a distance of

____ inches, at approximately   ____ wpm.

❑ When reading this size print with or without prescribed eyeglasses or contact lenses the student experiences visual or physical fatigue after ____ minutes (as reported by student or teacher).

Comments: _____

_____

_____

From this point forward all items should be attempted with student's prescribed spectacles or contact lens in use.

2. Enlarged Print Produced on a Photocopier   Date completed   10/1/08

When accessing print information visually the student is able to read

NA ❑ materials enlarged to ___% on

❑ 8 ½ × 11 inch paper   ❑ 8 ½ × 14 inch paper   ❑ 11 × 17 inch paper

at approximately _____ inches and at approximately _____ words per minute (wpm).

When reading this size print with or without prescribed eyeglasses or contact lenses the student experiences visual or physical fatigue after _____ minutes (as reported by student or teacher).

The student is willing to use materials enlarged by a photocopying machine on

❑ 8 ½ × 11 inch paper   ❑ 8 ½ × 14 inch paper   ❑ 11 × 17 inch paper

❑ to complete assignments in the regular classroom.

❑ at home to complete school assignments.

❑ while working with the teacher of students with visual impairments.

Comments: _____
_____
_____

3. Large Print   **Date completed**   <u>10/1/08</u>

The student is able to identify the following pictures of common objects:

<u>4 x 6</u> -inch high color photograph at a distance of approximately <u> 3 </u> inches.
☑ 3-inch high black-and-white line drawing at a distance of approximately <u> 6 </u> inches.
☑ 2-inch high black-and-white line drawing at a distance of approximately <u> 3 </u> inches.
☑ 1-inch high black-and-white line drawing at a distance of approximately <u>1.5</u> inches.
✓
When accessing large print with prescribed eyeglasses or contact lenses (if appropriate) the student is able to read
☑ 72-point print at a distance of approximately <u> 13 </u> inches.
☑ 60-point print at a distance of approximately <u> 12 </u> inches.
☑ 48-point print at a distance of approximately <u> 10 </u> inches.
☑ 36-point print at a distance of approximately <u> 8 </u> inches.
☑ 30-point print at a distance of approximately <u> 7 </u> inches.
☑ 24-point print at a distance of approximately <u> 6 </u> inches.
☑ 18-point print at a distance of approximately <u> 4 </u> inches.
☑ 14-point print at a distance of approximately <u> 2 </u> inches.
❑ 12-point print at a distance of approximately <u> NA </u> inches.

The student's preferred font is ❑ Arial ❑ APHont ❑ Tahoma ☑ Verdana
     ❑ other (specify): _____

The student's preferred point size with prescribed eyeglasses or contact lenses is
     ❑ 14 ❑ 18 ☑ 24 ❑ 30 ❑ 36 ❑ 48 ❑ 60 ❑ 72

The student prefers text in
     ☑ regular style.
     ❑ bold style.

The student is able to read continuous text in preferred font and point size at approximately
     <u>105</u> words per minute.

When reading this size print with or without prescribed eyeglasses or contact lenses the student experiences visual or physical fatigue after <u>30</u> minutes (as reported by student or teacher).

The student is willing to use materials printed in the preferred font and point size on 8 ½ × 11 inch paper
     ✓ to complete assignments in the regular classroom.
     ✓ at home to complete school assignments.
     ✓ while working with the teacher of students with visual impairments.

(continued on next page)

Comments: _____
_____
_____

4. Nonoptical Devices   **Date completed** _10/1/08_____

When reading print information, the student prefers
- ☐ text written with a pen or pencil on standard lined notebook paper.
- ☐ text written with felt-tip pen on standard lined notebook paper.
- ☑ text written with felt-tip pen on bold-lined notebook paper.
- ☐ text written with felt-tip pen on unlined paper.
- ☐ other (specify): _____.

When reading handwritten information the student prefers
- ☑ manuscript (printed) writing.
- ☐ cursive writing.

When reading, the student
- ☑ prefers overhead lighting
  - ☐ from an incandescent bulb.
  - ☑ from a fluorescent bulb.
  - ☐ from a halogen bulb.
  - ☐ adjusted with a dimmer switch.
- ☑ prefers window lighting adjusted with
  - ☑ blinds.
  - ☐ shades.
  - ☐ other (specify): _____.
- ☑ experiences glare problems on
  - ☑ paper.
  - ☐ desktop.
  - ☑ computer or video magnifier monitor.
  - ☑ whiteboard.
  - ☐ chalkboard.
  - resulting from
    - ☑ overhead lighting.
    - ☑ window lighting (natural light, sunlight).
- ☐ prefers less lighting than currently available.
- ☑ prefers additional lighting from a
  - ☑ desk lamp with a/an
    - ☐ incandescent bulb.
    - ☐ fluorescent bulb.
    - ☐ halogen bulb.
    - ☑ LED bulb.

☑ floor lamp with a/an
    ❑ incandescent bulb.
    ❑ fluorescent bulb.
    ❑ halogen bulb.
    ☑ LED bulb.
☑ prefers the location of the lighting source to be
    ☑ over the left shoulder.
    ❑ over the right shoulder.
☑ prefers to have materials placed on a
    ❑ desktop reading stand.
    ☑ portable reading stand.
    ❑ floor-standing reading stand.

The student is willing to use these devices and accommodations (the examiner may wish to list them individually)
☑ to complete assignments in the regular classroom.
☑ at home to complete school assignments.
☑ while working with the teacher of students with visual impairments.

Comments: _____
_____
_____

5. Optical Devices

Date completed <u>10/1/08</u>

When accessing print materials with the use of a prescribed optical device, the student uses
❑ eyeglasses.
❑ contact lenses.
❑ handheld magnifier.
    type _____
    power _____
    ❑ illuminated   ❑ nonilluminated
☑ stand magnifier.
    type _____
    power <u>4x</u>
    ☑ illuminated   ❑ nonilluminated
❑ telescope.
    type _____
    power _____

(continued on next page)

❑ video magnifier (specify type):
 ❑ desktop video magnifier.
 ❑ flex-arm camera model.
 ❑ portable model with handheld camera.
 ❑ head-mounted display model.
 ❑ electronic pocket magnifier.
 ❑ digital imaging system.
 ❑ other (specify): <u>not prescribed</u>   .

The student is able to read continuous text using the prescribed optical device at approximately

 <u>60</u> words per minute without a reading stand.

 _____ words per minute with a reading stand.

When reading regular-size print with the prescribed optical device the student experiences visual or physical fatigue after <u>10</u> minutes (as reported by student or teacher).

The student is willing to use these devices (the examiner may wish to list these separately)
 ❑ to complete assignments in the regular classroom.
 ☑ at home to complete school assignments.
 ☑ while working with the teacher of students with visual impairments.

Comments: <u>The student only uses the prescribed 4x magnifier for spot reading.</u>
_____
_____

6. Video Magnifier (CCTV)   **Date completed** <u>10/8/08</u>

Desktop Video Magnifier

When accessing print materials with the use of a desktop video magnifier (closed-circuit television or CCTV), the student is able to view a (insert a number to indicate the size)

 <u>3</u>-inch-high graphic and <u>3</u>-inch-high text on a <u>21</u>-inch-monitor
 at a working distance of approximately 10–13 inches.

 ___-inch-high graphic and ___-inch-high text on a ___-inch-monitor
 at a working distance of approximately ___ inches.

The student's polarity preference when viewing text on a video magnifier is
 ☑ dark on light.
 ❑ light on dark.

The student's color preference is
 <u>black</u> text on a <u>white</u> background.

The student is able to manipulate the controls of the video magnifier, with instructions from the examiner, to

    ☑ adjust the size of the image.

NA ❑ focus the image if the unit does not have auto focus.

When using the video magnifier, the student is able to

NA write a short sentence legibly on regular notebook paper while
      ❑ looking at the screen or monitor.
      ☑ looking at the paper.

    write a short sentence legibly on bold-lined paper while
      ❑ looking at the screen or monitor.
      ☑ looking at the paper.

When using the video magnifier, the student is able to read a 3- to 5-day-old sample sentence of his or her handwriting on

    ☑ blue-lined notebook paper.
    ❑ bold-lined writing paper.

The student is able to

    ☑ independently use an X-Y table for viewing materials with friction brake and margin stops are adjusted by examiner.

    Comments: _Bill has adequate coordination for controlling the X-Y table._

    ☑ independently adjust friction brake and margin stops after demonstration by examiner.

    Comments: _Bill easily grasped the concept of adjusting the friction brake to decrease the up and down movement of the text._

    ☑ independently manipulate the controls of the unit (knobs, buttons, switches, etc.).

    Comments: _Bill had some initial difficulty adjusting the margin stops, but after practicing on four different types of reading material, he was able to effectively adjust the margin stops._

The student is able to read approximately _145_ words per minute (wpm) when the friction brake and margin stops are adjusted properly by the examiner.

When reading this size print with or without prescribed eyeglasses or contact lenses the student experiences visual or physical fatigue after _NA_ minutes (as reported by student or teacher).

The student is willing to use these devices (the examiner may wish to list these separately)

    ❑ to complete assignments in the regular classroom.
    ☑ at home to complete school assignments.
    ☑ while working with the teacher of students with visual impairments.

Comments: _Bill liked the desktop video magnifier and had used one in middle school, but he stated that he would not feel comfortable using it in his regular classes._

(continued on next page)

Flex-Arm Camera Video Magnifier

When accessing print materials with the use of a flex-arm camera model video magnifier, the student is able to

- ❑ locate and operate the controls.
- ❑ use the device's X-Y table or manipulate the reading material without a table.
- ❑ rotate and adjust the camera for distance viewing.
- ❑ locate the distance target.
- ❑ identify the distance target.

The student is able to read approximately ___ wpm when the friction brake and margin stops are adjusted properly by the examiner.

When reading this size print with or without prescribed eyeglasses or contact lenses the student experiences visual or physical fatigue after ___ minutes (as reported by student or teacher).

The student is willing to use these devices (the examiner may wish to list these separately)

- ❑ to complete assignments in the regular classroom.
- ❑ at home to complete school assignments.
- ❑ while working with the teacher of students with visual impairments.

Comments: _This specific device was not evaluated._ _____
_____
_____

Portable Video Magnifier with Handheld Camera

When accessing print materials through the use of a portable video magnifier with a handheld camera, the student is able to

- ❑ locate and operate the controls.
- ❑ maintain an angle of the camera with the text that is adequate for reading while moving the camera.

The student is able to read approximately ___ wpm when using this device.

When reading this size print with or without prescribed eyeglasses or contact lenses the student experiences visual or physical fatigue after ___ minutes (as reported by student or teacher).

The student is willing to use these devices (the examiner may wish to list these separately)

- ❑ to complete assignments in the regular classroom.
- ❑ at home to complete school assignments.
- ❑ while working with the teacher of students with visual impairments.

Comments: _This specific device was not evaluated._ _____
_____
_____

Head-Mounted Video Magnifier

When accessing print materials through the use of a video magnifier with a head-mounted display, the student is able to

- ☐ locate and operate the controls.
- ☐ locate the distance target.
- ☐ identify the distance target.

The student is willing to use these devices (the examiner may wish to list these separately)

- ☐ to complete assignments in the regular classroom.
- ☐ at home to complete school assignments.
- ☐ while working with the teacher of students with visual impairments.

Comments: _This specific device was not evaluated._ _____

_____

_____

Electronic Pocket Video Magnifier

When accessing print materials through the use of an electronic pocket video magnifier, the student is able to

- ☑ locate and operate the controls.
- ☑ maintain the camera at an adequate angle to the text for reading while moving the device.
- ☑ operate a model with the camera on the side of the unit.
- ☑ operate a model with the camera in the middle of the unit.

The student is able to read approximately _103_ wpm when using this type of device.

When reading this size print with or without prescribed eyeglasses or contact lenses the student experiences visual or physical fatigue after _NA_ minutes (as reported by student or teacher).

The student is willing to use these devices (the examiner may wish to list these separately)

- ☑ to complete assignments in the regular classroom.
- ☑ at home to complete school assignments.
- ☑ while working with the teacher of students with visual impairments.

Comments: _Bill did very well with this device, but he felt it was too slow for long reading tasks._

_____

_____

Digital Imaging System

When accessing print materials through the use of a digital imaging system video magnifier, the student is able to

- ☑ locate and operate the controls.

The student is able to read approximately _165_ wpm when using this type of device.

When reading this size print with or without prescribed eyeglasses or contact lenses the student experiences visual or physical fatigue after _NA_ minutes (as reported by student or teacher).

The student is willing to use these devices (the examiner may wish to list these separately)

- ☑ to complete assignments in the regular classroom.

(continued on next page)

☑ at home to complete school assignments.

☑ while working with the teacher of students with visual impairments.

Comments: _Bill preferred this system over the others. He stated that using it with the computer_ _and its distance viewing feature made it valuable enough that he would use it in class._

___

7. Scanning Systems for Accessing   **Date completed**   10/8/08
Print Information Visually

When viewing print materials scanned into the computer using a standard imaging program (Microsoft Imaging, PaperPort, etc.), the student is able to

☑ operate the scanner.

☑ navigate the enlarged screen with the

     ☑ keyboard.
     ☑ mouse.

When viewing printed materials scanned into the computer with a specialized scanning system (such as Kurzweil 1000 or 3000, OpenBook, or WYNN), the student is able to

☑ operate the scanner.

☑ adjust the magnification to the desired size using the

     ☑ keyboard.
     ☑ mouse.

☑ adjust the rate and other speech parameters.

☑ navigate the image horizontally and vertically using the

     ☑ keyboard.
     ☑ mouse.

☑ select items from the menus and tools from the toolbar with the

     ☑ keyboard.
     ☑ mouse.

The student is willing to use these devices (the examiner may wish to list these separately)

     ❑ to complete assignments in the regular classroom.
     ☑ at home to complete school assignments.
     ☑ while working with the teacher of students with visual impairments.

Comments: _Bill quickly grasped the concept of how to use scanning systems but stated that he_ _would not want to have all of this equipment in his class unless there was a smaller version._

___

8. Visual and Physical Fatigue   **Date completed**   10/8/08

The student experiences visual/physical fatigue after reading

     ❑ for ___ minutes **without** adaptations.
     ❑ for ___ minutes **with** adaptations.

Comments:
(Please indicate fatigue factors for each visual access tool used by the student.)
<u>Bill experienced the least visual fatigue when reading with the digital imaging video magnifier</u>
<u>system using its visual and synthesized speech features.</u>

B. Tactile Access and Braille

Date completed _____

When accessing graphical information the student is able to discriminate tactilely
- ❏ solid lines of various thickness.
- ❏ dashed lines.
- ❏ dotted lines.
- ❏ raised-line drawings of simple shapes.
- ❏ the boundary between two clearly defined textured fill patterns.
- ❏ the boundary between three clearly defined textured fill patterns.
- ❏ the boundary between four clearly defined textured fill patterns.

The student is able to identify tactile information most accurately when it is presented as a simple tactile graphic
- ❏ tooled onto braille paper.
- ❏ produced as a collage of varying textures.
- ❏ thermoformed onto plastic.
- ❏ embossed as dots and lines onto braille paper by a computer-controlled braille embosser.
- ❏ produced as raised lines and patterns on capsule paper.

The student is able to read materials in
- ❏ uncontracted braille.
- ❏ contracted braille.

- ❏ Results of formal or informal braille assessments conducted by the teacher of students with visual impairments are attached.
  Student's oral braille reading rate is _____ words per minute (wpm).
  Student's silent braille reading rate is _____ wpm.

When accessing print information with a refreshable braille display, the student is able to
- ❏ read instructional-level text.
- ❏ press correct key combination to issue forward and reverse navigation commands
  - ❏ with verbal prompt.
  - ❏ without verbal prompt.
- ❏ read _____ wpm orally and _____ wpm silently.

The student is willing to use these devices (the examiner may wish to list these separately)
- ❏ to complete assignments in the regular classroom.
- ❏ at home to complete school assignments.
- ❏ while working with the teacher of students with visual impairments.

Comments: _____
_____
_____

(continued on next page)

C. Auditory Access

1. Live Readers and Recorded Information   Date completed <u>10/15/08</u>

When listening to instructional level information read aloud by the evaluator, the student is able to
- ☑ repeat words and simple phrases without having them repeated more than twice.
- ☑ paraphrase the information (a sentence or story).
- ☑ answer simple comprehension questions.

When listening to an analog or digital recording of a story, the student is able to
- ☑ repeat words and simple phrases without having them repeated more than twice.
- ☑ paraphrase the information (a sentence or story).
- ☑ accurately answer simple comprehension questions.

When using an analog or digital player-recorder, the student is able to
- ☑ insert and remove a tape or CD from the player-recorder.
- ☑ inactivate play, pause, stop, fast forward, and rewind functions (underline those demonstrated).
- ☑ understand and comprehend compressed or "fast" speech.
- ☑ manipulate variable speed and pitch controls.
- ☑ identify index tones, bookmarks, and page locators.

The student is able to
- ☑ listen to recorded speech and follow along with a print copy of the text.
- ☐ listen to recorded speech and follow along with a braille copy of the text.
- ☑ listen to synthesized speech and follow along with a print copy of the text.
- ☐ listen to synthesized speech and follow along with a braille copy of the text.

The student is able to read approximately
<u>180</u> words per minute (wpm) when listening and reading print or braille.

The student is willing to use these devices (the examiner may wish to list these separately)
- ☑ to complete assignments in the regular classroom.
- ☑ at home to complete school assignments.
- ☑ while working with the teacher of students with visual impairments.

Comments: <u>Bill stated that he would like to have recorded books to use when his eyes get tired,</u>
<u>particularly for longer reading assignments that he does at home</u>

2. Specialized Scanning Systems for   Date completed <u>10/8/08</u>
Accessing Print Information Auditorily

When accessing print materials scanned into the computer with a specialized scanning system (such as Kurzweil 1000 and 3000, OpenBook, and WYNN), the student is able to
- ☑ adjust the rate and other speech parameters.
- ☑ navigate through the document when provided instruction by the evaluator.

☑ select items from the menus or tools from the toolbar when provided instruction by the evaluator.

When listening to text read by the program, the student is able to
☑ repeat words and simple phrases without having them repeated more than twice.
☑ paraphrase the information (sentence or story).
☑ accurately answer simple comprehension questions.

The student is willing to use these devices (the examiner may wish to list these separately)
❑ to complete assignments in the regular classroom.
☑ at home to complete school assignments.
☑ while working with the teacher of students with visual impairments.

When accessing printed materials using audio-assisted reading the student is able to read _180_ words per minute (wpm).

Comments: _Bill stated that he would use this system in class if it were smaller, but that he_ _would find it very helpful for completing longer reader assignments._

D. Reading Rates   Date completed _10/15/08_

Optional; may be used to support use of various adaptations.

When accessing print information, the student is able to read
_NA_ words per minute (wpm) orally when reading materials in 12-point type using prescribed spectacles or contact lenses.
_105_ wpm orally when reading materials in the optimum point size and font:
      _24_ -point print and _Verdana_ font.
_60_ wpm orally when reading with a prescribed optical device.
_145_ wpm orally when reading with a video magnifier (CCTV). *desktop model*
_NA_ wpm orally when reading braille.
_180_ wpm when using audio-assisted reading.

Comments: _*105 wpm orally when reading with an electronic pocket model video magnifier;_ _165 wpm orally when reading with a digital imaging system video magnifier. These reading_ _rates are all informal measures._

E. Accessing Information Presented at a Distance   Date completed _10/8/08_

When accessing information presented at a distance on a chalkboard or whiteboard or by an overhead or computer projector or TV/VCR/DVD, the student reported that he or she
❑ sits close enough to view the information, at a working distance of approximately ____ feet.

(continued on next page)

❑ uses a handheld or spectacle-mounted telescope.
❑ uses a video magnifier with distance-viewing capabilities.
☑ gets an accessible copy from the teacher.
☑ uses a peer notetaker.
❑ uses an electronic whiteboard connected to an accessible computer.
☑ has information read aloud by a peer or paraeducator and
    ❑ brailles information on a braillewriter.
    ☑ writes information on paper.
    ❑ inputs information into computer or accessible personal digital assistant.
    ❑ records information on tape recorder or digital recorder.

❑ other (specify): _____.

Are these options working adequately?

❑ Yes
☑ No

Explain briefly:
Bill states that his teachers often forget to make him an accessible copy of the information
and the handwritten notes taken by his friends are often difficult to read. He is unable to see
PowerPoint presentations, videos, and teacher demonstrations. Bill would like some other way
to get access to this information.

The student is willing to use these devices and accommodations (the examiner may wish to list them individually)

☑ to complete assignments in the regular classroom.

Comments: _Bill stated that he would like a device that would allow him to see things at a_
distance. When shown the distance feature of a video magnifier he said he would use such a device
in class.

Section II: Accessing Electronic Information

A. Computer Access: Output Devices

1. Visual Access   **Date completed** _10/15/08_

The student is able to view electronic information on a desktop computer or in the computer lab without additional adaptations and identify or read

❑ text ❑ icon titles ❑ menus ❑ dialog boxes ❑ other system items on a

    ❑ 17-inch monitor at approximately ___ inches.
    ❑ 19-inch monitor at approximately ___ inches.
    ❑ 21-inch monitor at approximately ___ inches.
    ❑ other (specify): _____

The student prefers viewing text in a word-processing program on the computer in
_36_-point type in ❑ regular ☑ bold print

- ❑ Arial
- ❑ APHont
- ❑ Tahoma
- ☑ Verdana
- ❑ other (specify): _____

displayed on a <u>19</u> -inch monitor at approximately <u>3</u> inches.

The student is able to view electronic information on a
<u>NA</u> -inch computer monitor with the use of
- ❑ screen magnification hardware at approximately ____ inches.
- ❑ an articulated flexible monitor stand at approximately ___ inches.

The student is able to view electronic information using the computer operating system's screen enhancements such as
- ☑ screen resolution (specify): <u>800 x 600</u>.
- ❑ Windows Display Appearance Scheme (specify): _____.
- ☑ Windows Display Appearance Settings. *(Record specific settings selected on the Windows Display Properties Appearance Checklist appendix to this form.)*
- ☑ Microsoft Magnifier
  - ❑ magnification level: <u>3x</u>
  - ❑ other setting (specify): _____

  The student is able to use the Microsoft Magnifier to
  - ☑ identify screen elements.
  - ☑ read text in menus, dialog boxes, and text documents.
  - ☑ navigate around the screen. *with difficulty*
  - ☑ locate the file names listed in the Open file dialog box. *with difficulty*
  - ☑ select a requested file to open. *with difficulty*

(If the school district uses Macintosh computers, complete the previous sections for the accessibility features provided in the computer's operating system.)

When using a dedicated screen magnification program, the student is able to
- ☑ read 12-point print enlarged to <u>4x</u> magnification at a working distance of approximately 13 inches.
- ☑ locate and select menu items, buttons, and other screen elements with the mouse or other pointing device.
- ❑ locate and select menu items, buttons, and other screen elements using keyboard commands.
- ☑ navigate around the screen and maintain orientation.
- ☑ use an automatic reading feature at a speed setting of <u>55</u>.

The student's color preference is <u>black</u> text on a <u>white</u> background.

❑ The student is unable to access the computer visually.

(continued on next page)

The student is willing to use these devices (the examiner may wish to list these separately)
- ☑ to complete assignments in the regular classroom.
- ☑ at home to complete school assignments.
- ☑ while working with the teacher of students with visual impairments.

Comments: _Bill stated that he would use screen magnification software when needed._

2. Tactile Access   Date completed _NA_

When accessing electronic or computer-based information tactilely, the student is able to
- ☐ read braille text displayed on a dedicated braille display connected to a computer.
- ☐ read braille text displayed on an accessible PDA braille display connected to a computer.
- ☐ execute navigation commands with instruction.
- ☐ enter text through the braille keyboard, if available.

The student is willing to use these devices (the examiner may wish to list these separately)
- ☐ to complete assignments in the regular classroom.
- ☐ at home to complete school assignments.
- ☐ while working with the teacher of students with visual impairments.

Comments: _____

3. Auditory Access   Date completed _10/15/08_

When accessing electronic information auditorily, the student is able to understand synthesized speech produced by

software synthesizers:
- ☑ Intellitalk
- ☑ Write:Outloud
- ☑ Kurzweil
- ☑ TrueVoice
- ☐ DECTalk Access 32
- ☑ Eloquence (JAWS)
- ☐ OpenBook
- ☐ Microsoft Speech Engine
- ☐ Other (specify): _____

hardware synthesizers:
- ☐ Type 'n Speak, Braille 'n Speak, Braille Lite
- ☐ DECTalk Express
- ☐ Double Talk LT
- ☐ Other (specify): _____

When accessing electronic information auditorily through synthesized speech and a screen reader the student is able to understand and identify
- ☑ sentences and lines.
- ☑ words.
- ☑ distinctive sounding letters (such as *a, f, h, o, s, w*) when spelled in words.
- ☐ similar sounding letters (*b, c, d, e, p, t, z*) when spelled in words. *had some difficulty*

☑ distinctive sounding letters (such as *a, f, h, o, s, w*) when spelled in isolation.

❑ similar sounding letters *(b, c, d, e, p, t, z)* when spelled in isolation.
  had difficulty with some letters

When accessing electronic information auditorily through synthesized speech and a screen reader the student is able to execute navigation commands with instruction to

☑ read by characters. *had difficulty with some letters*

☑ read by words.

☑ read by sentence and lines.

☑ move forward (to the next character, word, line).

☑ move backward (to the prior character, word, line).

❑ When accessing electronic information auditorily, the student was **not** able to grasp the concept of navigation.

The student is willing to use these devices (the examiner may wish to list these separately)

❑ to complete assignments in the regular classroom.

☑ at home to complete school assignments.

☑ while working with the teacher of students with visual impairments.

Comments: <u>Bill stated that he didn't think he would need the speech program if he had the</u>
<u>screen magnification software tried earlier, although he did like having speech with the</u>
<u>magnification.</u>

B. Computer Access: Input Devices

1. Keyboard Use   Date completed <u>10/15/08</u>

☑ The student is able to use a standard keyboard without adaptation.

The student

☑ demonstrates keyboard awareness (has a general knowledge of the key locations).

❑ is able to search for keys and type individual letters.

☑ is able to locate and identify alphanumeric keys.

❑ is able to locate and identify function keys.

☑ is able to activate two keys simultaneously.

❑ is able to touch type while looking at his or her hands

  ☑ from dictation.

  ❑ from braille copy.

  ☑ from copy that is presented in the student's preferred font and point size and positioned on a flexible-arm copy holder.

❑ is able to touch type without looking at his or her hands

  ❑ from dictation.

  ❑ from braille copy.

  ❑ from copy that is presented in the student's preferred font and point size and positioned on a flexible-arm copy holder.

❑ does not demonstrate excessive miss-hits or key repeats. *makes numerous errors*

(continued on next page)

❑ uses good mechanics when typing (posture, wrist elevation, etc.). *has poor mechanics*
☑ types with _4_ fingers of right hand and _4_ fingers of left hand. *and posture*
☑ is able to type approximately _10_ words per minute (wpm)
    ☑ from dictation.
    ❑ from braille copy.
    ❑ from copy that is presented in the student's preferred font and point size and positioned on a flexible-arm copy holder.

❑ The student is able to utilize a standard computer keyboard with the following adaptations: *(Seek assistance from an occupational or physical therapist as needed.)*
    ❑ zoom caps   ❑ keyguard   ❑ tactile locator dots
    ❑ other (specify): _NA_____

❑ The student is able to utilize a standard computer keyboard with the following keyboard utilities: *(Seek assistance from an assistive technology specialist, occupational therapist, or physical therapist to complete this section.)*
    ❑ sticky keys   ❑ repeat keys   ❑ slow keys   NA
    ❑ mouse keys   ❑ toggle keys

❑ The student is **not** able to utilize a standard keyboard with or without adaptations. *(If checked, refer student for a computer access evaluation.)*

Comments: _Bill has a basic knowledge of the keyboard but types slowly and inefficiently. He is_ _often unaware of mistakes that he makes. He is unable to accurately see the text on the screen_ _when he types, even when he bends over and gets very close._

2. Pointing Device (Mouse)   **Date completed** _10/15/08_

The student is able to visually locate the pointer on the screen when it is set to
    ❑ standard size
    ❑ standard large
    ❑ standard extra large
at approximately ___ inches on a ___-inch monitor.

The student is able to visually locate the pointer on the screen when it is set to
    ❑ black
    ❑ black large
    ☑ black extra large *after searching*
at approximately _2_ inches on a _19_-inch monitor.

The student is able to visually locate the pointer on the screen set to
    ❑ inverted
    ❑ inverted large
    ❑ inverted extra large
at approximately ___ inches on a ___-inch monitor.
    ❑ other enlarged pointer (specify): _____
at approximately ___ inches on a ___-inch monitor.

The student is able to
- ☑ use the mouse to navigate the desktop and place the pointer on the desired screen element. *very slow*
- ☑ maintain the mouse or pointer position while clicking or double-clicking.
- ☑ maintain eye contact with the mouse or pointer while navigating the desktop. *not always*

The student is able to select the following items with the mouse:
- ☑ pull-down menus
- ☐ toolbar buttons
- ☐ scroll bars
- ☐ tabs in multipage dialog boxes
- ☐ radio buttons
- ☐ edit fields
- ☐ edit combo box
- ☐ combo box
- ☐ edit spin box
- ☐ left-right slider
- ☐ checkbox
- ☐ other controls

☑ The student is able to perform most mouse functions using keyboard commands.

☐ The student is **not** able to physically use a standard mouse. (*If checked for a student with low vision using an enlarged pointer or screen magnification software, refer student for a computer access evaluation to determine a more accessible pointing device.*)

Comments: _Bill can use the mouse to interact with the computer, but he is very slow and often selects unintended objects. He spends a good deal of time visually searching for the pointer and other objects even when using screen magnification software._

C. Personal Digital Assistants (PDAs)   Date completed _10/15/08_

The student is able to

☐ read the text displayed on a standard PDA.

☐ read the text displayed on a portable word processor with scalable fonts.
   Specify font _____NA_____ and point size _____.

☑ understand speech produced by a talking PDA, including
- ☑ sentences or lines.
- ☑ words.
- ☑ distinctive sounding letters (such as *a, f, h, o, s, w*).
- ☑ similar sounding letters (*b, c, d, e, p, t, z*). *some but not all*

☐ read the braille produced by a PDA with a refreshable braille display. *NA*

(continued on next page)

☑ execute navigation commands with instruction.

☑ execute navigation commands without instruction.   *once he became familiar with them*

☑ enter text through the   ☐ braille   or   ☑ QWERTY keyboard.

The student prefers using a/an
- ☐ portable word processor with scalable fonts.
- ☑ accessible PDA with speech output only.
- ☐ accessible PDA with refreshable braille display and speech output.

The student was able to answer simple comprehension questions about information presented on a/an
- ☐ portable word processor with scalable fonts.
- ☑ accessible PDA with speech output only.
- ☐ accessible PDA with refreshable braille display and speech output.

The student was able to read approximately   NA
- _____ words per minute (wpm) when using a portable word processor with scalable fonts.
- _____ wpm when using an accessible PDA with speech output only.
- _____ wpm when using an accessible PDA with refreshable braille display and speech output.

The student is willing to use these devices (the examiner may wish to list these separately)
- ☐ to complete assignments in the regular classroom.
- ☐ at home to complete school assignments.
- ☐ while working with the teacher of students with visual impairments.

Comments: _Bill stated that he would prefer to use a laptop with the screen magnification software for note taking._

D. Electronic Calculators and Dictionaries   Date completed _10/15/08_

The student is able to

☐ use a calculator with an enlarged display containing ___-inch numerals.

☐ accurately locate and press the keys on the calculator keypad.

☐ perform basic operations
- ☐ with prompting.
- ☐ without prompting.

☑ use a talking calculator and
- ☑ demonstrate understanding of the synthesized speech by repeating
  - ☑ single digits spoken by the calculator.
  - ☑ whole numbers spoken by the calculator.
- ☑ accurately locate and press the keys on the calculator keypad.

☑ perform basic functions
  ☑ with prompting.
  ☑ without prompting. When using a talking dictionary, the student is able to
☑ understand and identify distinctive sounding letters (such as *a, f, h, o, s, w*).
☑ understand and identify similar sounding letters (*b, c, d, e, p, t, z*).   *most letters*
☑ understand and identify individual words.
☑ understand definitions spoken as continuous speech.
☑ accurately locate and press the keys on the dictionary's keyboard. *when provided direction*
☑ perform basic functions
  ☑ with prompting.
  ☑ without prompting.

The student is willing to use these devices (the examiner may wish to list these separately)
  ☑ to complete assignments in the regular classroom.
  ☑ at home to complete school assignments.
  ☑ while working with the teacher of students with visual impairments.

Comments: _Bill's ability to understand the synthesized speech on the talking dictionary_
improved as he had the opportunity to hear more and more words and letters.

Section III: Communicating Through Writing

A. Nonelectronic Tools for Producing Written Communication

1. Writing Tools for Students Using Visual Access   Date completed _10/15/08_

When using standard writing tools (pencil, pen, etc.), the student is able to

❑ write manuscript (print) legibly at the rate of   NA
  _____ words per minute (wpm) from dictation,
  _____ wpm from copy, and
    ❑ read his or her handwriting.
    ❑ read a sample of his or her handwriting from 3 to 5 days earlier.

❑ write cursive legibly at the rate of   NA
  _____ wpm from dictation,
  _____ wpm from copy, and
    ❑ read his or her handwriting.
    ❑ read a sample of his or her handwriting from 3 to 5 days earlier.

❑ space appropriately between letters and words.

❑ sign his or her name legibly in cursive using
  ❑ a signature guide.
  ❑ the edge of a card, ruler, or some other similar device.

(continued on next page)

❑ The student produces legible writing **laboriously** and **with great difficulty** when using standard writing tools.

Comments: _____

_____

_____

The student is able to produce legible **manuscript** (print) writing using

☑ bold-lined paper at the rate of
___16___ wpm from dictation,
_____ wpm from copy, and:
   ☑ read his or her handwriting.
   ❑ read a sample of his or her handwriting from 3 to 5 days earlier.
❑ raised-lined paper at the rate of   NA
_____ wpm from dictation,
_____ wpm from copy, and
   ❑ read his or her handwriting.
   ❑ read a sample of his or her handwriting from 3 to 5 days earlier.

❑ an erasable pen or   ❑ a thick, dark pencil such as a primary pencil at the rate of   NA
_____ wpm from dictation,
_____ wpm from copy, and
   ❑ read his or her handwriting.
   ❑ read a sample of his or her handwriting from 3 to 5 days earlier.

☑ a felt-tip pen at the rate of
___16___ wpm from dictation,
_____ wpm from copy, and
   ☑ read his or her handwriting.
   ❑ read a sample of his or her handwriting from 3 to 5 days earlier.

❑ a whiteboard and erasable marker at the rate of
_____ wpm from dictation,
_____ wpm from copy, and
   ❑ read his or her handwriting.
   ❑ read a sample of his or her handwriting from 3 to 5 days earlier.

☑ a video magnifier (specify writing tools and adaptations being used)
   _desktop video magnifier_____   at the rate of
___20___ wpm from dictation,
_____ wpm from copy, and
   ☑ read his or her handwriting.
   ❑ read a sample of his or her handwriting from 3 to 5 days earlier.

_____ other (specify): _____

The student is able to produce legible **cursive** writing using   NA

☐ bold-lined paper at the rate of
___wpm from dictation,
___wpm from copy, and
   ☐ read his or her handwriting.
   ☐ read a sample of his or her handwriting from 3 to 5 days earlier.

☐ raised-lined paper at the rate of
___wpm from dictation,
___wpm from copy, and:
   ☐ read his or her handwriting.
   ☐ read a sample of his or her handwriting from 3 to 5 days earlier.

☐ an erasable pen or   ☐ a thick, dark pencil such as a primary pencil at the rate of
___wpm from dictation,
___wpm from copy, and
   ☐ read his or her handwriting.
   ☐ read a sample of his or her handwriting from 3 to 5 days earlier.

☐ a felt-tip pen at the rate of
___wpm from dictation,
___wpm from copy, and
   ☐ read his or her handwriting.
   ☐ read a sample of his or her handwriting from 3 to 5 days earlier.

☐ a whiteboard and erasable marker at the rate of
___wpm from dictation,
___wpm from copy, and
   ☐ read his or her handwriting.
   ☐ read a sample of his or her handwriting from 3 to 5 days earlier.

☐ a video magnifier (specify writing tools and adaptations being used)
_____ at the rate of
___wpm from dictation,
___wpm from copy, and
   ☐ read his or her handwriting.
   ☐ read a sample of his or her handwriting from 3 to 5 days earlier.

☐ other (specify): _____

The student is willing to use these devices (the examiner may wish to list these separately)
   ☑ to complete assignments in the regular classroom.
   ☑ at home to complete school assignments.
   ☑ while working with the teacher of students with visual impairments.

Comments: _Bill's writing was slow and labored. Lengthy writing tasks will be very difficult for Bill to complete in a timely manner. He did best using a dark pen and bold-lined paper. He was able to sign his name adequately._

(continued on next page)

2. Writing Tools for Students Using Tactile Access   **Date completed** 10/15/08

When using a manual braille-writing device, the student is able to use

NA ❑ a standard Perkins Brailler to emboss characters, words, and sentences at the rate of
___ words per minute (wpm) from dictation.
___ wpm from copy.

❑ a manual brailler with extension keys to emboss characters, words, and sentences at the rate of
___ wpm from dictation.
___ wpm from copy.

❑ a unimanual brailler to emboss characters, words, and sentences at the rate of
___ wpm from dictation.
___ wpm from copy.

❑ a slate and stylus to emboss characters, words, and sentences at the rate of
___ wpm from dictation.
___ wpm from copy.

❑ The student is able to sign his or her name legibly in cursive using
❑ a signature guide.
❑ the edge of a card, ruler, or some other similar device.

The student is willing to use these devices (the examiner may wish to list these separately)
❑ to complete assignments in the regular classroom.
❑ at home to complete school assignments.
❑ while working with the teacher of students with visual impairments.

Comments: _____
_____
_____

B. Electronic Tools for Producing Written Communication

Date completed 10/15/08

When using a computer with a scanner and imaging software, the student is able to
☑ scan a worksheet or form.
❑ use the software text tool to insert text into the worksheet.

When using an accessible computer running a word-processing program, the student is able to enter characters, words, and sentences at the rate of
20 words per minute (wpm) from dictation.
13 wpm from copy.

When using the Mountbatten Brailler or another electronic braillewriter, the student is able to emboss characters, words, and sentences at the rate of
NA wpm from dictation.

___wpm from copy.

When using an accessible PDA with a QWERTY keyboard, the student is able to enter characters, words, and sentences at the rate of
___wpm from dictation.　　　　　　NA
___wpm from copy.

When using an accessible PDA with a braille keyboard, the student is able to enter characters, words, and sentences at the rate of
___wpm from dictation.　　　　　　NA
___wpm from copy.

Comments: _____
_____
_____

Additional Assessment Information:

_____
_____
_____

Appendix: Windows Display Properties Appearance Checklist

Items Adjusted

☐ 3D Objects
　　　Color _____

☑ Active Title Bar
　　　Size _____　　　Color _____
　　　Font _____
　　　　　_14_ Size _*black*_ Color _✔_ Bold ____ Italic

☐ Active Window Border *default*
　　　Size _____　　　Color _____

☐ Application Background *default*
　　　Color _____

☑ Caption Buttons
　　　Size _48_

☐ Desktop *default*
　　　Color _____

☑ Icons
　　　Size _165_
　　　Font _Tahoma_
　　　____ Size _✔_ Bold ____ Italic

☑ Icon Spacing (Vertical) *default*
　　　Size _75_

☑ Icon Spacing (Horizontal) *default*
　　　Size _110_

(continued on next page)

☑ Inactive Title Bar

        Size _default_   Color _default_

        Font _Verdana_

            _14_ Size _____ Color ✓ Bold ____ Italic

❑ Inactive Window Border *default*

        Size _____   Color _____

☑ Menu

        Size _default_   Color _default_

        Font _Verdana_

            _16_ Size _____ Color ____ Bold ____ Italic

☑ Message Box

        Font _Verdana_

            _16_ Size _____ Color ✓ Bold ____ Italic

❑ Palette Title *default*

        Size _____

        Font _____

           ____ Size ____ Bold ____ Italic

❑ Scrollbar *default*

        Size _____

❑ Selected Items *default*

        Size _____   Color _____

        Font _____

           ____ Size _____ Color ____ Bold ____ Italic

❑ ToolTip *default*

        Color _____

        Font _____

           ____ Size _____ Color ____ Bold ____ Italic

❑ Window *default*

        Color _____

ARIAL FONT

This is 72 point print.

This is 60 point print.

This is 48 point print.

This is 36 point print.

(continued on next page)

This is 30 point print.

This is 24 point print.

This is 18 point print.

This is 14 point print.

This is 12 point print.

Tom was on his way to see Bill.

72

He came to the door.

60

It was a little red door.

48

Bill came out the door.

36

(continued on next page)

Bill had a blue ball.	30
His dog came out the door.	24
The dog had black and brown spots.	18
Tom and Bill went to play with the ball and Spot.	18
They ran on the green grass.	14
Bill threw the ball to Tom.	14
Spot ran after the blue ball.	12

Arial, APHont, Tahoma, Verdana

(Arial)
Tom was on his way to see Jill.
She came to the door.

(APHont)
Tom was on his way to see Jill.
She came to the door.

(Tahoma)
Tom was on his way to see Jill.
She came to the door.

(Verdana)
Tom was on his way to see Jill.
She came to the door.

(All fonts are displayed at 30 point size)

- Position the student in a chair sitting up straight with feet on the floor.
- Adjust the student's distance from the monitor of the video magnifier so that student's eyes are approximately 10–13 inches from the viewing screen. *(It is imperative that this working distance remain constant when measurements are made during the assessment.)*
- Adjust the height of the video magnifier monitor to the student's eye level or to the student's desired viewing position. (The examiner can obtain information about the best viewing position for the student from the ophthalmologic exam and the clinical low vision exam and consultation with the teacher of students with visual impairments will provide the examiner.)
- Lock the margin stops on the X-Y table. Turn on the unit and place a small object of interest to the student on the X-Y table under the camera. Adjust the magnification and focus so that the student can identify the object. Repeat this with several objects and allow the student to manipulate the magnification control to gain the student's interest and cooperation in working with the video magnifier.
- Place a 1-inch black-and-white line drawing under the camera. Adjust the zoom to maximum enlargement and focus the image. Adjust brightness and contrast if necessary. Reduce the image size to the lowest magnification.
- Ask the student to identify the object. If the student is able to identify the drawing at this level of magnification, measure the height of the image on the monitor and note it on the form.
- If the student is unable to identify the drawing at the lowest magnification level, gradually increase the magnification until the student can identify it. Be careful not to allow the student to lean closer to the monitor. Try to keep the student's working distance at 10–13 inches and use the system's size control to enlarge the target so that the student does not have to move closer to the monitor.
- If the student is unable to identify the target at the highest magnification level, then allow the student to move closer to the monitor. Measure the student's working distance and note it in the appropriate item on the form.
- Show the student how to control the zoom lens to adjust the magnification.
- Ask the student to adjust the size of the image to the largest magnification and then the smallest magnification.
- Ask the student to make the drawing fill up the screen.
- Finally, ask the student to adjust the magnification to the setting that allows him or her to see the object best. This gives the student a chance to observe the effects of using the camera's zoom lens and get some practice in adjusting it.

- If only part of the drawing is visible at the student's selected setting, ask the student if he or she can see the entire object and why he or she chose that setting. Note the student's comments in the comments section, because they will offer insight into whether the student has the cognitive and perceptual abilities to cope with being able to view only a portion of an object or image when it is highly magnified.
- Ask the student to adjust the size of the image to the smallest magnification. Place a different 1-inch line drawing under the camera. (The image should remain in focus because the distance between the camera lens and the image has not changed.)
- Ask the student to adjust the magnification to the best viewing size for him or her. Make sure he or she does not lean forward. Ask him or her to identify the drawing.
- Measure the approximate height of the image on the screen (not the image on paper) that he or she is able to identify and note it on the form. Also note the size of the video magnifier's monitor or screen.
- Repeat these steps with text. Be sure to measure the actual height of the text on the screen and note it on the form.

Focus

- If the video magnifier being used for the assessment has auto focus, skip the Focus section.
- Adjust the magnification to its maximum. Adjust the focus to put the image out of focus. Place a different image under the camera.
- Ask the student to adjust the focus until the image is clear and then adjust the magnification of the image until it is at the size he or she can see best. Note the student's ability to adjust the size and focus of the image on the form.

Polarity

- Show the student both polarity settings—black on white and white on black—with a line drawing and a sample reading passage at his or her independent reading level. Ask the student to read a few lines of the text. Note his or her preference on the form.

Color

- If the video magnifier being used has the feature that allows the user to set various color combinations of the image being enlarged, explore it with the student and note his or her color preference for text and background on the form.
- Note: Students will sometimes choose an unusual color combination because it looks "cool." After working with that combination for a while they often will choose another combination. If the student does choose a combination that seems unusual to the examiner, explore it further to determine if the selected combination is truly the best for the student or just an impulsive choice. Note this information in the comments section. However, some students will have a definite color preference and be able

(continued on next page)

to function more efficiently with that color combination. If the video magnifier being used for the assessment does not offer color and it is known that the student has a color preference when he or she works with a computer system offering that feature, contact the assistive technology specialist or rehabilitation engineer who will do the follow-up assessment to bring a color system for the follow-up or arrange with a vendor to borrow one.

Controls

- Place one of the tracking sample sheets under the camera and ask the student to adjust the magnification to his or her desired size.
- Adjust the friction brake so that the top-to-bottom movement of the page is stiff but movable. Set the left and right margin stops so that only the desired images are viewable on the screen.
- Ask the student to move the X-Y table to locate the target image and place his or her finger on it.
- Ask the student to move the X-Y table to view the next row and repeat the task.
- Repeat this process for several samples. Note how the student manipulates the table while viewing from right to left, and how he or she returns to the left edge and moves down to the next line. Many younger students will not be able to perform this task efficiently. However, the information gained

from observing this task will allow the examiner to determine if the student has the potential to master the physical and cognitive skills required to use the device. Note the observations on the form.

Writing

Even though this section of the assessment is primarily assessing the use of a video magnifier for reading or viewing print information, it is suggested that the student's potential for using this device to assist with writing also be assessed at this time.

- Place a regular sheet of notebook paper under the camera and readjust the margin stops so that the table does not move.
- Ask the student to write his or her name on one line while looking at the screen. Note if the student is able to look at the screen or looks at the paper instead.
- Repeat this task by asking the student to write a sentence on the next line. The margin stops will need to be readjusted to allow the student to complete the sentence or the student can simply move the paper.
- Replace the regular notebook paper with bold-lined paper and ask the student to write his or her name on one line and a different sentence on the next line. Record the results on the form.

Reading

- Remove the writing sample and replace it with a sample of the student's handwriting that is 3 to 5 days old. Ask the student to read it aloud.

- Remove the handwriting sample and replace it with a text selection at the student's independent reading level. Select a passage that is just one column of text. Ask the student to adjust the magnification to his or her desired size.
- Set the friction brake and the margin stops for this reading selection. Ask the student to read the selection aloud and record how long it takes to read the passage. Calculate the reading rate and record it on the form. Allow the student to practice reading with the device on several different reading samples and time each reading to determine if the student improves with practice. (This is not designed to be a formal reading measure, but the results may be compared to those obtained with other reading tools.)
- Note on the form if the student is able to use the X-Y table independently after demonstration and explanation. Add any necessary comments.
- Using several other reading samples of text in multiple columns, demonstrate to the student how to adjust the friction brake and margin stops.
- Return the margin stops to the outer edge of the X-Y table. Ask the student to make the adjustments with instruction and guidance from the examiner.
- Repeat the previous step but without guidance from the examiner. Note the student's performance on the form and add any necessary comments. (This will be valuable information for the teacher of students with visual impairments to use when designing instruction for efficient use of this device.)
- Place the student's writing samples completed earlier under the camera and ask the student to read them. Note the student's ability to read his or her own handwriting under the video magnifier with regular or bold line paper. Some students will remember exactly what they wrote and read it back quite quickly. If this occurs, ask the student to locate specific words and possibly spell some of the words. The goal here is to determine if the student is able to read the writing he or she created using the video magnifier.

These directions were derived from the operating system instructions for Windows 2000 and Windows XP. They will vary somewhat depending on the version of Windows you are using. However, they provide a guide to the types of features that will need to be addressed.

1. Access the Accessibility Wizard by opening the Start menu, choosing Programs, choosing Accessories; choosing Accessibility; and choosing Accessibility Wizard.
2. The first options offered by the Accessibility Wizard allow the user to select one of three choices of text size:

   • Use usual text size for Windows.
   • Use large window titles and menus.
   • Use Microsoft Magnifier and large titles and menus.

Ask the student to choose which of these is easiest to see. Select that option and then choose the Next button.

3. If the student chooses Microsoft Magnifier, skip to the assessment of Microsoft Magnifier (see Appendix 7H, "Assessing the Student's Ability to use Microsoft Magnifier"). If the student chooses either of the first two options, continue with the Accessibility Wizard assessment.
4. The next screen offers additional adjustments to determine the size of text and other items on the screen. There are three choices:

   • Change the font size.

   • Switch to a lower screen resolution.
   • Use Microsoft Magnifier.

Based on the font size selected on the previous screen, one or more preselected options may be recommended. Follow the recommendations and choose the Next button.

5. The next window, Set Wizard Options, offers choices to configure Windows for the user's vision, hearing, and mobility needs. These include the following options:

   • I am blind or have difficulty seeing things on screen.
   • I am deaf or have difficulty hearing sounds from the computer.
   • I have difficulty using the keyboard or mouse.
   • I want to set administrative options.

Select the options that are appropriate for the user. The first three options will lead to additional screens allowing adjustments in these areas. The fourth option, the administrative option, will provide an additional feature to turn off the accessibility features after the computer has been idle for a set period of time. The default setting is to turn off accessibility features after the computer has been idle for five minutes. This time setting can be adjusted for each individual user, or the user can choose always to leave accessibility features turned on.

6. Choose the Next button. Assuming that the first option was selected the next screen will offer the user four

choices for scroll bar and window border sizes.

7. Have the student choose the size that will be easiest to see and then select the Next button.

8. The Choose Icon Size dialog box will appear and display three choices for icon size: Normal, Large, and Extra Large. Ask the student to choose the one he or she can see the best and then select the Next button.

9. The Choose Color Settings dialog box will appear and display a list of color schemes. Have the student review each of the choices and select the one he or she can see best, and then select the Next button.

10. If the administrative option was selected earlier, then the Set Automatic Timeouts dialog box will be displayed. If more than one person will be using the computer it is a good idea to allow Windows to turn off the accessibility options after the system is idle for the specified amount of time. When these adjustments have been completed select the Next button. The Default Accessibility Settings dialog box appears and gives the user a chance to make his or her settings the active settings when the computer is turned on. If others will be using the computer it is best to choose No for this option. Select the Next button. The Save Settings to File dialog box will appear and provide the user the opportunity to save the settings to a file that can be used to configure other computers without having to go through the entire process again. When finished, select the Next button.

11. The Completing the Accessibility Wizard dialog box appears. It provides a summary of the adjustments that have been selected. These selections are displayed in the normal text size for Windows, not an enlarged size, but the examiner can review these settings with the student and then select the Finish button.

12. Demonstrate screen elements in several programs using the new settings and determine if these adjustments will allow the student to effectively view these elements.

13. Repeat the process and try other settings if necessary.

These directions were derived from the operating system instructions for Windows 2000 and Windows XP. They will vary somewhat depending on the version of Windows being used. However, they provide a guide to the types of features that will need to be addressed.

1. Find the Display Properties menu on the Control Panel or by right clicking on the desktop and selecting Properties from the pop-up menu.
2. The Display Properties dialog box will appear with tabs for multiple pages.
3. Select the tab for the Appearance page.
4. Select the Scheme option. A drop-down menu of different combinations of screen colors, sizes and formats or schemes will appear.
5. A number of these schemes have been designed to improve the appearance of the display for users with visual impairments. Demonstrate the various schemes to the student, starting with one of the high-contrast schemes. There are several other schemes providing enlarged text and other screen elements that will also need to be demonstrated to the student.
6. Ask the student to select the scheme he or she prefers. Select the Apply button.
7. Demonstrate how the appearance of the display is affected in various other applications by the new scheme.
8. Return to the Appearance page of the Display Properties dialog box.
9. Allow the student to try other schemes with different applications until he or she can decide which setting is best for him or her. Note this scheme selection on the checklist.
10. If none of the predefined schemes or combinations of screen colors, sizes, and formats improves the user's ability to see the display, then he or she can adjust these components of each screen element individually by selecting Items to open a list of individual screen elements that can be adjusted.
11. After adjusting one of the items, select Apply to view the change made by the new setting. Adjusting these elements individually can result in a combination or scheme that will benefit some users.
12. The resulting settings can be saved as a scheme using the student's name after each element is adjusted. This will eliminate the need to reselect all the settings if something goes wrong, or if the student wishes to cancel the most recent adjustments and try again. Also remember to save the settings again at the end of the session when all choices have been made.
13. If an effective combination is determined, be sure to note the setting for each item that has been adjusted.
14. Exit the Display Properties-Appearance dialog box after saving all settings.

Note that if the text displayed in menus and other items is set to 18 points or larger, parts of menus and menu items will not be fully displayed on the screen.

The final adjustments can be recorded in the Windows Display Properties Appearance Checklist in Figure 7.16.

Appendix 7H   Assessing the Student's Ability to Use Microsoft Magnifier

1. Access the Accessibility Wizard by opening the Start menu; choosing Programs, choosing Accessories; choosing Accessibility; and choosing Magnifier.

2. The Microsoft Magnifier program will appear at the top of the screen with the last magnification setting in effect. The remainder of the screen will be displayed unmagnified. The Magnifier Settings dialog box will also be displayed on the screen.

3. The first setting to adjust is the Magnification Level. Use the Up or Down Arrows to increase or decrease the magnification level, or click on the up and down triangles in the spin box.

4. Most of the other options for Tracking and Presentation will not need to be modified. If they are, note it on the assessment checklist.

5. If the student chooses a magnification level higher than 2, the size of the viewing window will need to be adjusted. To adjust the size of the viewing window, place the mouse pointer on the line border between the magnified and unmagnified sections of the screen. When it is in the proper position, it will turn into two small arrows pointing up and down.

6. Click and drag the line down to increase the size of the viewing window. The maximum size of the viewing window is approximately one-half the vertical height of the screen.

7. Ask the student to identify screen elements and read text from several applications to determine the effectiveness of this tool.

8. Guide the student through opening a file in a word-processing program using simple verbal instructions. Note how well the student is able to locate the necessary screen elements to accomplish this task.

9. Switch to the word-processing program.

10. Ask the student to use the mouse or keyboard to select the File menu.

11. Ask the student to use the mouse or keyboard to select the Open option.

12. Ask the student to locate the Title Bar.

13. Ask the student to locate the list of files that can be opened.

14. Ask the student to select a specified file to open.

15. Record the student's responses on the Assessment Checklist.

16. Exit the Microsoft Magnifier program.

1. Open a prepared word-processing file containing appropriate reading passages, with the text displayed in the student's preferred font at 12 points. This file will need to contain several paragraphs, enough to fill up about three-quarters of the screen.

2. Open an application that will display a graphic, picture, or map.

3. Open the screen magnification program. Start with the computer display open to the graphics application.

4. Have the student sit up straight in the chair with his or her back against the backrest.

5. Measure the working distance to ensure that the student is approximately 13 to 16 inches from the display.

6. When the student is ready, switch the computer to the word-processor application.

7. Adjust the magnification of the image until the student is able to read the text and view the material without having to lean forward.

8. Demonstrate the polarity options and ask the student if he or she prefers black text on a white background or white text on a black background.

9. Note the magnification size and any polarity preference on the checklist. Most screen magnification programs offer several different viewing modes or ways in which the enlarged image can be displayed (such as full, lens, area, or horizontal split). Demonstrate the different viewing modes offered by the program and explain to the student how these affect spatial orientation and the amount of text viewable on the screen.

10. Ask the student to move the mouse around to change the image being displayed and to notice how much of the paragraph is viewable at any one time.

11. Ask the student to move back to the left edge of the screen using the mouse and read a line of the text. Note if the student has any difficulty locating the left edge and how well he or she is able to track across the line of text.

12. Ask the student to find the beginning of the second paragraph. Note the strategy he or she uses to locate it and whether he or she gets lost or can get reoriented.

13. Move the mouse so that the display is in the middle of a line of text and about halfway down the unmagnified screen of text. Explain to the student how easy it is to get disoriented and that when using this type of computer access program the user must regain orientation by returning to a known point, such as the top left corner of the screen.

14. Ask the student to use this strategy and then move to the beginning of the third paragraph. Note the student's ability to maintain or regain his or her orientation.

15. Repeat steps 12 to 14 and ask the student to perform the tasks using keyboard commands that the examiner will supply.

16. Switch to the graphics application.

17. Ask the student to navigate around the image and verbally identify the information being displayed.

18. Ask the student to locate specific parts of the image: top right corner, bottom left corner, middle of image, and some specific feature of the graphic, etc. Again, note his or her ability to stay oriented.

19. Ask the student to repeat steps 17 and 18 using keyboard commands.

20. Change the screen magnification software to the lens setting. The lens mode will display the entire image, but only a small rectangular area will be enlarged. Point out to the student how much easier this is for navigating around the graphic image. Ask the student to locate specific features of the graphic.

21. Switch to the word-processor program and ask the student to read a line of text. Note how much more difficult it is for the student to stay on track.

22. Change the screen magnification software back to the full viewing mode.

23. Ask the student to open menus and select items from it, choose items in a dialog box, and select icons on a toolbar.

24. Set up the parameters for the review or panning mode for automatic reading and have the student read text with paragraphs. Adjust the speed so that the student can read the text easily. Note the speed setting for this option. (The examiner may wish to get assistance from an assistive technology specialist for this portion of the assessment.)

Writing the Recommendations Report

The job of the assistive technology team is not yet finished when it has completed its assessment of a student and documented its findings. The team now needs to decide what the data it has collected suggests about the technology that will best support the student, write a report that encompasses its recommendations, and help translate its findings into Individualized Education Program (IEP) goals. The Assistive Technology Recommendations Form included in this chapter can help organize the data from the assessment that will be used to write a final report. (An example of this form, as completed for Bill Alonso, whose assistive technology assessment checklist appears in Chapter 7, is presented in Appendix 8A to this chapter, and a blank version of the form appears in Appendix D at the back of this book. The report based on the recommendations for Bill is found in Appendix 8B.) The final assessment report should be submitted to the IEP team so that they can make plans for implementing the recommendations as part of the student's education program and write specific goals and objectives for the student. (Implementing the IEP is discussed in Chapter 9.)

It is important that the written report emphasize that the student will most probably need a combination of devices and other tools to accomplish his or her educational goals. It is unlikely that a comprehensive assistive technology assessment will find only one single device or method that will meet all the student's needs. Some technology will be appropriate for accomplishing certain tasks in specific environments, and other tools will be necessary to accomplish the same tasks, or others, in a different setting or under different circumstances.

GENERAL CONSIDERATIONS

The General Education Technology Plan
- Technology as an Instructional Tool
- Technology as a Productivity Tool

The Technology Continuum

Immediate and Future Needs

Parents' Concerns

Administrators' Concerns about Technology

Skills Training
- Students' Attitudes

A number of considerations need to be addressed by the assessment team in the formulation of its recommendations. Primary among them are the characterisitics of the student, including his or her needs and the sensory channels he or she uses to obtain information and interact with the environment, and the educational tasks the student needs to perform. In addition, several general considerations need to be taken into account. A comprehensive assessment is intended to ensure that all the educational needs of a student have been considered, as well as other issues that might affect the implementation of the recommendations. These considerations include the following:

- The general education technology plan for the local or state education agency
- The technology continuum for students who are blind or visually impaired, which would suggest the development and sequencing of certain skills
- The immediate and future needs of the student
- Parents' concerns about technology
- Administrators' concerns about technology
- Skills training
- The student's attitudes toward using various technologies

All these considerations, described in the following sections, need to be integrated into the specific recommendations for ways in which the student may access print, access electronic information, and produce written communication, and for ways in which materials in accessible formats may be provided.

THE GENERAL EDUCATION TECHNOLOGY PLAN

Most school systems have developed a general technology plan for their students, which usually indicates how students learn about technology—such as computers and the Internet—and how it is integrated into the general education curriculum. A simplified technology plan might look something like the one in Sidebar 8.1, "A School System's General Technology Plan: One Sample"; school districts may also develop a plan that lists expectations for technology-related learning for each specific grade level. Thus, in addition to addressing how the student will use technology to access information and produce written communication, the assistive technology assessment report needs to make recommendations about how the student will access the general education technology curriculum. For example, the report should envision how a first-grade student might use technology to practice basic skills in reading and math, when classmates are using inaccessible computer software, or

---

SIDEBAR 8.1

A SCHOOL SYSTEM'S GENERAL TECHNOLOGY PLAN: ONE SAMPLE

Many, if not most, school districts have developed a general technology plan for their students that may be similar to the one presented here, although probably more detailed. This is part of the general education curriculum, and students who are blind or visually impaired need to participate in and have access to the school system's plan. Thus, the recommendations stemming from the assistive technology assessment must address the ways that a student will access the technology curriculum.

Pre-K Through Second Grade

Computer software is used to reinforce and practice basic skills in reading and math.

Third Through Fifth Grade

Students begin learning keyboarding skills, basic word processing, and simple Internet searching and continue use of educational software.

Sixth Through Eighth Grade (Middle School)

Students refine keyboarding skills, word-processing skills, and research skills using the Internet and other electronic resources and begin to explore the use of other applications such as spreadsheet programs, database programs, and presentation software.

Ninth Through Twelfth Grade (High School)

Students use a variety of hardware (computers, printers, scanners, digital cameras, and so forth) in conjunction with software applications and online resources to develop and produce advanced reports, documents, and presentations containing text and graphics.

how a fifth-grade student will accomplish basic word-processing tasks and Internet searching. Whether technology is used in the general classroom or in a computer lab, its use generally has two broad objectives: as a tool for instruction and as a productivity tool for accessing information and producing written communication.

Technology as an Instructional Tool

Many technologies are used as instructional tools, particularly educational computer software that is used to teach, reinforce, and practice basic academic skills such as phonics skills or basic mathematics. Such programs are often inaccessible both to individuals who are blind or visually impaired and to those with additional disabilities, and few of the programs work with screen magnification or screen-reading programs.

When the objective is to use technology as an instructional tool and the technology is inaccessible, members of the student's IEP team will need to make suggestions about how the desired educational objectives can be accomplished through alternative activities and the use of materials in appropriate formats. So, for example, while classmates are using a computer program to practice spelling words, the student with visual impairments can be learning to use features on the Mountbatten to turn in spelling words in both print and braille. Recommendations in the final assistive technology assessment report will need to include assistive technology tools and services that will allow the student to accomplish these educational objectives.

Technology as a Productivity Tool

If the objective of an educational activity is to learn to use technology as a productivity tool—that is, to produce or access information—then the technology recommendations for a student need to include appropriate tools, adaptations and modifications, and training in the use of computer accessibility software to accomplish this same goal. These recommendations need to explain clearly how the student will access

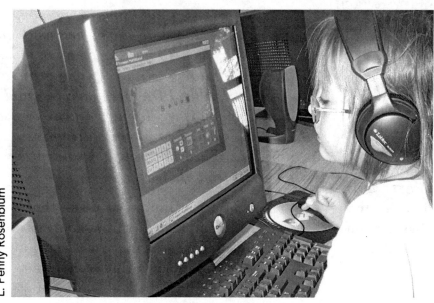

L. Penny Rosenblum

Although this student with low vision is able to make use of an educational computer program to practice basic mathematics skills, few such programs work with screen magnification or screen readers.

print information, including textbooks, various educational materials used in class, and print information presented at a visual distance (such as on a chalkboard or whiteboard or using an overhead projector). These may be issues that the team has not considered in addressing classroom access because these concerns are generally not part of the school district's technology plan, but in fact they are critically important for students with visual impairments. Additional recommendations need to be made about how the student will access electronic information provided by computers, personal digital assistants (PDAs), and other technological devices and software. Low-tech and high-tech devices also need to be recommended to assist the student in written communication. And, finally, recommendations need to be made about tools needed to provide educational materials for the student in the appropriate format, such as the use of print with optical devices, large print, braille, tactile graphics, and audio. These may be tools and services used by the student or by service providers who will produce materials in alternate formats for the student.

Each of these recommendations will need to be provided with a rationale and justification in the final report that emphasize the appropriate use of the recommended technology. Special care needs to be taken to make sure it is apparent how each of the devices or technology specified fits into the student's educational program and assists the student in accomplishing educational objectives. As mentioned earlier, the report should make clear that a given device can be right for accomplishing some tasks, but not appropriate for others, so that a variety of solutions are needed by the student.

THE TECHNOLOGY CONTINUUM

Students' technology needs are not static. They progress along a continuum throughout the student's educational career. Most students will begin learning to use low-tech tools and then gradually be introduced to a continuum of higher-tech tools as their skills increase. As some students move on to higher grades in school and need more powerful tools, they will spend less time using technology that provides fewer features. As older students begin using more technologically advanced tools, the technology they began using early in their education can be reallocated to younger students who still have need of its features. The example of Tamara illustrates the idea of a *continuum of assistive technology* for students who are blind or visually impaired:

Tamara is a fourth-grade student who has been using the Mountbatten Brailler since kindergarten as an assistive technology tool to facilitate her written communication. She has greatly benefited from the hard copy of braille text produced by this device, but she and her teacher of students with visual impairments feel that Tamara no longer needs to have access to all of her work in hard copy. In fact, Tamara is ready to move up the continuum of technology and begin to use an accessible PDA with a refreshable braille display. Once Tamara learns to use this new device, her Mountbatten Brailler can be reassigned to a younger student who can benefit from its features.

There is a continuum of tasks that are typically accomplished throughout a student's schooling, just as there is a continuum of assistive technology that can assist in accomplishing these tasks. The technology continuum for students who are blind or visually impaired is based on the students' needs, skills, and in some cases, age. Some technology tools are designed to complete tasks required in the early years of a student's educational program, while others are more appropriate for advanced tasks required later. As a student's educational tasks become more and more complex, he or she is likely to need more complex technology.

This technology continuum includes tools that assist students in accessing printed information, completing writing tasks, accessing electronic information, and converting print information into electronic information, as well as tools for producing materials in alternate formats. Students may need some or all of these types of tools throughout their educational journey, but the sophistication of these tools will vary by age group depending on the complexity of the tasks the student needs to accomplish. As the assessment team writes the assistive technology assessment report, it needs to consider whether its recommendations need to be geared toward moving the student through this continuum and into higher levels of technology use and skills. Understanding the continuum is important for students, parents, administrators, and teachers. One of the objectives of the recommendations and the final assessment report is to help these individuals and others understand this continuum and where the student being assessed fits on the continuum. This awareness is especially important with regard to moving to new and more complex technology as his or her needs become more complex.

The final report of a student's assistive technology assessment can serve as a guide for the IEP team in understanding how the recommendations fit into the student's individual needs and can indicate how they can contribute to an informal assistive technology plan for all the students in the system who are blind or visually impaired. By looking at a technology continuum for these students, such an informal plan can be enormously helpful to a school system as it addresses the general technology needs of students who are braille readers and students with low vision.

IMMEDIATE AND FUTURE NEEDS

Sometimes technology is available that can assist a student in meeting his or her immediate needs, such as providing print materials in the student's desired font and point size. However, there are many other technologies that will be useful to the student, but will require instruction and training for the student, the service providers working with the student, and, at times, the student's parents and other family members. These technologies can meet the student's needs, but it may be months or years before the student will use the devices, strategies, or features independently. Thus, it is important to plan ahead so that the student will be prepared to make use of the appropriate technology at the appropriate time. When making recommendations for immediate and future needs, it is important for an assessment report to emphasize that the student cannot be expected to learn to use all the relevant technology tools in the near future. Many of the technology solutions available to individuals who are blind or visually impaired require a complex set of cognitive, motor, visual, tactile, and auditory skills that will develop as the student grows and matures. In addition, the teacher may need time to develop his or her own technology skills before being ready to learn how to teach some of the newer, more complicated technology tools to students. Thus, in many cases the assessment team will need to make long-term recommendations that address the student's future needs as well as those that can be implemented immediately.

Determining a student's future needs can be difficult. Changes in the student's vision and changes in technology are often unpredictable. However, although the evaluators may not be able to make recommendations for specific pieces of technology that will be needed in the future, they certainly can highlight the needs that have to be addressed. Assessment reports for students whose eye conditions are progressive or who are dual print and braille users, for example, need to indicate how the student's needs are likely to change and offer suggestions for meeting them. Recommendations for follow-up assessment to monitor future needs are also important. In general, as students progress through the school system, their future needs will involve accessing larger quantities of print and electronic information, completing longer and more complex writing tasks, and requiring a wider variety of materials in alternate formats. The assistive technology recommendations made can help guide the IEP team in planning how the student will obtain the skills necessary to take full advantage of current and future technology devices and strategies. Therefore, the recommendations will need to explain how the student will start using certain technology tools, develop skills with them, and then progress to more advanced techniques and the timeline for introducing, practicing, and mastering their independent use. For example, Bill Alonso will start using a screen magnification program to do simple tasks but will learn to use its more advanced features as he becomes more familiar with the technology and receives additional training.

PARENTS' CONCERNS

It is to be expected that parents have a number of concerns about the assistive technology that their child will use, and the technology assessment report needs to address these concerns. Parents often worry that their child will not receive equal access to the technology curriculum in which their child's classmates participate. Often, however, it is not within the power of a school system to make accessible to a student with visual impairments the exact same software or technology devices that other students are using.

However, what the school system *can* offer, as already indicated, is alternative activities with accessible materials that will ensure that the visually impaired student will meet the same educational objectives as his or her classmates. In addition, the educational program can provide a student with the opportunity to develop technology skills that will be necessary for success in education, employment, and daily life. The recommendations report can address any concerns parents may have by making these alternatives clear and in this way ensuring that the student becomes as adept in the use of technology as his or her classmates. In addition, members of the IEP team, such as the teacher of students with visual impairments, can help parents—who are also members of the team—clearly understand the role of technology in their child's educational and daily life and encourage them to support the student's development of technology literacy and skills.

ADMINISTRATORS' CONCERNS

Although school system administrators in general try to do what is best for all students, they must also make difficult decisions about the expenditure of limited resources. Administrators may be surprised when they receive an assistive technology assessment report for a student who is blind or visually impaired and begin to investigate the cost of implementing the recommendations, since many of the technology tools needed by students who are blind or visually impaired can be quite expensive. In almost every assistive technology assessment report, it will be necessary to point out the rationale and justification for the tools recommended. Several points can be underscored to make these expensive recommendations more palatable.

First, some administrators may be overwhelmed by the sheer quantity of the assistive technology tools and services needed by a student who is blind or visually impaired and their cost. In addition, in a school district in which visually impaired students are uncommon, questions can arise about the equity and appropriateness of devoting what seems like a disproportionate share of resources for a single student. An explanation of the technology continuum described earlier can help by stressing that some of the recommendations address future needs, not all the recommended devices and services need to be purchased immediately, and some of the equipment may be useful for multiple students over time.

A second point to emphasize when formulating the rationale and justification for the recommendations is that purchasing assistive technology is often a better value than using other options. In many cases, as shown in several examples later in this chapter, it is simply more cost effective to purchase the new technology. Providing a student with appropriate equipment that he or she can use independently, for example, can save staff time in making numerous photocopies of materials for the student, which in fact may not be an effective accommodation.

A third point to note is the flexibility offered by many technology tools, especially if they can be used with multiple students. For instance, a specialized scanning system in a middle school recommended for one particular student would not be used by that student continuously throughout the school day. This same system could be used by the teacher of students with visual impairments or other staff members to convert printed information into electronic information, which eventually could be produced in braille or large print for another student, or put to other important uses within the school.

The final point to make is that most of the technology recommended for students who are blind or visually impaired can be recycled to younger students. A typical desktop video magnifier purchased for a second-grade student may be used by that student until she moves into middle school and begins changing classes, when she will need a system that offers more portability. The desktop system can then be assigned to a younger student who does the majority of his or her reading in a single location. This ability to recycle technology can help stretch limited budgets further.

The bottom line is that the school system is responsible for providing the assistive technology devices and services that the student requires to take advantage of the free and appropriate public education provided for in the Individuals with Disabilities Education Act (IDEA). Explanations and reasoning may help some administrators realize the overall financial benefit of doing the right thing in addition to meeting the statutory requirements.

SKILLS TRAINING

Training in the skills needed to use assistive technology is covered by the definition of assistive technology services that must be provided to students who need them under IDEA (see Appendix A, "It's the Law"). The importance of including training in skills needed to use the recommended devices and strategies in the recommendations and final report cannot be overemphasized. Without training, the technology may be of little use to the student and will not accomplish the ultimate goal of maximizing the student's potential. In the report written for Bill (Appendix 8B), training is recommended numerous times for the use of a video magnifier, reader, recorded textbooks and audio-assisted reading, talking scientific calculator, talking dictionary, word-processing program, and keyboarding.

Emphasizing training and specifying the skills that need to be developed in the recommendations for a student helps to ensure that training will be included in the student's IEP and therefore that the teacher of students with visual impairments will be able to allocate sufficient service time for this item. IEPs must be written based on the needs of students as determined by evaluation. By increasing and improving instructional time to meet those documented needs, IEPs can help students who are blind or visually impaired acquire the knowledge and skills to take advantage of the tools provided by technology.

Students' Attitudes

A final important issue to consider when making recommendations for assistive technology is the student's attitude about using

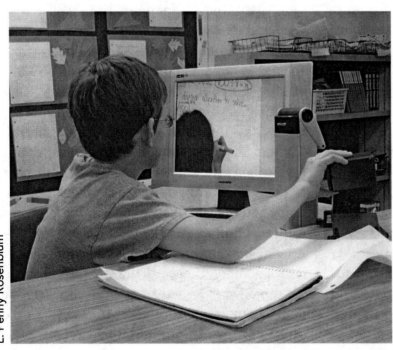

L. Penny Rosenblum

Some students are reluctant to use any technology they perceive as making them "look different." Effective instruction that allows the student to experience immediate benefit from using the device can often overcome the initial reluctance.

it. Some students are reluctant to use anything that they perceive as making them "look different." For this reason, this question needs to be addressed repeatedly throughout the assistive technology assessment, and assessment team members need to be alert to a student's possible discomfort about using certain devices. If the evaluator believes that a particular technology tool will benefit a student and the student does not want to use it, the support team may need to find ways to convince the student to use the technology. In some cases, students are hesitant to use a new technology because they have not learned to use it efficiently. It may seem more trouble than it is worth at first, especially devices that are complex to use or have many features. In such instances, good instruction is critical so that the student can experience immediate benefit from using the device. This, in turn, will improve the student's motivation to use the technology, and increased practice will increase the student's skills. The comments recorded during Bill's assessment (see Appendix 7A in Chapter 7) indicate that he was reluctant to use a desktop video magnifier in class, but when he experienced the benefits of the digital imaging system's features, especially the distance-viewing capability, the device's usefulness overcame his reluctance.

Supportive discussions with the student and family may also be helpful. Instances in which students can be helped to see themselves as "power users" of "cool" technology may also sway the direction of the situation. These and other strategies to address this issue are discussed in Chapter 9. Before completing its final report, the assessment team may need to discuss whether the student's attitude toward the technology will be an obstacle and whether there is a way to encourage and convince the student to use the technology being recommended.

WRITING THE RECOMMENDATIONS

The Assistive Technology Recommendations Form provided in this book is intended as a guide for synthesizing the information from the assistive technology assessment. The recommendations should address the student's needs in the general areas highlighted throughout this book and be part of a final report submitted to the IEP team:

- Accessing print information
- Accessing electronic information
- Producing written communication
- Producing materials in accessible formats for the student

There is also space on the form to indicate any additional hardware or software needed. The form is designed to be a quick tool that the evaluator can use to note possible devices and strategies to recommend in the final assistive technology assessment report. Different specialists on the assessment team will have recommendations based on their areas of expertise and the areas of the assessment they were involved in evaluating. When completing each section of the recommendations form, the team members may want to review the related sections of Chapters 2–5 that describe various technologies and their uses. The report itself should clearly explain the rationale for the recommendations based on the student's performance during the assessment, as illustrated in the sample report provided in Appendix 8B.

As stated throughout this book, the results of the learning media assessment will guide the team in making recommendations related to the student's primary learning medium—the sense of vision, touch, or hearing. It is important to bear in mind, however, that the student may not always choose to use his or her primary literacy medium. Depending on the quantity of material to be accessed and the location in which it must be accessed, the student may choose to use a secondary medium. Most students will need to use a variety of tools to access print information. Some of these tools will be appropriate at certain times of the day and not at others, depending on the student's level of fatigue and other factors. Other tools will be useful for short reading tasks, but not longer ones.

The issue of fatigue will need to be addressed on an ongoing basis. Fatigue can be caused by such factors as poor posture or working in a cramped or uncomfortable position for long periods of time. Students with low vision may experience visual fatigue because the materials they need to read may contain print that is too small or print with poor contrast, and there may be too much or too little lighting. Fatigue may be an issue with the use of most of the technology tools recommended in the assistive technology assessment report. Attempting to avoid fatigue is one of the rationales for recommending multiple tools to accomplish similar tasks by using different sensory modalities, depending on the length and complexity of the task.

COMPILING THE REPORT

After completing the Assistive Technology Recommendations form, the assistive technology assessment team will need to collaborate in writing the final report. Some teams have each member contribute content for various sections of the assessment and recommendations that he or she completed and then have the coordinator of the team combine them into one final report. Other teams may choose to submit the information to the coordinator and have the coordinator write the final report to ensure consistency in the writing style and presentation. Each team needs to choose the approach that will best help its members provide the information that must be communicated to the IEP team to meet the student's needs.

The final report should contain a short descriptive summary about the student, his or her current and future needs, and a list of recommendations with rationales and justifications. The report should also be accompanied by the team's assistive technology considerations checklist, background summary, assessment results, and assessment recommendations (the forms provided in Chapters 6, 7, and 8, if they were used), and possibly a resource list of vendors that produce the recommended hardware and software.

The descriptive summary about the student should include any information that the team feels will be relevant to the reader's understanding of the report, such as pertinent information from the background materials discussed in Chapter 6. A paragraph about the student's current levels of functioning will be needed to highlight the tasks that the student has difficulty completing. Modifications and adaptations that have already been made to the educational program, including any assistive technology that has been used with the student, should be described along with a statement about their effectiveness. The student's acceptance or rejection of these interventions should also be noted.

One approach to organizing the recommendations along with their rationale and justification in the final report is to use the four main sections of the Assistive Technology Recommendations Form. The items that have been recommended and are checked on the form can be numbered in sequence, and the paragraphs in the report discussing each item can be given the corresponding numbers. The discussion of each item will give details about the tasks and settings in which it will be appropriate for the student to use the particular technology. In many cases, it will also be necessary to describe the tasks and settings for which this tool will *not* be appropriate. Explanations of the recommendations will need to include the rationale and justification for recommending each type of assistive technology.

It is strongly recommended that the explanations given in the final report emphasize the features of the different types of technology rather than recommend a specific brand of device or software to allow current and future IEP teams to meet the student's assistive technology needs without being tied to one particular brand. However, it can be useful to include an appendix containing information about the recommended devices and services and where they can be procured (as was done in the report for Bill in Appendix 8B). In many cases, members of the assistive technology assessment team themselves will be asked to locate vendors and submit purchase orders for the recommended devices, so such an appendix may not be necessary. If other school system personnel will be responsible for acquiring the recommended assistive technology, then a more detailed appendix may be helpful. If members of the assessment team are not

doing the purchasing, it is recommended that they be contacted when decisions about specific models and types of devices are made, since deciphering the descriptions of the wide variety of models available for some types of assistive technology can be challenging. (Among the sources for such information are the technology section of the web site of the American Foundation for the Blind [www.afb.org/technology] and the online technology magazine *AccessWorld* [www.afb.org/aw]. See the Resources section, Appendix B, at the back of the book, for suppliers of various technologies and other sources of information about products.)

The recommendations will need to emphasize repeatedly that a combination of solutions and a variety of tools will be required to give the student maximum flexibility in accomplishing required educational tasks. Students, parents, teachers, and administrators need to realize that there is no one perfect solution to meet all a student's needs for access to information, just as there is no one single solution for all low vision students or for all braille readers. Moreover, assessment is not an exact science, and students may need a trial period with many technologies. Therefore, the school may want to rent or lease expensive equipment, when possible, until it can be determined that the recommended technology will truly meet the student's needs.

One final point bears repeating: in many cases, the recommendations made in the report do not all have to be implemented immediately. That is because some of the recommendations are designed to be proactive and look ahead to future needs and skills that will be taught over time. For example, the final report for Bill Alonso suggests that, in view of his future needs, he should be trained to make appropriate use of a human reader. The student's IEP team will need to determine which of the student's needs are most critical and begin implementing the assistive technology recommendations associated with those needs as soon as possible, and to indicate those needs in the form of specific IEP objectives. In some cases, various suggestions can be designed as part of a two- to three-year plan in which the student masters certain skills and is provided with access to additional technologies that can facilitate his or her educational program. During that time, new products and technologies will in all likelihood become available that will enhance the student's ability to maximize his or her educational potential. It is also sometimes the case that specific devices recommended may no longer be the most appropriate, but the student will continue to need the assistance that they provide. For this reason, regular monitoring of a student's progress and follow-up assessments are an essential part of the work of the IEP team. Overall, the assessment report should encourage the IEP team to implement the recommendations that can be put in place in the near future, while taking the steps necessary to implement the remaining recommendations in a timely manner. Chapter 9 contains more information about implementing the recommendations.

ACCESSING PRINT INFORMATION

Accessing Print Visually
- Low-Tech Solutions
- Enlarged Materials
- Large Print
- Scanned Materials
- Nonoptical Devices
- Video Magnifiers
- Scanners and Specialized Scanning Systems

Accessing Print Tactilely
- Braille
- Accessing Graphical Information Tactilely

Accessing Print Auditorily

Accessing Information Presented from a Distance
- Information in the Student's Preferred Medium
- Optical Devices
- Digital Video Cameras
- Electronic Whiteboards
- Audio-Described Videos

ACCESSING PRINT VISUALLY

Many students who access information visually use prescribed eyeglasses, contact lens, or optical devices for near and distance viewing. Recommendations for all students need to reinforce and support the use of the optical devices prescribed in the clinical low vision evaluation. In Bill's case, continued use of his 4× magnifier is recommended. Details about these prescribed devices and their recommended use should be noted on the recommendations form and in the final report. The recommendations should ensure that the student has access to the prescribed optical devices as well as training in their use and should provide opportunities to encourage their use. Although prescribed optical devices are essential for many students, the use of other technologies will also need to be recommended along with suggestions on how and when to use combinations of the recommended tools.

Low-Tech Solutions

One low-tech solution that can be recommended for some students is the use of teacher-made materials printed with a dark felt-tip pen or marker on bold-lined paper. This is a labor-intensive option for providing visual access to print information, however, and should be recommended sparingly. It is generally appropriate for materials such as a list of spelling or vocabulary words, simple math problems, fill-in-the-blank statements or questions, or perhaps text to be copied for writing practice. It's still important to list this recommendation, however, especially for children in early grades such as kindergarten and first grade, where teachers often create brief, ephemeral materials and may not know that special dark-lined paper is commercially available. Dark or bold writing instruments and bold- or raised-line paper also often serve as a good tools for producing written communication.

Enlarged Materials

Enlarging materials on a photocopying machine is another option that can be recommended for limited use in providing visual access to print information. As discussed in Chapter 5, this option serves only as a partial solution at best and should be used sparingly, but it is used all too often because of its availability and presumed low cost. However, a cost analysis that takes into consideration the cost of staff time to make the copies and the cost per page to operate and maintain the copying machine usually demonstrates that the low cost of this practice is an illusion.

Aside from the issue of expense, and equally if not more important, the use of photocopied materials is usually not an effective accommodation for a student who is visually impaired. The use of a photocopier to enlarge materials therefore should only be recommended in situations in which no other acceptable alternative is available, as in the following situation:

A high school social studies teacher reads an article in a magazine at breakfast and decides that it would be useful for his students to read it in economics class that morning. The teacher knows that his student with low vision in the class does not have access to an optical device that allows her to read the size print used in the magazine. The teacher also knows that there is not enough time to have the article produced in an accessible format. Based on information that has been provided in the recommendations from the assistive technology evaluation and from consultations with the teacher of students with visual impairments, the teacher knows that enlarging the article on the photocopying machine 160 percent on 11 × 17 inch paper will be adequate for the student to read in the class. For this situation, the enlarged photocopy will be adequate, but it is not acceptable for most of the materials the student will need to access for this and other classes.

It is imperative that the final assessment report for a student explain in great detail the appropriate and inappropriate use of photocopiers to enlarge materials and include examples of when it is acceptable and unacceptable.

Large Print

Another tool that can be recommended for some students to access printed information visually is large print. Although large print is often the first accommodation thought of for students who are visually impaired in some school systems, it is often not the most effective or flexible way in which to meet students' needs, and in fact can limit their access to information, given the relatively small number of materials available in large print as a matter of course. For this reason, any recommendations in the assessment report that mention large print need to specify the appropriate circumstances for its use.

When is large print useful, and what considerations relate to its use? For some students, the use of handheld optical devices may not be practical for longer reading tasks, and commercially available large-print books and locally produced large-print materials can offer adequate enlargement in some cases. However, large-print books are often too big to be of practical use at a student's desk and are awkward to handle, so they may not be the most appropriate tool for the student to use in class and many students refuse to use them. Thus, although large-print books are often recommended because they seem like a logical solution, they frequently go unused by students. In general, if commercially available large-print books (in an 18- or 24-point font) provide the student with an adequate image size that can be viewed at a comfortable reading distance and position, it may be recommended that the student use them in certain settings. For example, using a large-print book or other large-print materials with a reading stand or book stand and a controllable lighting source may be an effective and efficient tool for reading longer passages at home where there may be more room to work and the student is not restricted by the constraints of a typical classroom desk. Some students are uncomfortable using large-print materials at school because they feel the books make them look "different" from their classmates, but may choose to use them at home or in the privacy provided by a resource room setting for students who are blind or visually impaired. As with the other tools for accessing printed information already discussed, the appropriate circumstances for using large print must be clearly defined in the assistive technology assessment final report. It is unlikely that large-print books will be the only adaptation and accommodation that a student will need, as their use restricts the student to textbooks only and does not allow access to the myriad other educational materials found in modern classrooms.

Scanned Materials

If students are able to read enlarged text at a comfortable working distance, it may be recommended that some educational materials and even books be scanned into a computer, converted to text, and printed in the student's preferred font and point size on 8½ × 11 inch paper, as described in Chapter 5. Although unauthorized copying and scanning can raise copyright concerns in some quarters, consideration has been given in the United States to the allowable creation of accessible materials specifically for individuals who are visually impaired. This option can prove to be one of the most flexible and useful for many students who access print information visually, particularly for nontextbook materials. Large-print materials created in this way can be contained in regular-sized notebooks, file folders, and other common binding options, which makes the material easier to use and less obtrusive than large-print books or materials photocopied on large paper. Scanned text is also flexible and can be printed in different fonts and sizes, depending on the student's needs. The following example illustrates the importance of applying this flexibility:

Toby is comfortable reading several pages of text in 18-point print at a viewing distance of approximately 6 inches when he is holding the material or it is placed on a reading stand. In a class activity, Toby needs to read information on one page and write his responses on a separate piece of paper. Toby reads some of the information on the page in the 18-point print at approximately 6 inches and then moves his head until his gaze is 6 inches from the other piece of paper to write. He could complete the task more efficiently, however, if he could maintain his head position at approximately 6 to 8 inches from the 24-point writing paper and just glance over at the reading material, which is positioned farther away, without moving his head.

For these types of activities and situations, it would have been helpful if the assistive technology recommendations for Toby had indicated the desirability of providing him with reading material in a point size that he can read at a 10- to 12-inch distance for certain classroom activities. This would allow him to accomplish a variety of tasks without having to constantly move his head back and forth between the two papers or assignments, as in the situation described. The data recorded during an assistive technology assessment concerning the viewing distance at which a student can read various sizes of large print will guide the recommendations made by the assessment team.

Nonoptical Devices

Assistive technology assessment recommendations should also suggest nonoptical devices that can greatly enhance a student's efficiency and stamina. Lighting is one of the most obvious nonoptical solutions that is too often overlooked. The recommendations in the final assessment report should emphasize how lighting can affect the student's performance and stamina. Students who have to strain because of too little light, too much light, or excessive glare are going to have difficulty reading and writing visually, whether using print or electronic means. The report should describe the ideal lighting environment for the student while reflecting the realities found in classrooms, such as overhead fluorescent lights and sunshine coming in windows. The recommendations will need to point out how seat placement in relation to a light source can affect the student's ability to access print information visually. In most cases, a student's desk should not face the windows or have the student's back to the windows. The light should fall on the student's desk from the left side if the student is right handed and from the right side if the student is left handed. If available, blinds or shades should be recommended to control direct sunlight entering the room. There may not be time in the assistive technology assessment to determine the ideal lighting recommendations for all the learning environments in which the student works. If this is the case, recommendations for lighting can be written as suggestions that need to be investigated by the student and the teacher of students with visual impairments (see recommendations #4 and #5 for Bill in Appendix 8B for examples).

Recommendations about the use of supplemental lighting sources should also be made in the final report as appropriate. Special emphasis should be given to the use of desk lamps and floor lamps with explanations of how various types of lighting (incandescent, fluorescent, halogen, LEDs) can affect the student's completion of educational tasks (see recommendation #6 in Appendix 8B). Careful attention will need to be given to placement of lights for spot reading and for continuous text reading. If there is no time during the assistive technology assessment process to determine the best lighting tools for specific tasks, the report should recommend that this vital issue be addressed at a later date and a follow-up report provided to the IEP team for future implementation.

Another often overlooked nonoptical tool that can be a great benefit to many students who are blind or visually impaired is a book stand or reading stand. Several types are available commercially, which can be recommended, or stands can easily be made. Some students simply use a closed three-ring binder as a stand to prop up a book or other reading material, but in many cases it will not raise the height of the material enough to allow the student to read without having to bend over, which can cause fatigue (see recommendation #7 for Bill in Appendix 8B). A comprehensive recommendation might include a desktop, portable, and floor model reading stand or book stand. The written report will need to give the details about each style of stand and recommendations for the most appropriate setting for its use. If stands are to be made by volunteers, the teacher of students with visual impairments will need to consider carefully the setting in which each stand will be used and make careful calculations about its dimensions and design. (Braille readers also find reading stands helpful; see the next section on Accessing Print Tactilely.)

Video Magnifiers

In general, the recommendation that can be made most often for students with low vision who wish to access printed information visually is the use of a video magnifier. This technology offers a wide variety of models that can assist individuals in accomplishing educational, employment, and independent living activities as described in Chapter 2. The cost of video magnifiers can be considerable, but this is not a good reason for the assessment team to avoid recommending them, as they are one of the most useful tools for students with low vision and can be cost-effective in the long run (see

Sidebar 8.2, "Justifying the Expense of a Video Magnifier," and recommendation #8 for Bill in Appendix 8B).

A desktop model video magnifier is frequently recommended because it allows an individual to access almost any printed information as well as objects, three-dimensional models, and other items. Its color and polarity features can be recommended as tools to assist students with accessing text and graphics. Several variables must be taken into consideration when recommending this device. Although desktop video magnifiers provide the greatest number of features that can assist a student when completing tasks requiring continuous text reading for several pages or more, they are rather large and require a work area separate from the student's desk. If adequate space is available for the device and for the student to work with it, a desktop video magnifier can be a very valuable tool for the student's educational program. In settings where insufficient space is available in the classroom, or if the student changes classes during the day, a desktop video magnifier may not be practical. However, if one can be placed in a nearby location such as a media center, resource room, or study hall, it can still function as an extremely valuable tool for the student. Recommendations for the use of a video magnifier that will not be located in the student's classroom will need to be accompanied by recommendations for instruction in organizational skills, time management skills, and responsible use of privileges.

The decision to recommend a desktop video magnifier is further affected by how the student chooses to access print information displayed on a chalkboard or a whiteboard. In classroom settings with adequate space for a student to use a desktop video magnifier, a system with distance viewing

JUSTIFYING THE EXPENSE OF A VIDEO MAGNIFIER

Although video magnifiers can be expensive, the assessment team should not shrink from recommending their use. The rationale and justification provided with the recommendation for a video magnification system should emphasize both the benefits such a system provides to the user and the long-term economic benefit it provides to the school system. Some of the benefits of a video magnifier that should be noted include the following:

- The ability to magnify almost all printed and handwritten materials: books, magazines, worksheets, and so on
- The ability to magnify most objects and items
- The ability to choose a wide range of magnification
- The ability to select the polarity of the display (light on dark, or dark on light)
- The ability to select the color of text and background
- The ability to view the information in an ergonomically correct position

The economic benefit to the school system, both short term and long term, lies in the fact that any printed material that the individual needs to access is accessible with a video magnifier. This will considerably decrease—but not totally eliminate—the need for materials to be scanned into a computer and printed in a student's desired font and point size or enlarged on a photocopying machine and the need to purchase large-print books, making a video magnifier a cost-effective solution, as in the following example:

Robert is a rising fourth-grade student with low vision. In previous years his teacher of students with visual impairments has enlarged numerous classroom materials—and sometimes entire books—on a color photocopying machine. Robert's assistive technology assessment has recommended a video magnifier with both near and distance capabilities that costs approximately $3,500. Some administrators might be reluctant to make such a major purchase. A clear explanation about the cost of staff time to produce the enlarged copies (which in most cases, as explained in Chapter 2, is not an adequate solution), the price per page of the copies, the maintenance of the copying machine, and the number of years over which these expenses will be incurred will help the administrator realize that the recommended video magnifier is a better long-term investment. And, the device may also be recycled to other students should Robert later switch to other, more portable types of technology.

capabilities in the form of a flex-arm camera (see Chapter 2) can be recommended, which will allow the student to rotate the camera 90 degrees to view the board and then rotate it back down to view reading materials on the desk. If the student will also be using a computer system in this setting, then selecting a video magnifier that has computer compatibility will allow the computer and the video magnifier to share the same monitor. As with all of the devices and services recommended, the written report will need to give detailed descriptions of the activities in which the technology will be of assistance to the student.

An alternative recommendation that can be made for students who need to use a video magnifier in multiple locations is one of the numerous portable models or electronic pocket models discussed in Chapter 2. A recommendation for a portable video magnifier requires careful consultation among the examiner, the teacher of students with visual impairments, and the student, to make sure the student has the strength and coordination to use such a device. Most portable units require the user to maneuver a small handheld camera over the material to be enlarged, which entails a certain level of physical coordination. Most students can master this skill, but those with motor impairments may find it too time consuming and inefficient to use such a system, and students who are able to successfully manipulate the handheld camera may find it tiring to use for extended periods of time. This fatigue factor limits the usefulness of these devices for students who need to read lengthy passages of text that may take more than 20 or 30 minutes. The main advantage of these devices—their portability—may be offset by their inefficiency when using them for lengthy reading

passages. However, these devices can be excellent tools to recommend for activities that require short reading tasks.

In some cases the assessment team may recommend both a desktop and a portable video magnification system. The portable system gives the user immediate access to print information that requires relatively short reading time, while the desktop model meets the need to accomplish larger and longer reading tasks. Before making the final recommendation on such an important and expensive device, the coordinator of the assessment team and the teacher of students with visual impairments will need to investigate the latest models and features of video magnifiers. Digital imaging models (see Chapter 2) offer both near and distance viewing, computer compatibility, and most of the features found on desktop models, and some even offer the transportability of portable models. However, these features may come at the expense of image quality and may require the use of a computer system. It can be difficult to find the perfect video magnifier to meet all of a student's print access needs, and in many cases, the recommendations will have to be for a device that can meet some needs, while others are met through different methods.

Scanners and Specialized Scanning Systems

In addition to the use of scanners and imaging software for teachers to create materials for students (as discussed in Chapter 2), scanners can also be used by some students to access print information for themselves. However, the poor navigational and magnification controls available in imaging software are not sufficient for most users, and they will therefore need to use the navigational features of a screen magnification program while the imaging program is left in an "un-zoomed" mode. Therefore, imaging software may be more useful for producing written communication than as a tool for accessing print information. (See the section in this chapter on written communication for additional details.)

Some students can benefit from specialized scanning systems that convert printed information into electronic information in the form of editable text. This text can then be displayed on a computer in the student's desired font, point size, and color combination (such as yellow text on a black background or blue text on a white background). When recommending such a system, the assessment report should clearly identify the features of such a system. For a student with low vision, emphasis should be placed on systems that also provide an image of the page, including graphical information that can be enlarged and easily manipulated by the user. In this way, the student can have immediate access to any graphical material in textbooks or other materials, such as maps, charts, or graphs, and can also use the program's features to complete scanned worksheets and produce written copies for the classroom teacher, as explained in Chapter 2.

In conclusion, it is particularly important to stress in the recommendations for accessing print visually that the student may use some or all of these options for different tasks. Too often a student's access to print will be restricted to what can be provided by an enlarging photocopying machine, and in most cases this is not adequate. For example, in the sample report provided for Bill in Appendix 8B, a magnifier is recommended for short reading tasks and a portable video magnifier is recommended for textbooks, classroom handouts, and information presented at a distance in the classroom. And, when the video magnifier is not available, printing on bold-lined paper with a black felt-tip pen is suggested for handwritten information and for classroom materials, which can be scanned into a computer and printed in his preferred format. In addition, recorded textbooks are recommended for times when Bill is too visually fatigued to read visually.

ACCESSING PRINT TACTILELY

Braille

Recommending the use of braille for a student is part of a larger assessment process that involves the family and other IEP team members. In particular, the learning media assessment will guide the assessment team in recommending technologies that can assist the student in the use of materials in braille as his or her primary or secondary medium. However, the assistive technology assessment is another important document that should be considered by the IEP team in addition to the other assessments and documents mentioned at the beginning of Chapter 6. Data collected during the assistive technology assessment about a student with low vision who is primarily using sight as a learning medium may indicate that braille should also be considered as an additional tool to assist the student in accessing the educational program.

Although it may seem that compiling recommendations regarding braille for students who already use braille is stating the obvious, it is always important to document the specific needs of an individual student. Tools that can be used by the student and school system personnel to produce materials in braille will need to be recommended and can be discussed at various points in the assessment report, such as when discussing the support of tactile access or the need for additional hardware and software.

It is important to emphasize that individuals who access print information tactilely will use a combination of tools, as do those who access information visually. Although electronic braille (electronic files that are used to send braille to an embosser or refreshable braille display) for textual material is becoming more readily available, it will not eliminate the need for text produced in hard-copy braille and graphical information produced as tactile graphics. The assessment report should reiterate that accessing information via a refreshable braille display will not eliminate the need for paper braille any more than e-books and other electronic information are likely to eliminate the need for hard-copy books and other print materials.

As noted earlier, reading stands are a low-tech solution for many students. When students need to read from a braille book or other document and write information using a braillewriter or keyboard, they may find it helpful to have the book placed on a stand above the writing device. This placement allows them to read the braille material and shift their hands efficiently down to their writing device when needed. In addition to indicating the use of a bookstand in the report's recommendations, the evaluator will need to explain in the report what this type of bookstand might look like, including its dimensions, and how and when the student might find this tool useful. It will be desirable to have several of these stands so that they will not have to be transported between classes and between school and home. The student may also need a stand that is the correct dimensions for a manual braillewriter,

one that is appropriate for a computer keyboard, and perhaps one that is best for an electronic braillewriter. Depending on the size of the student's desk or work surface, one stand could be made that would be big enough for all of these needs. Commercial versions of this type of book stand are not readily available, but they can be made from relatively inexpensive materials. This type of book stand can be a project for an industrial arts class or woodworking class, or the teacher of students with visual impairments might be able to contact a local civic organization that has members who do woodworking projects and would be available to help out. (If a stand is made for the student, team members need to remind the builder to sand all the surfaces to prevent him or her from being injured by a splinter.)

Accessing Graphical Information Tactilely

Access to information that is displayed graphically has always been limited for students with a visual impairment. The assistive technology assessment and recommendations can address this issue in two ways. The first approach is to recommend that the student receive instruction in the use of tactile graphics from a very early age, while the use of real objects, when possible, is recommended for every age. Instruction in the transition from real objects to models and two-dimensional tactile graphics is recommended for students in kindergarten and early elementary grades. This transitional instruction is also recommended for older students who may have lost vision and for those who have not received previous instruction in the use of tactile graphic materials.

The second way to address the issue of tactile graphics is to recommend that the teacher of students with visual impairments be provided with resources, equipment, materials, and training to produce or purchase the tactile graphics that will be needed by the student at the time of the assessment and in the future. Technology and new techniques for tactile graphics production are expanding the availability of this type of information, as described in Chapters 2 and 5. This justifies the expenditure in technology and the instructor's time for the production of these materials in an accessible format. The recommendation for the use of tactile graphics should include a discussion of the various options for the production of these materials and the ones that might be most effective for the student both now and in the future. This recommendation, like others in the report, may require the assistive technology assessment team to conduct extensive investigations into the availability and options for purchasing these technologies. (See the completed recommendations form and sample report for Semena in Appendix C at the back of this book for an example of how to incorporate this into the recommendations.)

ACCESSING PRINT AUDITORILY

A recommendation that a student access print information auditorily often initiates considerable discussion among professionals, many of whom might be concerned that recommending the use of speech access means the assessment team is "giving up" on the student's use of braille or print. However, choosing a learning medium is not an "either/or" situation, and the goal of an assistive technology assessment is to determine which tools work best for which tasks. Once literacy skills are firmly established, speech access can be a useful tool to support learning. For example, many students may find that reading a 30-page chapter of an American history textbook with compressed speech can be quicker than reading the same material in print, large print, or braille, but this approach would most likely be totally inadequate for a chapter in a math textbook. Time and efficiency are the factors that often determine which tool a student will use. Students need to learn how to use all the tools that are appropriate as well as strategies to use when choosing a tool for a particular task.

In many situations, the easiest and fastest way for students who are blind or visually impaired to obtain access to print information is to have someone read the information aloud. Although this is a good solution with some materials, it is not appropriate in many other situations. Therefore, when recommending the use of a live reader, the recommendations report needs to be very clear about the circumstances under which this arrangement can be a useful tool for the student. For example, a teacher may write a homework assignment on the board that says, "Read pages 38–44 in our history textbook and answer questions 1–7." A student who is blind or visually impaired might naturally ask the teacher or a fellow student to read aloud what the teacher has written. The student would then write, braille, type, or record the information. This would be an appropriate and efficient use of a reader as a tool for accessing information (although the student could also get the information using other means, such as using a telescope or other distance viewing option). However, if the teacher asks the class to read pages 21–23 in class, this would most likely not be a task that the student would want to use a reader to complete. It would be more appropriate for the student to have an accessible copy of the information in his or her desired reading format.

The use of live readers and acquisition of the skills needed to use a reader efficiently and effectively is an appropriate recommendation for many students who are blind or visually impaired, particularly if they are going on to college. The sheer bulk of reading material that needs to be digested in most college courses and the speed with which the student needs to go through the material make using a reader a helpful option in addition to other technology solutions. The final report ought to explain the necessity for instruction in the skills needed to use a reader appropriately and can emphasize that the definition of assistive technology in IDEA specifies that services such as these are legitimate items under the category of assistive technology.

Recommending the use of audio recordings of print information requires a detailed explanation of the necessary hardware and software and the issues associated with training individuals in the use of these tools. Textbooks recorded on audio cassettes have been replaced by digitally recorded books on compact discs and other delivery and storage options, but many library books are still available on tapes that can be used for training. Both cassette tapes and CDs are being replaced by digitally recorded books and other information provided as electronic files that will be accessed through digital e-book readers and accessible computer software. The recommendations provided in this regard need to address both immediate and future needs for accessing print information auditorily—for example, by indicating that the student be provided with training in the use of the hardware and software to access

all three of these formats because some of the books needed by the student will be available in only one format.

One area of training that will need to be emphasized in the assessment report recommendations is the development of listening comprehension skills so that students learn to determine the significant aspects of the information they are listening to. The IEP team should not assume that the student will automatically be able to use auditory books and information without instruction. Recommendations for training services in this area are appropriate for students of all ages, beginning in a simple way with preschool students. Another area for skills training to be recommended is notetaking, so that the student learns to capture the significant details of the information he or she is listening to for later review. This type of training will need to be recommended for most individuals who are blind or visually impaired, unless there are other disabilities that prevent the student from accessing information in an auditory format.

Technologies that allow text to be scanned into a computer and then accessed through synthesized speech can be recommended for many students as a useful tool for accessing print information. This type of technology is usually recommended for older students who have already developed good literacy skills in their primary learning media. Successful users of this technology will in all likelihood also have developed basic keyboarding and computer skills. This type of specialized software can also be recommended for students who access information visually, such as Bill in the example in the appendixes to this chapter, because they provide features that allow the user to select the font, point size, and the text and background colors of the information being displayed. The text can be simultaneously read aloud to the user and displayed in his or her preferred visual format (referred to as *audio-assisted reading;* see Chapter 2). Recommendations that combine this type of system with braille translation software and a braille embosser, or a refreshable braille display, can provide the student with an additional tool that can be used to access print information tactilely as well as auditorily. (See also the recommendations and sample report for Semena in Appendix C at the back of this book for an example of how to incorporate this methodology into the assessment recommendations and final report.)

ACCESSING INFORMATION PRESENTED FROM A DISTANCE

A great deal of learning in classrooms occurs in group activities that may take place some distance from the students' desks or work tables. Any recommendations for tools and strategies for students who are blind or visually impaired will therefore need to address the provision of access to text and graphics written on chalkboards or whiteboards, projected onto screens by overhead projectors or computer projection systems, or displayed in other locations in the classroom. Determining the most appropriate recommendation to meet a student's needs in this regard requires in-depth consultation with the classroom teacher. For most students, recommendations for accessing information presented at a distance have to include a variety of tools and strategies, depending on the type of information being displayed, the classroom circumstances, and the abilities of the student.

Information in the Student's Preferred Medium

The first recommendation to consider, as in most situations in which a student needs access to print, is providing the information in the student's primary learning medium in a format that can be made available at his or her desk. This course of action works in situations in which adequate time is available to have the information produced in braille, print or large print, an auditory format, or an electronic version if the student has the appropriate access tools. A recommendation for this type of solution should state that the teacher of students with visual impairments and the classroom teacher need to work out a system that allows the information to be supplied far enough in advance to allow for the production of the material in the student's primary learning medium (see recommendation #3 for Bill in Appendix 7B). This recommendation cannot always be carried out, particularly in subjects such as math and science, in which the instructor usually writes information on the board during class.

If information cannot be provided ahead of time in the student's preferred medium, some students may be provided access by having the information spoken or dictated and having ample time to braille, write, or type it using an appropriate tool. If this option is recommended, the assessment report should state clearly that this solution is appropriate only for small amounts of information.

Optical Devices

For students with low vision, recommendations for viewing information at a distance can include the use of an optical device such as a handheld telescope (if one has been prescribed by a low vision specialist), a video magnifier with distance viewing capabilities, or a digital video camera. Such recommendations need to include detailed explanations of the tools, the strategies for using them, and the settings and situations in which they are appropriate.

Handheld Telescopes

A recommendation for the use of a prescribed handheld telescope would need to make clear how the student would use the device to view information on a chalkboard or whiteboard and then copy it or respond to it in writing. The importance of skills training also needs to be mentioned (see Sidebar 8.3, "Considerations for Recommending a Handheld Telescope"). However, a handheld telescope is generally not the best tool for tasks such as reading an entire board full of information. Bill's Considerations Checklist presented in Chapter 6 indicated that he had found that the constant need to switch between far and near viewing when trying to copy work from the board using a telescope was too time consuming. Monocular telescopes can also be difficult to use for students with visual field losses and certain eye conditions, and some students have difficulty with the motor coordination required to use a handheld telescope; the low vision specialist's recommendations will be helpful to the team.

Desktop Video Magnifiers

For lengthy distance-viewing tasks involving larger amounts of print information or for students who cannot use a telescope efficiently, a desktop video magnifier with distance viewing capabilities might be recommended. Using this device requires less physical coordination than using a handheld telescope and allows the individual to view

text on the unit's monitor while copying it by writing or typing. However, this device might not be appropriate if there is not sufficient space for it in the classroom.

Portable Video Magnifiers

If the student needs to access information in several different locations, a portable video magnifier with distance viewing capabilities can be recommended. With these models, the camera section of the video magnifier can be easily disconnected from the monitor and transported to various locations. This arrangement can be time consuming and is not practical in some settings, since a monitor must then be made available in each location. However, some newer portable video magnifiers can use the screen of a laptop computer as the display monitor, so this may be a viable solution for some older students who are already using an accessible laptop computer. This was the recommendation for Bill. The digital imaging model recommended also has the ability to create electronic copies of Bill's textbooks or other print materials used in his classes, so it is a very versatile device.

Digital Video Cameras

Use of a digital video camera can be an affordable solution that might be recommended for accessing information presented at a distance. Many students with low vision can be trained to use a regular, commercially available digital video camera mounted on a tripod. This device, which allows the student to both view and record activity at a distance using the camera's zoom feature, can be beneficial for students in math, science, and other classes where the instructor often writes or presents complex information during class, such as the explanation of how to complete a complicated physics problem.

SIDEBAR 8.3

CONSIDERATIONS FOR RECOMMENDING A HANDHELD TELESCOPE

Before a student can make use of a handheld telescope, the device must be prescribed for the individual by a low vision specialist. Its use is generally appropriate only for viewing small amounts of information in accomplishing tasks such as the following:

- Copying lists of words or short phrases for spelling or vocabulary, important dates, famous people, and the like
- Reading short questions to be answered immediately by writing or typing

- Reading questions or statements to be used in classroom discussion
- Reading and copying short items such as class assignments, homework assignments, and due dates

Students with appropriate motor and cognitive skills can use a handheld telescope successfully if they have had sufficient training and practice. The recommendations in the final assessment report need to provide for training in the necessary skills, such as the following:

- Spotting and locating desired information on the board
- Holding the telescope steady while tracking across a line of text
- Holding a group of words or a phrase in short-term memory
- Learning to operate the telescope with the nondominant hand to increase efficiency

---

Not only can the recording be reviewed as often as the student likes, but it can also be paused at important points in the process to allow the student to spend more time viewing the various steps than is possible when viewing it as it is taking place. For example, a student might record a science demonstration and review it later at home, pausing to examine each detail of the experiment.

With the correct configuration and cables, the screen of a laptop computer can be used as the monitor for a video camera provide the added benefit of allowing the student to save and view the information on the laptop. Screen magnification software on the laptop can also be used to further

magnify parts of the video to allow the student to see greater details of a demonstration or action.

Many educators will be familiar with digital video cameras, but most will in all probability not have investigated the benefits that such technology can provide to students with low vision. Moreover, some may be concerned about the legal issues involved with videotaping in the classroom (see Sidebar 8.4, "Issues in Using a Video Camera in the Classroom"). Therefore, recommending the use of a video camera requires a detailed explanation of its benefits and the circumstances under which the student will use it, as well as a logical justification for using this technology, to overcome any reluctance that may be exhibited by some members of the IEP team, particularly in relation to legal issues.

Electronic Whiteboards

A last strategy to recommend for accessing information written on a board is the use of an electronic whiteboard. As discussed in Chapter 2, this technology can either be a stand-alone electronic whiteboard or a device that attaches to an existing whiteboard that provides the same capabilities. A recommendation for this type of device would need to include both the hardware and the software necessary to transfer the information written on the board to an accessible laptop or desktop computer for the student. This option is a very viable recommendation for many students with low

vision in settings in which whiteboards are used extensively. It is particularly effective for helping students who need to understand the explanation of math and science problems. The rationale and justification for this recommendation in the final assessment report needs to emphasize that the image displayed on the computer screen of the information presented on the whiteboard can be enlarged using screen magnification software, and that snapshots of this information can be saved periodically and reviewed whenever the student desires.

Handwriting recognition software is available for electronic whiteboards that converts the handwritten text into editable text for a word processor. However, the accuracy of this conversion is not sufficient to be used by students who cannot access the image of the text on the computer screen.

SIDEBAR 8.4

ISSUES IN USING A VIDEO CAMERA IN THE CLASSROOM

Two major concerns are often raised about the recommendation for a student with low vision to use a video camera in the classroom. Some educators may object to having a video recording made of the activities in their classroom and may worry that the presence of the camera might have a negative impact on the interactions between the teacher and students. The other objection often cited is the "right to

privacy" of the teacher and the other students in the classroom. Similar issues have arisen concerning the audio recording of class presentations over the years. In most cases, a compromise can be arranged that balances the rights of the student to access the educational curriculum and the privacy rights of others. The teacher may request that the recording be turned off at certain times, or the student may be instructed to point the camera only at the instructor or the board. A video camera may also be used just as an electronic telescope without using the record feature. In this mode, the student can still zoom in to view the classroom demonstration at the same time as classmates are viewing it.

This technology, therefore, is not generally recommended for students who use tactile or auditory access, but can be of benefit to some students with low vision who have learned to use a computer with the appropriate access software.

Audio-Described Videos

One recommendation that can be made for all students who are blind or visually impaired is the classroom use of videos that provide an audio description, which are becoming increasingly available (see Chapter 2). The explanation for this recommendation should encourage the school system to seek out and select video materials that are audio described. (See recommendation #13 in appendix 8B.) Most new video display systems will be able to support the secondary audio track that is part of these videos, but the recommendation should note that video equipment will need to include this feature. Although not all movies and presentations are available in this format, this recommendation will alert classroom teachers to use them when possible.

Determining which of these various options to recommend for distance viewing in the classroom requires careful consideration and consultation between the student and the members of the assistive technology assessment team, particularly with regard to the student's attitude toward using the technology, as well as a careful review of the notations made by the evaluators during the student's assessment. As elsewhere, justification in the final assessment report for the technologies recommended for accessing information displayed at a distance is an important part of the report.

ACCESSING ELECTRONIC INFORMATION

Computer Access
- Output Devices
- Input Devices

Other Types of Electronic Information
- Specialized Scanning Systems
- Accessible PDAs and Laptop Computers
- Other Electronic Tools

COMPUTER ACCESS

Since learning to use the computer is now such an essential skill in most schools and for most employment, one fundamental goal of the assistive technology assessment is to determine the most effective way for the student to access this important device. In making recommendations for how a student who is blind or visually impaired will access electronic information made available by computers, the technology assessment team needs to consider that in many schools, students use computers in the classroom, the media center, and the school's computer lab. Many of these computers may be connected to a Local Area Network (LAN) that allows the individual computers to share printers, Internet connections, and various files and programs. In most cases, recommendations that will allow students to access a classroom or personal computer can also be made for accessing computers connected to the school's network, but it will be necessary to confer with the school system's network administrator and to work with support staff from access technology vendors to resolve any technical issues that might arise.

As discussed earlier, it may not always be possible to provide the student with complete access to every activity conducted with computers throughout the school, but acceptable alternatives can be recommended, sometimes using a different medium or learning tool, that will allow the student the opportunity to learn the same content as his or her classmates. In many schools, computers are used as a tool or medium to introduce, review, or practice academic skills in subjects such as language arts, math, and science, and many of the computer programs used for these activities rely on information and content presented in a graphical format that is not penetrable to students using braille or speech as an access medium. In such situations, the recommendation is for the teacher of students with visual impairments to confer with the academic instructor about the educational objective for the computer-based activity. Together they can determine if the objective can be met through adaptations, such as having someone describe the graphical information in meaningful terms or creating tactile graphics that will convey the essential information. If not, the teacher of students with visual impairments and the classroom teacher will need to devise an alternative accessible activity to achieve the educational objective.

Specific recommendations will need to be provided for how a student will interact with computers to access electronic information, along with ample explanations. These explanations will need to include rationales and justifications that highlight how access to computers provides students who are blind or visually impaired both the ability to complete the same technology curriculum and use the same tools as their classmates and the opportunity to accomplish educational tasks that other students are able to complete with more common tools. The recommendations can begin by exploring the options available to the student for accessing the computer's output and then follow up with the options for how the student will input information into the computer.

Output Devices

Recommendations concerning how a student accesses computer output need to be guided by the students' predilection for accessing the information visually, tactilely, or auditorily, with the assessment team keeping in mind that the student may use a combination of approaches. As always, the issue of fatigue must be addressed when recommendations are made for accessing electronic information and may lead to suggestions for making more than one device or method available to accomplish a particular task. For example, a student with low vision may use screen magnification software efficiently to read and complete a written assignment in the morning. By the afternoon, however, the student may be experiencing visual fatigue and may choose to use a tactile or auditory tool to access the information and complete a similar assignment.

Visual Computer Access

Recommendations for students with low vision who need to access a computer visually may relate to one of four options: use of a larger monitor, use of a fully adjustable monitor stand, use of a physical screen magnifier, or use of screen magnification software, as described in Chapter 3. A key factor in determining which of these is appropriate for the student is to identify which solutions will allow the student to sit in an ergonomically correct position in relation to the computer monitor and comfortably view the information displayed on the computer screen. The recommendations for Bill Alonso (see recommendation #15 in Appendix 8B) include screen magnification software with a screen-reading feature that can be used when he is visually fatigued.

Large Monitors. A recommendation for a large monitor (19 inches or larger) will allow some students to achieve correct posture and maintain a comfortable viewing distance. However, careful consideration should be given to making this recommendation, since, as explained in Chapter 3, large monitors can be expensive and require additional space on the desktop or work surface. In addition, they restrict the student to using only the computer that has the larger monitor. Therefore, a large monitor would not be indicated for a student who needs to access computers in various locations throughout the school and at home. However, this option is sometimes chosen for a student's home or work computer, because it allows the student to access software applications directly, such as word-processing programs, and does not require him or her to learn to use additional software or hardware.

Adjustable Monitor Stands. One option that is often overlooked is the recommendation that a student use an adjustable monitor stand or arm to hold the computer monitor. This option is indicated when the student is able to read 12-point text on a monitor at a viewing distance of less than 10 inches. Mounting the monitor on a fully adjustable stand or arm allows the student to place the monitor at the optimum viewing position in terms of height, viewing distance,

and angle of tilt. Stands of this type can be recommended for either CRT (cathode-ray tube) or LCD (liquid crystal display) monitors, although LCD monitors are generally the better option because they are significantly lighter than a CRT monitor of comparable screen size. This weight differential can be an important point to emphasize because it will affect the feasibility of moving the monitor to different locations within the school. CRT monitors do provide a sharper and brighter image than LCD monitors of equal size, but in most cases the image on an LCD monitor will be sufficient for the student to see comfortably.

It is important to specify the type of mounting system to use for the monitor stand, as this system will affect the type of desk or other furniture needed, how easy it is to move to another location, and the stability of the monitor when making adjustments. Attention needs to be paid to where on the desk the stand should be mounted to allow the monitor to be situated for the student's optimum position. The most frequently recommended option is an LCD monitor using a fully adjustable *clamp-mounted* monitor stand, because it is the most versatile and will meet the needs of many different users. This standard office accessory does an excellent job of allowing the user to place the monitor at eye level and at a comfortable viewing distance. The student is then able to sit up correctly in his or her chair and operate the keyboard and mouse without having to lean over his or her hands to see the screen. However, if there is plenty of desktop space, a *stand mount* with a heavy base will prevent the monitor from tipping over. A *permanent mount* that is bolted to a desk is the most stable and is virtually theft-proof, but offers no portability.

Screen-Magnifying Lenses. Screen magnifying hardware, in the form of a magnifying lens that fits over a standard CRT monitor, is recommended only if the student can benefit from a small amount of magnification, from 1.25× to 2×. Recommending this option would allow the student to increase his or her viewing distance by a few inches. In some cases, this adaptation will be enough to improve the overall ergonomics of the student's work station. However, most students will need a greater degree of magnification than can be provided by this type of magnifying lens.

Operating System Accessibility Options. The accessibility options offered by some Macintosh and Windows operating systems (discussed in Chapter 3) can be recommended as an adequate adaptation for some students. When used in conjunction with the enlarged fonts available in most word-processing programs, these features can provide an acceptable solution for those who use the computer exclusively as a writing tool (see recommendation #14 in Appendix 8B).

These options constitute only a partial solution for computer access, however, because they still do not provide a way for the student to access information from the Internet and other resources. These standard accessibility options may work for some students in combination with the three hardware options just discussed— larger monitors, fully adjustable monitor stands, and hardware screen magnifiers. If operating system accessibility features are recommended, the final assessment report will need to emphasize the limitations of this option and the likelihood of needing other tools for tasks on the computer other than word processing.

Screen Magnification Software. The use of dedicated screen magnification software, described in Chapter 3, is recommended for students who wish to access the computer visually and can work effectively with magnifications of 3× to 5× but are unable to use any of the options already discussed. The recommendations should include suggestions for magnification size, color and polarity options and the use of the synthesized speech feature of the screen magnification program. A realistic recommendation for some students would be to access text-based information auditorily through the speech option and to access graphical information visually through the screen magnification features.

The rationale and justification for this recommendation can stress the screen magnification program's ability to customize the text in this way to meet the student's needs and to highlight each word as it is spoken by the software-based speech synthesizer. Recommendations can also emphasize the benefit for some students of the combined auditory and enhanced visual output, because they do not have to rely solely on either their vision or hearing to access information (see Chapter 3). In addition, recommendations can mention the usefulness of synthesized speech for reading extended text passages. These powerful features can be used to justify the added expense of a dedicated screen magnification program over the accessibility options offered through the computer's operating system. In addition, this type of software makes all of the computer's resources available to the student, not just those that can be enlarged with the operating system's accessibility options. As with other technologies, the key to successful implementation is to include recommendations for appropriate training for the student and school system personnel in the use of all suggested technologies.

When recommending the use of screen magnification, the assistive technology assessment team needs to consider the degree of magnification needed by the student and the student's potential to use this access technology efficiently. Displaying materials at a magnification level of 5× or higher severely limits the amount of information that will appear on the screen at any one time. The recommendation must consider this fact and explain when and how it will be more helpful for the student to use other features of the program. The limited amount of information on the screen may not be a problem for some students, but others find the amount of screen navigation required confusing, and they waste valuable time maintaining screen orientation in order to locate the material they are trying to view. If the student is spending more time finding the information than actually reading or learning it, this is an indication that additional access methods such as tactile or auditory options will need to be recommended.

Tactile Computer Access

For students whose primary learning channel is tactile, a refreshable braille display may be the appropriate tool to recommend for accessing information presented by a computer. A braille reader might also use speech access. As with most recommendations for assistive technology, this is not an "either/or" decision. The main consideration in deciding which option to recommend is efficiency—how efficiently can the student access the information and how well is the student able to understand and comprehend it? Speech access may potentially be a faster method of obtaining information, but tactile access may be necessary for the development of students' basic literacy comprehension and for them to grasp the concepts of text formatting in a written document. For example, when students are able to read the braille display, they can see how words and names are spelled, how punctuation is used, and other information found in the hard-copy braille text that is not immediately evident when speech access is being used.

For most students who are braille readers, an assistive technology device that has a braille display will be essential. Determining whether to recommend a refreshable braille display for a particular student depends first and foremost on the student's ability to read braille. This information is normally obtained by the assessment team about the student's braille skills from the teacher of students with visual impairments based on current braille reading assessments. Students who are competent and efficient braille readers will benefit from access to refreshable braille, which can reinforce and expand braille literacy skills such as spelling and punctuation. Students who are not advanced braille readers can also benefit, however. For an individual who is struggling with braille reading, refreshable braille can be an instructional and motivational tool that can provide practice and reinforce skills. A recommendation for a trial use of refreshable braille would be indicated for such a student if the technology were available within the school system or through some type of loan program. A recommendation for a braille display will also need to include a recommendation for a screen-reading program, which is the software required to control the braille display.

As discussed in Chapter 3, there are two types of refreshable braille displays: dedicated units that connect directly to a computer and displays that are incorporated into accessible personal digital assistants (PDAs). Because dedicated braille displays are expensive, recommendations for them would need to be explained and justified in great detail. The benefit of a dedicated braille display is the larger number of cells these devices generally have. For high school students interested in computer programming or other tasks that require a line-by-line correspondence between what's on the computer screen and what's under one's fingers, a 40- or 80-cell display can be very helpful. Overall, however, an accessible PDA with a refreshable braille display is usually the most cost-effective recommendation to meet a student's need for tactile access to the computer. (For more information on this option, see the section in this chapter on recommending accessible PDAs under "Accessing Other Types of Electronic Information.)

Auditory Computer Access

For students whose primary means of accessing the computer will be through their sense of hearing, the typical recommendation is for screen-reading software, but some students can benefit from a talking word processor (see Chapter 3). In particular, young students who are not quite ready to deal with the complexity and numerous commands required by a dedicated screen magnification or screen-reading program can find this type of software helpful. It can be an extremely beneficial tool for assisting students in learning keyboarding skills and can effectively serve students with varying degrees of vision loss as they are developing basic computer skills (see the discussion of talking word processors in the section on "Input Devices").

A dedicated screen-reading program can be recommended for many different students, but before making this recommendation, the assessment team should consider both the student's abilities to understand synthesized speech and to comprehend the concepts of navigating around the screen. If the student demonstrates these abilities during the assessment, then recommending the use of screen-reading software with the appropriate training is indicated.

Justification for purchasing a dedicated screen reader can emphasize that although it is more expensive than simply using the speech options built into a computer operating system, screen-reading software is much more versatile and works with a greater variety of application programs. Moreover, a dedicated screen-reading program not only provides the student with a way to access the computer as a productivity tool, but also opens up the vast world of information that is available on the Internet and as electronic files. Access to such a large body of information is in itself justification enough for providing this tool to students. Supporting access to information through the use of screen-reading software and a computer is also relatively inexpensive when compared to the costs of other accessible formats, although there are times when information in alternate formats will still be needed.

Input Devices

Chapter 4 outlines the various options that students can use for inputting information into a computer, such as keyboards or pointing devices. Recommendations for tools or methods that a student will use to interact with the computer will be greatly influenced by the student's physical and cognitive abilities. Consequently, the use of inputting devices is an area in which other members of the assistive technology assessment team may need to be particularly involved. Although many students can learn to use a standard computer (QWERTY) keyboard and possibly a mouse, others will need adaptive or alternative keyboards and pointing devices, and still others will need to use voice recognition systems or combinations of these various options.

Keyboard Use

Most students will receive a recommendation to use a standard keyboard and pointing device. Because taking advantage of computer-based technology tools requires students to become as proficient as possible in keyboarding skills, it is crucial to also recommend that the student receive training to develop or improve his or her keyboarding. The explanation for this recommendation needs to be clear about how the instruction should take place and about the various roles of the service providers working with the student and the need for individualized or small-group instruction. The recommendations should also be clear about which staff members will be responsible for direct instruction and which ones will be responsible for supervising practice on days when instruction does not occur.

Keyboarding instruction should in general be conducted with the use of a talking word processor, which has the following advantages:

- Talking word processors provide the student immediate feedback about the accuracy of each keystroke.
- These programs allow students with low vision the opportunity to have the text displayed in various fonts and point sizes, thus encouraging the student to monitor his or her accuracy through sight and sound and become less dependent on looking at the keyboard.
- They allow students to print their work and share it with classmates, teachers, parents, and families.
- As students progress, they can begin to learn some of the basic skills of word processing, such as printing, saving, editing, and eventually formatting documents.
- The programs also provide the instructor with tools for collecting, printing, and saving data about the student's progress.

The rationale for the assessment team's recommendation should additionally discuss the use of a talking typing tutorial. It should be emphasized that these tools serve the student best when used for practice and reinforcement of skills, rather than as initial instruction in keyboarding.

Any recommendation for keyboarding instruction also needs to address the issue of how students will locate the desired keys on the keyboard, as detailed in Chapter 4. Extreme caution should be taken in recommending large-print or braille labels on the keys. Using such labels generally slows down students' progress in developing the tactile and motor skills and muscle memory to support efficient keyboarding skills and deters the students' progress in becoming proficient touch typists. As noted in Chapter 4, a better recommendation for most students is the use of locator dots to label new keys as they are being learned and then the removal of these dots as appropriate. Recommending the labeling of keys in high-contrast print or in braille is indicated for students who have physical or cognitive difficulties that may prevent them from developing the skills needed for touch typing.

Some students will not be able to function efficiently with a standard computer keyboard. There are numerous adaptations to the standard keyboard that can be recommended, such as those available in the Windows and Macintosh operating systems accessibility features, as well as alternative keyboards. The appropriateness of a recommendation for software or hardware adaptations or the use of alternative keyboards will need to be determined by the physical or occupational therapist assigned to the assistive technology assessment team.

Pointing Devices and Other Tools

Recommendations for the use of a pointing device to interact with a computer can include a standard mouse, cordless mouse, trackball, joystick, or any one of numerous other input devices. Students who have no usable vision will most likely not use a pointing device to interact with the computer, but many students with low vision will be able to do so. Students with visual impairments should generally be instructed in the use of keyboard commands, as using these can often be more efficient than using a mouse or other pointing device (see Chapter 3). However, many software programs do not offer keyboard commands for all of their functions, which makes these applications inaccessible to most people who use screen readers and braille displays. Therefore, recommendations for an appropriate pointing device and training in its use should be included in the report for students with low vision who have enough usable vision to use a pointing device to interact with these programs (see recommendation #17 for Bill in Appendix 8B).

The assessment team coordinator may wish to recommend that the teacher of students with visual impairments or the assistive technology specialist explore the student's ability to use a pointing device other than the standard mouse, since some students may not be able to use a conventional pointing device because of physical limitations. Determining the most appropriate pointing device to recommend for these individuals should be made through consultations with the occupational or physical therapist assigned to the assistive technology assessment team.

Although voice recognition software that allows the user to control the computer and dictate text is becoming more widely available and reliable, recommendation of a voice recognition system is only indicated for individuals who are unable to use other options efficiently and should be done only after careful consultation and consideration by all members of the assistive technology assessment team and an assessment of how this software will interact with other access programs. A voice recognition system can be recommended for students who access the computer's output through synthesized speech and screen-reading software and have difficulty with the writing process as a result of conditions such as dysgraphia. This recommendation should typically be accompanied by the suggestion that the student consider using keyboard input for editing text to overcome the difficulties associated with using a voice recognition system in conjunction with screen-reading software to accomplish this task in a word processor. Until voice recognition systems become more efficient, students with visual impairments will need to master keyboarding skills, with the use of adaptations as needed, as discussed previously, to take full advantage of current and future technology tools designed to work with a computer.

An additional recommendation concerning computer input is the use of a copyholder. Many students can benefit from using a clamp-on copyholder with a flexible arm that allows them to place information in a comfortable location for reading and copying. These are generally inexpensive and readily available in most office supply stores. The rationale can describe how materials placed on the copyholder can be adjusted to the ideal height and viewing distance for the student (see recommendation #18 in Appendix 8B).

OTHER TYPES OF ELECTRONIC INFORMATION

Students in general need to access other types of electronic information in addition to that generated or output by a computer. This electronic information is often material that was originally available in print form and then converted into electronic files, for example, as a result of scanning. The recommendations report will need to address the student's need to access various types of electronic information, including, but not limited to, print that has been scanned into a computer and converted into electronic text, information entered into or electronically transferred to an accessible PDA, data provided by electronic calculators, and the contents of electronic dictionaries. The assessment team may wish to recommend that the student's IEP team consider the student's needs and explore the available devices as they both change in the future.

Specialized Scanning Systems

Specialized scanning systems, described in Chapter 2, are often recommended as a tool for accessing printed information, but as mentioned earlier in this chapter, most of these systems also allow the user to access a wide variety of electronic files. This technology tool is appropriate to recommend for most high school students and many middle school students who are blind or visually impaired, such as Bill Alonso (whose scanning system is incorporated into his digital imaging video magnifier). The multipurpose aspect of these systems is an important justification for their recommendation. In addition to the ability to access print information, these systems can provide visual and auditory access to online book depositories (such as Bookshare and Project Gutenberg), as well as many others (see the Resources section at the end of this book). The final assessment report can emphasize the value of the various features of these systems as well as the ability of these systems to convert some electronic files into formats that can be accessed by portable devices such as accessible PDAs and various e-book readers, so the student may use the information provided in situations in which there is no computer access.

Accessible PDAs and Laptop Computers

Accessible PDAs and accessible laptop computers are tools that can both be used to accomplish multiple tasks in the categories of accessing information and producing written communication.

Accessible PDAs are one of the more versatile devices available for students who are blind or visually impaired. They are available in a variety of models and offer visual, tactile, and auditory access. Recommending an accessible PDA involves a good deal of careful consideration. In addition to recommending a device with the appropriate output mode, it is essential for the assessment

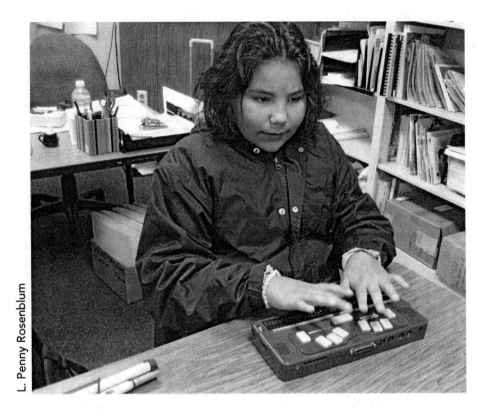

L. Penny Rosenblum

Accessible PDAs are one of the more versatile devices available for students who are blind or visually impaired.

team to provide a detailed list of the features that are available on the device to meet the student's needs. Many of the options found on accessible PDAs can also be found on laptop computers with the appropriate access technology, such as screen magnification software, screen-reading software, and a refreshable braille display. Choosing between recommending an accessible PDA or an accessible laptop computer can be a difficult decision because there are many types of both devices available, offering many different features; both PDAs and laptops can be used for accessing print and electronic information; and both can serve as a tool for producing written communication. The assessment team will need to closely examine all of the student's needs and the environments in which these needs must be met in order to determine which device offers the most effective and appropriate options for a student.

Accessible PDAs are often recommended for students in high school and middle school. The access to information that these tools provide can also be of benefit to many elementary school students if they are provided with the appropriate instruction. Currently there is no research that indicates the "best" age to introduce these versatile devices. Although some students may not need a PDA for notetaking until middle school or even high school, there are still several reasons to recommend an accessible PDA for a younger student:

- Students may need one to two years to learn the operation of an accessible PDA before they can be expected to use it efficiently to take notes in class.
- Students can benefit from learning organizational skills using the device's calendar and address book.

- Students can use the device to access electronic information and print information that has been converted into electronic form that is not available in other formats.
- Students can also benefit from the device's calculator and clock features.

In formulating their recommendations, the assessment team will need to carefully review the various features, advantages, and disadvantages of the respective devices (the information in Chapters 2, 3, and 4 of this book will be helpful in this regard) and gather information about the latest developments in accessible PDAs before deciding to suggest either an accessible PDA or accessible laptop computer and writing the rationale and justification for the recommendation. Sidebar 8.5, "PDAs versus Accessible Laptops: Deciding Factors," lists some of the considerations in selecting one device over the other.

Accessing a PDA or Laptop Visually

There are a few models of PDAs that can be accessed visually by a student with low vision. The ones that are available require additional screen magnification software and a portable keyboard if the built-in keyboard is too small or ergonomically uncomfortable for the student who wishes to use it for notetaking. A PDA whose output can be displayed at various magnification levels can offer a student access to electronic files and print information that has been converted into electronic files. However, the display screens on these devices are small, limiting the amount of information that can be presented, especially if the information has been enlarged or magnified. Many of these devices can also present information in an audio format. Thus, it might be

recommended that the student use such a device as a tool to access electronic files auditorily and use the visual display only when needed to confirm spelling or other features of the information provided. A portable QWERTY keyboard can also be recommended with this device to enter data, take notes, and produce written communications.

Another choice to consider is an accessible PDA with speech output. This option will provide a student with a device containing multiple tools that can be used to complete educational tasks. Before recommending a device of this type, the assessment team will need to determine the student's ability to access information auditorily and the student's potential to acquire the necessary listening skills to take advantage of this type of information. Recommending this type of accessible PDA can be particularly useful to students with low vision who have a degenerative condition that may require them to rely more upon auditory access to electronic information while they learn braille. Having access to a PDA with speech output can be a good transition tool for students who may be moving from accessing material visually to doing so auditorily and eventually to tactile access.

For some students with low vision, such as Bill Alonso, an accessible laptop computer might be a better recommendation. The accessible laptop can assist the student in accomplishing all the same tasks as an accessible PDA with a visual display. A laptop can display all the same types of information as the PDA, but on a much larger screen. With the additional recommendation of screen magnification software, a student would be able to view the information at his or her desired degree of magnification and see much more of that information on the screen at one time than would be possible on a PDA. A laptop computer not only provides all the features found on most PDAs, but can also serve as the foundation for many other tools that the student can use to access his or her educational program. For example, a portable video magnifier

SIDEBAR 8.5

PDAS VERSUS ACCESSIBLE LAPTOPS: DECIDING FACTORS

Deciding whether an accessible personal digital assistant (PDA) or an accessible laptop is most appropriate for a student involves the consideration of a number of factors. In general, the following points should be addressed when recommending an accessible PDA or accessible laptop computer for a student who is blind or visually impaired:

- *Battery life.* Batteries used in accessible PDAs last longer than batteries used in laptop computers.
- *Weight.* Laptop computers are usually heavier than accessible PDAs, particularly if the laptop has a larger screen (usually 17"), which might be preferred by a student with low vision.
- *Training.* Many students have already learned how to operate an accessible computer system. Some accessible PDAs use a different operating system than computers, so students will need additional instruction to use them. Some accessible PDAs use a mobile version of a standard computer operating system, which can shorten the learning curve for many students. However, these devices may not offer all of the features that the student needs.
- *Price.* The prices for accessible laptop computers and accessible PDAs can vary greatly depending on the features that are needed. The assessment team coordinator will need to determine the essential features needed in each system and investigate the pricing available.
- *Tasks to be completed.* Accessible PDAs and accessible laptop computers can both be used to accomplish many tasks, including accessing print information that has been converted into electronic form; accessing electronic information such as electronic books, the Internet, and e-mail; producing written communications; and in some cases navigation with the addition of an optional GPS (global positioning satellite) system. One device may perform these tasks more easily, while the other may offer additional features and the flexibility to connect to a wider variety of other devices. For students with low vision, a laptop may be used to support visual displays for other technology, such as a video magnifier or screen magnifier, whereas the small display screen of a PDA may be insufficient for such functions.

with near and distance capabilities can be connected to a laptop to provide a way to access print documents handed out in class and to access information displayed at a distance for group viewing. It might also serve as the receiver for information from an electronic whiteboard. With the addition of an external keyboard, a larger monitor, and a printer, it can serve as an excellent writing tool for longer assignments. The disadvantages of an accessible laptop are the extra weight and the shorter battery life (although battery life is getting longer as the technology improves), but for many students these characteristics will not significantly affect the tool's usefulness.

If the student needs a simple writing tool, the assessment team may want to consider recommending one of the dedicated word processors discussed in Chapter 4 that has scalable fonts. These programs are comparatively inexpensive and can meet several of the writing needs of some students. A dedicated word processor might be an appropriate recommendation for an elementary school student who only needs a portable writing tool. However, the other features available on these devices are not accessible, and recommending such a tool for a single task may not be the best use of limited resources for a middle or high school student. For these students, an accessible PDA with speech output or an accessible laptop computer might be more appropriate recommendations.

Accessing a PDA or Laptop Tactilely

The decision to recommend an accessible PDA versus an accessible laptop computer is a bit easier to make when a student accesses information tactilely. Many of the same considerations that apply for students who use visual access must be addressed in weighing the features of these two types of devices against a student's needs and circumstances, but the need for a refreshable braille display for a student makes a big difference. To be workable for tactile access, an accessible laptop computer will need to be augmented with a separate braille display, whose purchase will involve additional expense as well as additional time and effort to set up and break down the resulting system for transport. Therefore, in most cases, an accessible PDA with a refreshable braille display will be the more appropriate recommendation. It should be noted, however, that accessible PDAs with refreshable braille displays are expensive. The assistive technology assessment team will need solid data to persuade administrators to support this technology recommendation (see Sidebar 8.6, "Rationales for an Accessible PDA"). If school administrators balk at the price of a PDA with a braille display, they may be swayed by the argument that the greatest economic benefit will be in the decreased (but not eliminated) need to purchase, store, transport, and produce hard-copy braille. These benefits will be realized and increased over the course of a student's educational program and will outweigh the initial cost and maintenance of an accessible PDA with a refreshable braille display. (See the example of Semena in Appendix C at the back of this book for an example of how to incorporate this into the recommendations.)

Accessing a PDA or Laptop Auditorily

For a student who accesses information auditorily, making the decision to recommend an accessible PDA with speech output or an accessible laptop computer will also require a great deal of investigating and consideration by the assessment team.

RATIONALES FOR AN ACCESSIBLE PDA

When making recommendations for computer access for students who read braille, the advantages of an accessible PDA with a braille display that need to be emphasized are both educational and economic. An accessible PDA offers a student a tremendous increase in his or her access to print and electronic information through the use of braille. The expansion of the student's access to print will allow him or her to fully develop the literacy skills necessary to succeed in educational and employment endeavors. And, the frequent use of electronic files instead of braille in hard copy can be a tremendous cost saver in the long run. These advantages include the following:

- Information in the form of data files can be easily transferred between the accessible PDA and a computer.
- While connected to a computer, the accessible PDA's braille display can serve as a braille display for the computer.
- Supplemental educational materials created using word-processing software on a computer (such as review sheets, worksheets, quizzes, and tests) can be provided directly to the student, reducing the amount of material that must be transcribed and produced in braille on paper.
- Numerous books, including textbooks, are becoming available as electronic files that can be accessed using the braille display of an accessible PDA. The number of available titles is increasing every day.
- Obtaining these electronic books (e-books) is becoming easier and significantly less expensive than paper braille books to produce and distribute to students in a timely manner.
- E-books and other electronic information that would normally be produced in hard-copy paper braille require significantly less space for storage.
- PDAs are lightweight and can easily be transported from class to class and from school to home.
- Books and other materials as electronic files can be easily stored and transported in the accessible PDA, providing access to the information in various locations, including school, home, and work.
- Most information stored as electronic files can be navigated and searched much more quickly and easily than information in hard-copy braille.
- Accessible PDAs with refreshable braille displays offer numerous other features that are valuable to braille readers for educational, employment, and personal tasks, including the following:
  - A standard and scientific talking calculator
  - An address book
  - A calendar function for tracking assignment due dates and other events
  - An onboard word-processing program with a spell checker that can be used for notetaking and other writing tasks
- Files can be printed directly to a printer.
- A PDA can be connected to a modem and used to access the Internet.
- A PDA can be used as a braille instructional tool for beginning braille readers.

Many of the pros and cons will be similar to those discussed for students with low vision who use visual access. In addition to those concerns, the assessment team will need to consider that the student will not benefit from the visual display provided by an accessible laptop. Therefore, the extra weight and battery power required to operate a computer display screen, which may be an acceptable trade-off for a student with low vision, are not needed by a student with no usable vision. For this student, the increased portability of the PDA may be a more important consideration than the extra features found on the laptop.

An additional factor that needs to be taken into account when making this recommendation is the student's general circumstances and need for computer access. If the student will have access to a desktop computer at school and possibly at home, then the accessible PDA may be the better recommendation. Its portability will allow the student to complete tasks in settings where it may not be practical to use a laptop computer. However, if the student does not have access to a desktop computer, the flexibility of the laptop to serve other functions may make it a better choice. This is seldom an easy decision, but with careful consideration of the tasks that need to be completed and in which settings, the assessment team can make a recommendation that will provide the student with the necessary tools to take advantage of his or her educational program.

Other Electronic Tools

Talking Calculators

Because accessing mathematical and scientific information can be difficult for many students who are blind or visually impaired, recommendations for tools that can assist with these tasks are particularly important. Although the first level of intervention should be providing the information in the student's primary learning medium, recommendations are also needed for how students will use common math tools such as calculators. The recommendation of a talking calculator or a calculator with an enlarged display that performs basic mathematical operations usually needs little justification. However, scientific calculators that talk or have an enlarged display have typically been expensive. Recommendations for these models may therefore need additional rationales and justification, although newer models have become available that are more reasonably priced and offer the features necessary for advanced math classes. Recommendations for these calculators should be based on the student's need for the specific features and functions, his or her ability to see or hear the display, and his or her physical ability to manipulate the controls of the device.

Recommendations for the use of basic and scientific calculator programs that are part of a computer's operating systems are appropriate for students who have readily available access to computers and have developed skills using them with screen magnification software or screen-reading software. Careful consideration must be given to this recommendation, however, because the student may only be able to take advantage of the technology where there is an accessible computer. In many cases it will be necessary to make an additional recommendation for an accessible calculator that is transportable and can be used in any location.

One additional recommendation that can be made for calculator access is the use of an accessible PDA that has a scientific calculator as one of its features. This suggestion can be a financially attractive option because it provides the calculator along with the other features found in these portable devices and eliminates the need to purchase an expensive scientific talking calculator.

Talking Dictionaries

Recommendations for tools that provide access to dictionaries and other reference materials are important to include in a final assessment report, as these materials are widely used in classrooms. Available large-print dictionaries are generally bulky and limited in scope; and, although braille dictionaries may still be available in some places (such as in the libraries of specialized schools for students who are blind), they typically exceed 30 volumes and are generally out of date. To provide students a more efficient portable tool for accessing information, an elementary- or high school-level talking dictionary is highly recommended.

The rationale and justification for recommending a talking dictionary will need to emphasize that the device needs to be fully speaking; that is, it should speak each letter entered into the device, speak the word entered, speak the entire definition for an entry, speak menus and options, and speak all the instructions and text displayed on the screen. The following advantages should be included in the justification to highlight the value of this type of tool:

- The ability to quickly locate a desired word, eliminating time wasted in trying to locate words in print or braille dictionaries and thesauruses
- The ability to quickly determine the correct spelling of unknown or suspect words

- Increased independence and efficiency in gaining access to reference materials
- Additional features (grammar guide, word games, and others detailed in Chapter 3) that can be used to accomplish other language arts tasks and practice skills
- Portability, allowing use in a wide variety of locations and settings

The use of dictionaries and other reference materials that are available as computer programs or as resources on the Internet can also be recommended for individuals who have accessible computers and Internet connections readily available. The assessment team should be cautious about recommending this option as the only tool to address this need, however, because it is viable only when and where an accessible computer system is available.

COMMUNICATING THROUGH WRITING

Writing Manually

Writing Math

Completing Worksheets

Accessible Computer Systems

Writing Tools for Braille Readers

Accessible PDAs

As indicated throughout Part 1 of this book, technology provides excellent tools, both high-tech and low-tech, to help students who are blind or visually impaired to communicate effectively through the written word. Some tools are appropriate to recommend for students with low vision, while others are better suited for students with no usable vision. Certain strategies and options will be feasible for short writing assignments, while longer assignments will require different adaptations. In addition to students' varying needs and the varying nature of writing tasks, the potential for fatigue creates a need for multiple methods of accomplishing the same tasks, as well. Recommendations relating to producing written communications, just as those relating to accessing print, should emphasize that the student will need to use a variety of tools and strategies, as is done in the final report for Bill Alonso (see Appendix 8B), and the final report must provide a logical rationale and justification for each recommendation.

WRITING MANUALLY

Many students have a need to produce written communications in print. Some students with low vision can use standard writing tools, that is, a pen or pencil and paper. It is reasonable to recommend that the teacher of students with visual impairments explore a wide variety of writing instruments (pencils, pens, and markers) and various types of paper (unlined, lined, bold-lined, raised-lined, and bold-lined graph paper) to be used for short writing tasks, including both text and math. Recommending the use of raised-lined or bold-lined writing paper and a felt-tip pen or some other dark marker may be all that is required to improve a student's writing in some cases. The length of a writing task or assignment, and sometimes the location in which it is to be completed are the main factors determining whether standard writing tools can be recommended. The assessment report must explain the types of writing tasks for which these tools will be appropriate.

Students who are blind need to learn to sign their name, regardless of whether or not they learn how to shape print letters. A screen board and crayons and raised-line

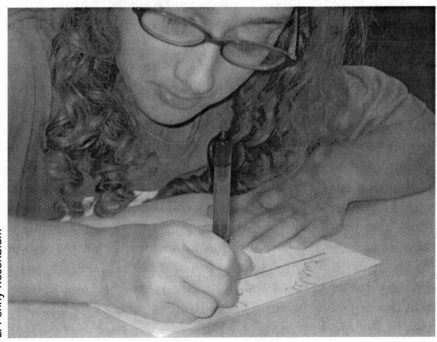

L. Penny Rosenblum

Students who are blind need to learn to sign their name, regardless of whether or not they learn how to shape print letters.

paper can be recommended to assist these students in learning to write their signature. These materials can be used to produce tactile feedback during the writing process and create a raised representation of the writing that can be felt by the student. These often overlooked tools can also be recommended for any beginning writer. Recommendations such as these are indicated for short writing assignments and while the student is learning handwriting.

WRITING MATH

Writing math problems and equations legibly on paper can be difficult for some students with low vision. Maintaining vertical alignment is also often a difficult task. In such cases, a recommendation for the use of bold-line graph paper is indicated to help the student keep numbers properly aligned, which assists the student in completing these types of tasks.

Students with low vision may also find the use of a small whiteboard helpful in completing math problems. The rationale provided in the assessment report can point out how the larger surface, broader lines provided by markers, and excellent contrast between the colored markers and the whiteboard help the student to independently and successfully complete math assignments. This strategy works best in situations where the teacher or a paraeducator is able to view a math problem as soon as it is completed so that the student can then erase the problem and continue on to the next one. However, because use of a whiteboard does not produce a permanent copy of the student's work, arrangements need to be made with the math instructor if it is to be used successfully. It is important to note in the report that this methodology is effective in certain situations, but it is limited and cannot be used for a variety of written assignments.

Recommendations for assistive technology to assist with writing math can include an accessible computer and math writing and editing software, which was recommended for Bill Alonso (see recommendation #23 in Appendix 8B). A program can be recommended that allows the instructor to input math problems into the computer that the student can complete by entering his or her answers into the computer. These programs allow the student to access the problems presented through synthesized speech, embossed braille, enlarged numerals on the computer monitor, or a printout in the student's preferred font and point size. Such a recommendation requires a detailed explanation of how both the student and teacher will use the technology to accomplish the desired task.

COMPLETING WORKSHEETS

Making worksheets accessible for students with low vision should also be addressed in the recommendations report. Although these materials can be enlarged using the methods discussed earlier in this chapter and in Chapter 5, students have to be able to write information legibly on the lines and to read back their own writing. An excellent recommendation for this task is the use of an accessible computer with an optical scanner, imaging software, and a printer, a solution discussed in Chapter 4. The worksheet can be scanned into the computer with the scanner and the imaging software. Materials can be prepared in an electronic format and provided to the student at the time of the assignment, or the student can be taught how to perform the scanning process for himself or herself. All lines, blanks, check boxes, words to circle, or pictures to connect are viewable on the computer screen. Screen magnification software can also be used with the imaging file created by the imaging program. The student then places the cursor at the desired location and types in the answer or draws the requested circle or line. Once the task is completed, the student can print a copy of the document for the teacher. This arrangement constitutes an extremely powerful tool. The rationale and justification for the recommendation will need to include an explanation of how this process works and for which educational tasks it will be appropriate.

Imaging software was discussed earlier in this chapter as a method for accessing print information. Although its features are not as user friendly for reading as those of a video magnifier, its options for writing are different. Using a video magnifier system for writing requires the student to write in a horizontal plane while viewing the material in a vertical plane. Many students find this difficult and time consuming, and others are unable to do it at all. Imaging software, with its option for entering text from the keyboard to complete forms instead of writing by hand, can prove to be a more efficient writing tool for some students.

ACCESSIBLE COMPUTER SYSTEMS

A computer system with the appropriate accessibility options, a word-processing program, and a printer are the writing tools that will be most appropriate for the majority of people who are blind or visually impaired, because of their ability to increase the efficiency, quantity, and quality of a student's writing. Indeed, an accessible computer system may be the single most beneficial tool offered by current technology.

It is recommended that students learn to use the word-processing program that is most widely used at their school. Doing so will provide them with additional resources for technical support, because there will be individuals on site who can answer general questions.

The rationale for recommending a computer for writing tasks should explain that, in addition to improving the student's overall efficiency while engaged in the educational process, this tool solves two additional problems: Teachers and students no longer have to struggle to decipher illegible handwriting, and teachers no longer have to wait for a student's work done in braille to be "interlined" or reverse translated into print. Computer access will not only offer the student more timely feedback from his or her teachers, but will also provide opportunities for him or her to develop writing and other skills that will be of benefit through the entire educational process and later on in the world of work.

WRITING TOOLS FOR BRAILLE READERS

A variety of writing tools can also be recommended for braille readers. These students need two types of writing tools: one to produce information in braille for the student himself or herself to read, and one to produce information in print when the student wishes to communicate with others who do not read braille.

A slate and stylus and a manual braillewriter can be recommended for most braille readers. These tools are effective for many students to use when writing information that they will refer to later or information that will be translated from braille into print for the classroom teacher. The use of the slate and stylus is the most portable option for writing braille, and slates are available in a variety of sizes, with a model for nearly every task. It is vital that students learn to use this portable writing tool and that the assistive technology assessment team recommend it along with instruction in its use. The slate and stylus can be recommended for tasks such as jotting down telephone numbers, noting assignments and due dates, making labels, and other short writing tasks, while the manual braillewriter usually works best for longer writing tasks.

For students who do not have the finger strength to operate the keys of a standard braillewriter, the use of extension keys (see Chapter 4) should be recommended if the assessment indicates that this adaptation would allow the student to operate the device successfully. Another option that can be recommended for these students is an electric braillewriter. Explanations will also need to be provided in the recommendation highlighting the tasks for which these devices are adequate and the tasks that will require other writing tools. Recommendations for braille-writing tools for students who only have the use of one hand should include the unimanual (one-handed) braillewriter. Extension keys can be recommended with the unimanual braillewriter for those students who also have inadequate finger strength for pressing the keys.

The Mountbatten Brailler can also be a good recommendation for students who have difficulty operating a standard braillewriter. The Mountbatten has numerous features and benefits that make it worth recommending for many other braille readers as well. In particular, it allows students to emboss text and then have it back translated and printed for the classroom teacher, thus providing more immediate communication between the student and teacher. Because of the expense of this equipment, the recommendation will need to include detailed explanation of its various features and how they will allow the student to accomplish required writing tasks and participate more independently in the educational program. When making this recommendation, the assessment team must take care to include mention of all of the accessories necessary to take advantage of these features.

ACCESSIBLE PDAS

Both braille readers and students with low vision can benefit from using accessible PDAs for producing written communication, accessing print information that has been turned into electronic information, and notetaking. These devices are available with either a braille or QWERTY keyboard for input and synthesized speech or refreshable braille display for output. As noted earlier in the discussion on using accessible PDAs for accessing electronic information, recommendations for this device must be emphatic that they are one of the most cost-effective pieces of technology available for students who are blind or visually impaired (see Sidebar 8.6). An accessible PDA can be recommended as an extremely valuable and efficient writing tool for notetaking and other short writing tasks. However, it should also be noted that the device lacks the sophisticated formatting options necessary for completing research papers and reports. A computer system with the appropriate access options will need to be recommended for such activities.

ADDITIONAL HARDWARE AND SOFTWARE

Supporting Hardware and Software

Producing Materials in Alternate Formats

SUPPORTING HARDWARE AND SOFTWARE

Input from both the general technology specialist and the assistive technology specialist will be needed to determine what additional hardware and software might be necessary to carry out the rest of the recommendations put forward in a final assessment report. For example, recommendations will need to be made for the student to have access to a computer system with the hardware specifications required to operate the adaptive software that has been recommended. Additional hardware, such as a flatbed scanner and printer, may be necessary. Technical specialists will be most effectively able to write out the specifications for this equipment. The explanation provided with these recommendations can detail how often the student will need to use the computer system to justify the need for a separate system for the student or the feasibility of the student's using a computer available in the school with the appropriate access hardware and software. (See the suggestions made for Bill in recommendation #27 in Appendix 8B for an example of how this might be handled.)

This point in the final report is a good place to address the issue of making other computers in the school accessible to the student. That is, although not every computer in the school has to be completely accessible with all the needed adaptations, if the student needs to use a computer in the media center or the computer lab, for example, the school district or local education agency is responsible for providing access to those computer systems. In many cases, the accessibility software needed by a student can be installed on more than one computer. Sidebar 8.7, "Copyright Issues and Accessibility Software," explains the situations in which this practice is acceptable.

PRODUCING MATERIALS IN ALTERNATE FORMATS

The recommendations contained in the final assessment report also need to consider the technology that will be needed for the school system to meet its responsibility to provide accessible materials to the student in a timely manner. Providing access to materials used in educational programs has traditionally been extremely time consuming for teachers of students with visual impairments. Technology offers a great deal of help with this difficulty, as Chapter 5 indicates. With the appropriate hardware and software, the teacher of students with visual impairments can produce many classroom materials in the appropriate format for students who are blind or visually impaired. For example, supplemental classroom materials can be keyboarded into a computer, scanned in with a scanner and optical character recognition (OCR) software, retrieved from an Internet site, or loaded from the original electronic file. Once the information is in the computer, it can be edited and formatted with a word-processing program. Depending on a student's needs, the information can be formatted and translated with braille translation software and

COPYRIGHT ISSUES AND ACCESSIBILITY SOFTWARE

Most software applications and other materials require purchasers to accede to a user's agreement designed to uphold the copyright protecting the material to be used. In general, copyrighted software can be installed on several computers if only one student is using the access software at any one time. For example, it is permissible to install a screen-reading program on all the computers that a student might need, including his or her home computer, if that student will be the only person using that piece of software. It is also permissible for more than one student to use the same piece of accessibility software on the same computer. The easiest way to determine whether a situation or use is violating U.S. copyright law is to consider whether it is possible for more than one person to use the software at the same time. If two students share one accessibility program on different computers, this practice would be of concern because both students would be able to use the software at the same time—a violation of the law.

The issue of copyright has become so important that some school systems will not allow software to be installed on more than one computer, even when it may be permissible to do so. It may be necessary to have the school system's computer administrator communicate directly with the software company, along with the teacher of students with visual impairments or another member of the assistive technology team who can explain how a student will use the program. Most access software vendors are willing to accommodate their customers and work out the situation with the school to the benefit of the student and protection of the vendor's concerns.

embossed on a braille embosser, or the text can be printed on 8½ × 11 inch paper in the student's preferred font and point size. The devices and software appropriate for a particular student need to be included in the recommendations.

Braille embossers and ink printers are available in a variety of styles and models. Recommending the correct model to meet the student's needs and the need of the school system to supply materials in alternate formats for other students is extremely important. A personal braille embosser to meet the needs of a single student can be recommended, or a professional or heavy-duty braille embosser (or more than one) can be suggested if braille will need to be produced for multiple students or if the need for additional braille production is anticipated. The explanation accompanying this recommendation can emphasize the fact that the higher production speed and the durability of a higher quality embosser will outweigh its extra expense. If the school system is providing a volume of braille materials for multiple students, it is often more cost effective and efficient to have it produced at a central location; text or braille-ready files can be e-mailed to the transcribers and the resulting hard-copy braille can be picked up by the teacher of students with visual impairments or delivered to the school via interschool mail.

Recommendations for equipment to produce materials in large print will also need an economic rationale to justify the initial expense. Inkjet printers are inexpensive and can produce materials in any desired font and point size. A high-quality inkjet printer can be recommended for the production needs of a single student. However, if large print will need to be produced for more than one student, a laser printer will be more economical in the long run, even though its initial cost will be greater. Printing large-print documents on an inkjet printer will take longer than printing regular print documents, and as the point size of the material increases, the production time increases dramatically. Using a laser printer will greatly reduce the time that the teacher of students with visual impairments or other school personnel will have to spend in producing the materials. The amount of ink used for large print is also much greater than that used to produce a document in regular print, and the overall cost per page to print on a laser printer is less than that for most inkjet printers. Thus, an immediate and direct savings can be realized by using a laser printer for large-print production. The recommendations for hardware and software for producing materials in alternate formats can be highly cost effective, because the equipment can be used to meet the needs of most of the students served by the teacher of students with visual impairments.

SUMMARY

Carefully considered recommendations and a final report that contains persuasive justifications and rationales for their implementation are critical outcomes of the assessment process. If compiled and presented comprehensively and thoughtfully, they will provide the student's IEP team with the information needed to implement recommendations that meet the student's needs, which in turn form an essential underpinning to the student's efforts and educational program. Indicating how the student will develop the skills to take advantage of the recommended technology and the specific goals and objectives for the student are an important part of these materials. Once the final recommendations have been formulated for a student, the next vital step is implementing the assistive technology plan in the student's IEP, a strategically decisive process discussed in the next chapter.

ASSISTIVE TECHNOLOGY RECOMMENDATIONS FORM

Student Name: <u>Bill Alonso</u>

Date(s) of Assessment: <u>10/1, 10/8, & 10/15/2008</u>

Based on the results of the assistive technology assessment, the following recommendations are made regarding assistive technology to support this student's educational objectives.

Section I: Accessing Print

Students with visual impairments will use a combination of tools and strategies to access printed information. Some will be appropriate for short reading passages and others will be necessary for longer assignments.

A. Accessing Print Visually

Check all that apply.

1 ☑ Student should use regular print materials with the following optical devices:
    ❑ prescribed eyeglasses or contact lenses
    ❑ prescribed handheld magnifier
       type: _____   _____ power   ❑ illuminated
    ☑ prescribed stand magnifier
       type: _____   __4__ power   ☑ illuminated
    ❑ prescribed handheld telescope
       type: _____   _____ power
    ❑ prescribed spectacle-mounted telescope
       type: _____   _____ power
    ❑ other optical devices recommended in clinical low vision evaluation
       Specify: _____
    ❑ Student should use materials written with felt-tip pen on regular blue-lined notebook paper.
2 ☑ Student should use materials written with felt-tip pen on bold-lined paper.
    ❑ Student should use materials written with felt-tip pen on unlined paper.
    ❑ Student should use regular print materials enlarged on a photocopying machine.
       Specify: _____times at _____% enlargement
    ❑ Student should use large-print books.
3 ☑ Student should use regular print materials scanned into a computer, edited, and printed in
    <u>24</u> point print in the <u>Verdana</u> font.
4 ☑ When possible, student should be provided with overhead lighting
    ❑ from an incandescent bulb.
    ☑ from a fluorescent bulb.
    ❑ from a halogen bulb.
    ❑ adjusted with a dimmer switch.

5 ☑ When possible, student should be provided with window lighting adjusted with
    ☑ blinds.
    ❑ shades.
    ❑ Other (specify): _____

6 ☑ When possible, student should be provided with additional lighting from
    ☑ desk lamp with a/an
        ❑ incandescent bulb.
        ❑ fluorescent bulb.
        ❑ halogen bulb.
        ☑ LED bulb.
    ☑ floor lamp with a/an
        ❑ incandescent bulb.
        ❑ fluorescent bulb.
        ❑ halogen bulb.
        ❑ LED bulb.

7 ☑ Student should use a book stand or reading stand (specify type):
    ❑ braille book stand
    ❑ desktop model
    ☑ portable model
    ❑ floor model

8 ❑ Student should use regular print materials with a video magnifier (CCTV) (specify type):
    ❑ desktop model
    ❑ flex-arm camera model
    ❑ head-mounted display model
    ❑ portable model
    ❑ electronic pocket model
    ☑ digital imaging model
    Specify essential features: _Portable system with near and distance viewing capability;_
    ability to take snapshots of information on boards and save as electronic file; ability to
    scan and convert print pages into electronic files; ability to present information on
    computer screen in student's preferred font, point size, and color combination, and as
    synthesized speech.

    ☑ Student should use regular print materials with the following type of scanner and imaging software:
    ❑ standard imaging program
    ☑ specialized scanning program

Additional comments or recommendations: _____
_____
_____
_____

(continued on next page)

B. Accessing Print Tactilely

Check all that apply.

- ❑ Student should use materials in braille.
- ❑ Student should use an electronic refreshable braille display to access print and electronic information.
- ❑ Student should be provided opportunities to use tactile graphics created by various production techniques and in a variety of media, including real objects, models, collage, tooling and stenciling, thermoform, capsule paper and fuser, computer-generated, and commercially produced.
- ❑ Student should use tactile graphics to access maps, charts, and diagrams.

Additional comments or recommendations: _____
_____
_____

C. Accessing Print Auditorily

Check all that apply.

9 ☑ Student should use a live reader for accessing certain materials (specify):
    See report _____

10 ☑ Student should use recorded materials for accessing some print information (specify):
     See report _____

11 ☑ Student should use a computer-assisted reading system such as Kurzweil 1000 or OpenBook.

Additional comments or recommendations: _____
_____
_____

D. Accessing Information Presented at a Distance

Check all that apply.

12 ☑ Student should be provided an accessible copy of information presented on chalkboards or whiteboards, overhead projectors, computer projection systems, and so forth.

   ❑ Student should use a handheld telescope for accessing chalkboards or whiteboards, overhead projectors, computer projection systems, and so forth.

12 ☑ Student should use a video magnifier with distance viewing capabilities for accessing chalkboards or whiteboards, overhead projectors, computer projection systems, and so forth.

   ❑ Student should use a digital video camera connected to an appropriate size monitor for accessing chalkboards or whiteboards, overhead projectors, computer projection systems, and so forth.

   ❑ Student should use an electronic whiteboard connected to an accessible computer.

13 ☑ Student should be provided audio-described videos when available.

13 ☑ Student should be provided a separate _20_-inch monitor for viewing DVDs, movies, and other video presentations.

Additional comments or recommendations: _____
_____
_____

Section II: Accessing Electronic Information

A. Computer Access—Output Devices

1. Visual Access

Check all that apply.

14 ☑ Student should use a standard computer monitor: Optimal size: _25" LCD_

14 ☑ Student should use a standard computer monitor with the following hardware adaptations:
  - ☑ adjustable monitor arm
  - ☐ hardware screen magnifier

14 ☑ Student should use a standard computer monitor with the following Windows or Macintosh Display Appearance Settings (list on separate page if needed): _600 X 800 pixels screen resolution, large icons, large fonts_
  - ☐ Student should use the following Accessibility options in the computer's operating system:
    - ☐ Macintosh   ☐ Windows Accessibility
  - ☐ Student should use the following screen magnification program provided in the computer's operating system:
    - ☐ Macintosh Zoom   ☐ Microsoft Magnifier

15 ☑ Student should use a dedicated screen magnification program.
  Specify essential features: _text-reading capability via synthetic speech_

2. Tactile Access

  - ☐ Student should use a refreshable braille display.
    Specify essential features: _____

3. Auditory Access

Check all that apply.

  - ☐ Student should use a talking word processor to develop basic computer skills.
  - ☐ Student should use the following screen-reading program provided in the computer's operating system:
    - ☐ Macintosh VoiceOver   ☐ Microsoft Narrator
  - ☐ Student should use a dedicated screen-reading program.
    Specify essential features: _____
  Additional comments or recommendations: _____
  _____
  _____

B. Computer Access—Input Devices

1. Keyboard Use

Check all that apply.

  - ☐ Student should use a standard keyboard.
  - ☐ Student should use a standard keyboard with
    - ☐ large-print labels, white text on black background.

(continued on next page)

    ❑ large-print labels, black text on white background.

    ❑ braille labels.

16 ☑ Student should use a standard keyboard with locator dots to develop or improve keyboarding skills.

16 ☑ Student should receive individual keyboarding instruction.

    ❑ Student should use a talking word processor for keyboarding instruction.

16 ☑ Student should use a talking typing program for keyboarding practice and reinforcement of skills taught by instructor.

    ❑ Student should use a standard keyboard with Windows Accessibility or Macintosh Universal Access options:

    ❑ StickyKeys

    ❑ FilterKeys

    ❑ ToggleKeys

    ❑ Other (specify): _____

    ❑ Student should use a standard keyboard with hardware adaptations.
    Specify:_____

    ❑ Student should use an alternative keyboard.
    Specify:_____

2. Pointing Devices and Other Tools

Check all that apply.

17 ☑ Student should use a standard pointing device like a mouse or trackball.

    ❑ Student should use an alternative pointing device.
    Specify:_____

    ❑ Student should use a voice recognition system to control the computer.

18 ☑ Student should have access to a copyholder that allows printed materials to be positioned at a comfortable viewing distance.

    Additional comments or recommendations: _____

    _____

    _____

C. Accessing Other Electronic Information

1. Specialized Scanning Systems

19 ☑ Student should have access to a specialized scanning system.

    Specify essential features: *See report* _____

2. Accessible Personal Digital Assistant (PDA)

    ❑ Student should have access to a personal digital assistant with the following features:

    ❑ scalable font display

    ❑ screen magnification capability

    ❑ synthesized speech output

    ❑ refreshable braille display

    Specify essential features: _____

3. Other Electronic Tools

20 ☑ Student should use a ☐ basic or ☑ scientific talking calculator.
　 ☐ Student should use a computer-based calculator program with
　　 ☐ screen magnification software.
　　 ☐ screen-reading software.
　 ☐ Student should use a dictionary or thesaurus program on a computer with
　　 ☐ screen magnification software.
　　 ☐ screen-reading software.
21 ☑ Student should use a portable talking dictionary.
　 Additional comments or recommendations: _____
　 _____
　 _____

Section III: Communicating Through Writing

Students who are blind or visually impaired will use a combination of tools and strategies to produce written communication. Some will be appropriate for short writing assignments and others will be necessary for longer assignments.

Check all that apply.

22 ☑ Student should use pen or pencil and paper
　　 ☑ for short writing assignments.
　　 ☐ for most writing assignments.
22 ☑ Student should use felt-tip pen or other bold marker.
22 ☑ Student should use ☑ bold-lined ☐ raised-lined notebook paper.
　 ☐ Student should use ☐ bold-lined ☐ raised-lined graph paper for math.
　 ☐ Student should use crayons and a screen board for beginning handwriting.
　 ☐ Student should use a whiteboard with erasable markers.
23 ☑ Student should use a computer with a math writing and editing program.
　 ☐ Student should use a computer with a scanner and imaging software to complete forms.
24 ☑ Student should use an accessible computer with word-processing software.
　 ☐ Student should use a manual braillewriter.
　 ☐ Student should use a manual braillewriter with extension keys.
　 ☐ Student should use a unimanual (one-handed) braillewriter.
　 ☐ Student should use a unimanual (one-handed) braillewriter with extension keys.
　 ☐ Student should use a slate and stylus.
　 ☐ Student should use an electronic braillewriter.
　　 Specify: _____
25 ☑ Student should use an adaptive analog or digital recorder for notetaking.
　 ☐ Student should use an accessible PDA for notetaking and other short writing tasks.
26 ☑ Student should use an accessible laptop or notebook computer for notetaking.
　 Additional comments or recommendations: _____
　 _____
　 _____

(continued on next page)

Section IV: Additional Hardware and Software

Student should be provided with access to the following hardware and software:

- ❑ Macintosh computer system with
  - ____MB memory ____ GB hard drive ❑ CD/DVD drive
- 27 ☑ Windows-compatible computer system with
  - _2_ MB memory _80_ GB hard drive ☑ CD/DVD drive
  - ☑ word processor ☑ printer
  - ☑ Internet access ☑ flatbed scanner
  - other: _centralized workstation; docking station with monitor and keyboard; separate_ _monitor and keyboard for home use; rolling carrying case for laptop and video magnifier;_ _work table in each classroom_

Equipment needed to produce materials for student in appropriate format:

- ❑ Macintosh or Windows-compatible computer system with
  - ____MB memory ____ GB hard drive ❑ CD/DVD drive
  - ❑ Internet access ❑ flatbed scanner ❑ OCR software
  - ❑ word-processing software ❑ braille translating software
  - ❑ inkjet or laser printer ❑ braille embosser or printer
  - ❑ tactile graphics production equipment:
    - Specify: _____

Additional comments or recommendations: _____
_____
_____

The recommendations made here do not all have to be implemented immediately. These suggestions are designed for a two- to three-year plan in which the student masters certain skills and is provided access to additional technologies that can facilitate his or her educational program. During that time, new technologies are likely to become available that will enhance the student's ability to maximize his or her educational potential. The specific devices recommended may no longer be the most appropriate, but the assistance that they provide will continue to be a need for this student.

Samantha Higgins   _Teacher of students with visual impairments_
Assessment Completed by (signature)   Position

Beatrice Collins   _Assistive Technology Specialist_
Assessment Completed by (signature)   Position

_____   _____
Assessment Completed by (signature)   Position

_____   _____
Assessment Completed by (signature)   Position

Student's Name: <u>Bill Alonso</u>

Date(s) of assessment: <u>10/1, 10/8, & 10/15/2008</u>

Bill is a 10th-grade student who is functioning on grade level in all regular classes and is receiving services from Samantha Higgins, a teacher of students with visual impairments. Bill has a visual impairment, which is stable, that makes it difficult for him to read standard print materials, access information presented at a distance (on a chalkboard, whiteboard, etc.), view and read information on the school's computers, and complete lengthy writing tasks in a timely manner. Bill was recommended for an assistive technology assessment because of the difficulties he is having in these areas.

This assessment was conducted in several sessions during the month of October 2008. Bill's needs were determined based on the tasks to be completed in his various classes, the school's media center, the computer lab, and the classroom where he receives services from the teacher of students with visual impairments. The attached Assistive Technology Assessment Checklist was used to determine Bill's potential for using of a wide variety of assistive technologies. The Assistive Technology Recommendations Form specifies the various technologies that will assist Bill with completing his educational goals. (The numbers on that form are keyed to the numbered items in this report.) This report will summarize these findings and provide the rationales and justification for the recommendations.

Accessing Print Information
Bill will use a combination of tools and strategies to access print information. Some will be appropriate for short reading passages and others will be necessary for longer assignments.

1. Bill should continue to use his prescribed 4× illuminated stand magnifier for short reading tasks such as a few lines of text in a paragraph, reviewing a map or diagram, or a short set of instructions for a homework assignment.
2. If information is provided to Bill in a handwritten format and a video magnification system (see recommendation in item #8) is not available, the information should be provided in manuscript (print) writing on bold-lined paper using a black felt-tip pen.
3. If classroom materials and other print information need to be used in locations where Bill does not have access to a video magnification system (see recommendation #8), these materials will need to be scanned or typed into a computer, edited with a word processor, and printed in a 24-point Verdana font on 8½ × 11 inch paper. The teacher of students who are visually impaired will need to work

(continued on next page)

closely with each of Bill's classroom teachers to establish an efficient procedure for providing these materials to her, which allows adequate time for production, so that Bill will have them in an accessible format at the same time they are provided to his classmates.

4. Whenever possible, Bill should be provided with overhead lighting for reading and completing schoolwork. Overhead lighting provides the best illumination for general activities, but there will be some activities for which Bill will need additional lighting (see recommendations #5 and #6).

5. Whenever possible, Bill should have the option to control the natural lighting through windows with blinds. Bill and Ms. Higgins should visit each of Bill's classrooms to determine the most appropriate seating for Bill, with lighting in mind. Special consideration must be given to the lighting conditions at various locations throughout the room and the assistive technology that Bill will be using when selecting the ideal location. Appropriate seating and the option to control blinds or shades will allow Bill to minimize the glare and reflection caused by natural and artificial lighting. (See item #27 for additional considerations.)

6. At his request, Bill should have access to an LED desk or floor lamp. Access to a desk or floor lamp will provide the additional light needed for some educational tasks, such as science labs and the manipulation of small objects.

7. When reading regular print with his magnifier or in large print, Bill should have access to a portable reading stand or book stand. The book stand will allow Bill to place reading materials in a position that will be more comfortable and will minimize physical fatigue.

8. Bill will need to have access to a portable video magnification system that can be easily transported to all of his classes and that provides both near and distance viewing features to access his textbooks, classroom handouts, and information presented at a distance. The most appropriate video magnification system to meet these needs is a digital imaging model that connects to a laptop or notebook computer. (See item #27 below for details of the laptop recommendation. The laptop should be a model with a 17-inch monitor. This is necessary to provide more viewing area for the enlarged image presented by the video magnification system.) This type of system will provide the greatest flexibility and independence for Bill. This system can eliminate the expense of buying large-print books for Bill. Large-print books for a typical high school student such as Bill cost approximately $500–$1,500 per subject. Over the course of Bill's high school years, eliminating the need for these books could easily result in a savings of $10,000–$15,000. The digital imaging video magnifier system recommended costs approximately $3,500, and the required laptop computer costs approximately $1,000. (See item #27 for additional details.)

Bill will be able to use the distance viewing feature to capture information presented on chalkboards or whiteboards as image files that can be saved to a portable electronic storage medium such as a flash drive. He can then review these files on the laptop computer, his home computer, or any other computer with the appropriate accessibility features. This can be an ideal tool for Bill to access the explanation of math and science problems.

This type of digital imaging model video magnifier can also be used to create electronic copies of Bill's textbooks and other print materials used in his classes. These documents can be scanned and files can be created by Bill, his teachers, or any staff member with basic computer skills and saved to Bill's flash drive. Accessing these files on Bill's home computer with the appropriate software can eliminate the need to transport the system between school and home each day. These files can also be used to produce documents for Bill in his preferred font and point size.

Bill will need to receive extensive training in the use of the features of this digital imaging video magnifier. This training should be provided by Ms. Higgins outside the regular classroom using materials of high interest to Bill and should include specific instruction in the proper care of the technology. Bill should demonstrate effective use of the device before being asked to use it in class.

A device of this type is highly recommended for Bill because of its ability to meet multiple needs and the cost savings achieved by not having to purchase separate technologies to meet those additional needs.

9. Later in Bill's education and future employment there will be occasions when he will experience visual fatigue and will not be able to adequately access information visually even with his assistive technology. At other times, print information may not be available in a format that is accessible for him. In these situations Bill will need to use the services of a human reader. Bill will need to receive training in the appropriate use of a reader for both short and long reading tasks.

10. Bill will need to be provided with recorded textbooks as a supplement to his printed textbooks and as an alternative method of access to textbook materials when he experiences visual fatigue. Bill needs to learn to use recorded textbooks and other materials, including instruction in the use of the recording and playback equipment. Additional instruction will need to be provided to Bill by the teacher of students with visual impairments in how to absorb information presented auditorily and in the use of the audio-assisted reading strategy in which the student simultaneously reads the text along with the recording. This training should be provided with materials of high interest to Bill before attempting textbooks or other school-related materials.

11. Bill will need to be provided with a specialized scanning system to assist with reading some printed text. The school can meet this need by means of the scanning and speech features available in the video magnification system recommended in item #8.

(continued on next page)

12. Whenever possible Bill should be provided with an accessible print copy (in 20-point Verdana type) of information presented on a chalkboard or whiteboard, overhead projector, or computer projection system. When this is not possible, Bill can use the distance viewing feature of the video magnification system recommended in item #8.

13. Bill will need to use two types of technology to access videos presented in class for group viewing. Whenever possible, these videos should include audio description, and school staff should begin to look for this feature when selecting videos to be used for educational purposes. The second tool that Bill will need is a separate 20-inch or larger TV or monitor. This TV or monitor will need to be connected to the video display system and placed at a convenient height and location that will allow Bill to obtain a viewing distance of approximately 24–30 inches.

Accessing Electronic Information

Bill will use a combination of tools for accessing electronic information. These will include tools for working with computers and other devices that provide electronic information.

14. Bill should be provided with access to a desktop computer system with a 25-inch LCD monitor. (See recommendation #27 for additional details about Bill's computer needs.) This monitor should be mounted on a fully articulating adjustable monitor arm stand. At the time of this report, the best model is the LCD Monitor Arm from Access Ingenuity (which can be seen at www.accessingenuity.com/lcd-monitor-arm-0). This stand will allow Bill to position the monitor at the correct height and distance for optimal viewing.

    Bill will also need to have the opportunity to adjust several of the basic display property settings of the computer. These should include, but not be limited to, setting the screen resolution to 800 × 600 pixels, selecting larger icons, and selecting large fonts.

15. Some computer applications and programs do not have any options for adjusting how they display information on the computer screen, and the technologies recommended in item #14 will not be adequate for Bill to work effectively with these programs. To complete tasks using these programs, Bill will need to have a screen magnification program installed on the computers he will be using. The screen magnification software will need to have a feature that reads text to the user via synthesized speech. There will be many times when Bill will experience visual fatigue, having exhausted his visual energy. At these times he will need to rely on this text-reading feature to complete tasks using the computer.

    The screen magnification program will also assist Bill when using the laptop computer for notetaking and other short classroom assignments.

    Bill will need to receive specific instruction in the use of the screen magnification software that goes beyond the basic level. Instruction in the more advanced features of the program will help him become more efficient in its use as he progresses on to more complicated tasks. Learning these more advanced features should not delay Bill's use of the technology to accomplish simple tasks, but they should be gradually added as he develops more familiarity with the program and the types of tasks required by his educational objectives.

16. Bill should use a standard keyboard for inputting text to the computer, with some type of locator dots marking specific keys to assist with orientation to the keyboard. Bill and Ms. Higgins can determine the exact placement of these dots.

   Bill is currently able to enter text on a standard keyboard. Due to the increased quantity of computer work in his educational program and that he will encounter in later employment, Bill will need to greatly improve his speed and accuracy in keyboarding skills. To accomplish this, Bill will need to receive some individualized keyboarding instruction from the teacher of students with visual impairments. This instruction should be conducted with a talking word-processor program or with the speech feature of the Screen magnification program recommended in item #15 and a standard word-processing program. It is also recommended that he be provided with an accessible typing tutor or keyboarding program to practice and reinforce these skills. It is extremely important that Bill develop efficient keyboarding skills to take advantage of current and future technologies.

17. Bill should be strongly encouraged to learn to use keyboard commands to control the computer and most of the programs he will be using. However, some programs that Bill may need to use to achieve his educational objectives may not be fully controllable via keyboard commands. For these programs Bill should use a standard mouse or pointing device of his choice. He should also be provided with pointer enhancement software that is part of the screen magnification program recommended in item #15 or one available as shareware or freeware downloaded from the Internet.

18. To complete some educational tasks, Bill will need to read text from a printed source and type it into the computer. Bill will need a clamp-on copy holder with a fully flexible arm to accomplish this task. This type of device will hold the material at the appropriate height and viewing distance to allow Bill to maintain correct posture while typing in the information.

19. Bill will need access to a specialized scanning system to convert print information into electronic information that will be accessible to him. This can be accomplished with the features of the video magnification system recommended in item #8.

20. Bill will need to be provided with a talking scientific calculator to complete tasks in his math and science classes, and he will need to receive training in the efficient use of this device.

(continued on next page)

21. Bill will need to have access to a portable talking dictionary and thesaurus to assist in completing reading and writing objectives. At the time of this report, the only talking dictionary and thesaurus that is fully accessible is the Franklin Speaking Language Master Special Edition. Bill will need to receive some initial training in the use of this device, but he will be able to explore many of its features independently.

Communication Through Writing

Bill will use a combination of tools and strategies to produce written communication. Some will be appropriate for short writing assignments and others will be necessary for longer assignments.

22. Bill should use a felt-tip pen and bold-lined writing paper for short writing assignments and for personal writing tasks. These tools will only be adequate for writing tasks less than one-half of an 8½ × 11 inch page.
23. Bill, his math teachers, and his teacher of students with visual impairments will need to investigate the use of math writing and editing programs that he can use on the computer with the screen magnification software recommended in item #15.
24. Bill should be provided access to a desktop computer with the accessibility features described in recommendations #14 and #15 and a full-featured word processor to complete most writing tasks. This need can be met with a separate desktop computer or by using the laptop computer required for the video magnification system recommended in item #8. (See item #27 for further explanation.) Bill will need to receive ongoing training in the use of the word-processing program, starting with the basic features and then moving on to the more advanced features as his skills increase.
25. Bill should use an accessible analog or digital recorder as a backup notetaking system in his classes. This device should have a bookmark or tone indexing feature. This is necessary for Bill to be able to mark important points in the recording or to mark locations in the recorded presentation that he might need to find in order to fill in missing information in his written notes.
26. Bill should use an accessible laptop or notebook computer as his primary notetaking tool. As Bill's keyboarding skills continue to improve, he will be able to use this tool to take class notes effectively and efficiently. Using manual writing tools (paper and pencil) will never be fast or efficient enough for Bill to absorb all of the information presented (see recommendation #27 for additional details).

Additional Hardware and Software

27. Bill will need an accessible computer to complete many of his educational objectives related to accessing print information, electronic information, and writing using the hardware, software, and training described in the preceding recommendations.

The ideal situation for Bill will be to have access to an accessible desktop computer at a central location in the school, an accessible laptop or notebook computer, and an accessible computer at home. This arrangement would provide the greatest flexibility and reduce the need for transporting equipment.

Another alternative is to provide Bill with an accessible laptop computer and a centralized workstation where the laptop could be connected to a docking station containing the 25-inch monitor (see recommendation #14), a separate keyboard, a printer, and Internet access. This arrangement could meet multiple needs for Bill. It would supply Bill with the tools he needs to access a wide variety of printed information requiring longer reading times, to prepare longer written documents for class assignments, and to conduct Internet research. The accessible laptop is excellent for classroom work and shorter assignments, but its keyboard and smaller screen are not conducive to efficient completion of longer reading and writing activities. Therefore a workstation with the larger monitor and keyboard will be necessary to assist Bill in completing many required assignments.

The portability of the laptop and the video magnification system recommended in item #8 will provide Bill with tools to access various types of information presented in class, produce short written assignments, and take notes.

Bill will also have assignments to complete outside class that will require the use of assistive technology. This need can be met by the use of the laptop computer, the digital imaging video magnification system, and a larger monitor and keyboard. The school system should be able to provide an older 19-inch or larger CRT monitor that is still in good working order and a separate keyboard that Bill can connect to the laptop for the extended reading and writing tasks that will need to be completed at home.

A high-quality rolling case or backpack case will be needed to protect the computer and the video magnification system during transport. This will allow Bill to safely carry the equipment to classes and home when needed.

For this portable system to work effectively, Bill will need a worktable in each classroom. The laptop and video magnification system are too large for most typical school desks and might easily fall off and be damaged. When selecting a location for Bill's worktable, the following factors must be considered, in addition to the lighting conditions discussed in recommendation #5:

Availability of electricity. The laptop and video magnification system can operate on the computer's battery, but there will be times during the day when the battery will need to be recharged.

Classroom traffic. Because of the video magnification system's light weight, it might be knocked off the work table. Placing the worktable in an area of the room that has a low traffic flow will be desirable.

(continued on next page)

Obstructions. The environment will need to be free of any obstructions that might block Bill's view when he is using the distance viewing feature of the video magnification system.

Selecting the best location for Bill's worktable in each classroom will require an evaluation of these three factors. The ideal location will be one in which each factor is optimized, but in many classrooms that may not be possible. In these classes, Bill and the teacher of students with visual impairments will need to consider their options carefully and select the location that will give Bill the best combination of these factors.

Plans to implement the recommendations in this report will need to be made as soon as possible. This will include purchasing the technologies, acquiring training for Ms. Higgins and other staff, and instructing Bill in the use of the technologies. It is very important that adequate instructional time for Bill be provided to ensure that he is comfortable using the technologies before he is asked to use them in class to complete assignments. The teacher of students with visual impairments will need to provide detailed instruction on how to use the technology. Using topics of high interest to Bill during the initial instruction, rather than current classroom topics, should increase his interest in learning how to use the technologies and help him understand their value and potential benefit. Once Bill becomes comfortable using the various technologies, instructional activities should simulate the general classroom environment in which he will be using the technologies.

Appendix: Sources of Recommended Technology

The following is a list of the devices and technology recommended in this report for Bill Alonso, along with some sources for obtaining them. This is not an exhaustive list.

(Note: Full contact information has not been provided in this example, but appears in the Resources section to this book.)

Accessible analog or digital recorder

Access Ingenuity
www.accessingenuity.com
(877) 579-4380 or (707) 579-4380

American Printing House for the Blind
www.aph.org
(800) 223-1839 or (502) 895-2405

Accessible typing tutor (Talking Typer for Windows)

American Printing House for the Blind
www.aph.org
(800) 223-1839 or (502) 895-2405

Adjustable monitor arm stand

Access Ingenuity
www.accessingenuity.com
(877) 579-4380 or (707) 579-4380

Bold-lined and raised-line writing paper

American Printing House for the Blind
www.aph.org
(800) 223-1839 or (502) 895-2405

Independent Living Aids
www.independentliving.com
(800) 537-2118 or (516) 937-1848

Desk or floor lamps

Access Ingenuity
www.accessingenuity.com
(877) 579-4380 or (707) 579-4380

Independent Living Aids
www.independentliving.com
(800) 537-2118 or (516) 937-1848

LS&S
www.lssgroup.com
(800) 468-4789 or (847) 498-9777

MaxiAids
www.maxiaids.com
(800) 522-6294 or (631) 752-0689

Felt-tip or bold pens

American Printing House for the Blind
www.aph.org
(800) 223-1839 or (502) 895-2405

Independent Living Aids
www.independentliving.com
(800) 537-2118 or (516) 937-1848

MaxiAids
www.maxiaids.com
(800) 522-6294 or (631) 752-0689

Shop Low Vision
www.shoplowvision.com
(800) 826-4200

Handheld and stand magnifiers

Independent Living Aids
www.independentliving.com
(800) 537-2118 or (516) 937-1848

LS&S
www.lssgroup.com
(800) 468-4789 or (847) 498-9777

MaxiAids
www.maxiaids.com
(800) 522-6294 or (631) 752-0689

Locator dots for computer keyboard

EnableMart
www.enablemart.com
(888) 640-1999 or (360) 695-4155

Independent Living Aids
www.independentliving.com
(800) 537-2118 or (516) 937-1848

MaxiAids
www.maxiaids.com
(800) 522-6294 or (631) 752-0689

Laptop, LCD, TV monitors

Local computer dealers and electronic appliance stores

Math writing/editing programs

Design Science
www.dessci.com/en/company/
(800) 827-0685

Henter Math, LLC
www.hentermath.com
(888) 533-6284 or (727) 347-1313

ViewPlus Technologies
www.viewplus.com
(541) 754-4002

Portable reading stand or book stand

Access Ingenuity
www.accessingenuity.com
(877) 579-4380 or (707) 579-4380

American Printing House for the Blind
www.aph.org
(800) 223-1839 or (502) 895-2405

(continued on next page)

Independent Living Aids
www.independentliving.com
(800) 537-2118 or (516) 937-1848

LS&S
www.lssgroup.com
(800) 468-4789 or (847) 498-9777

Portable talking dictionary/ thesaurus

Access Ingenuity
www.accessingenuity.com
(877) 579-4380 or (707) 579-4380

Franklin Electronic Publishers
www.franklin.com
(800) 266-5626

Independent Living Aids
www.independentliving.com
(800) 537-2118 or (516) 937-1848

LS&S
www.lssgroup.com
(800) 468-4789 or (847) 498-9777

Portable video magnification systems

ABISee
www.abisee.com
(800) 681-5909 or (978) 201-9302

Another Eye
www.anothereye.com
(888) 274-1862 or (866) 778-7523

Bierley Associates
www.bierley.com
(800) 985-0535 or (408) 365-8012

Bookbinder Group
(800) 535-9436 or (212) 369-5360

Christal Vision
www.christal-vision.com
(800) 299-0700 or (210) 666-0700

Clarity
www.clarityUSA.com
(800) 575-1456 or (775) 782-5611

Enhanced Vision Systems
www.enhancedvision.com
(888) 811-3161 or (714) 374-1829

Freedom Scientific
www.freedomscientific.com
(800) 444-4443 or (727) 803-8000

Freedom Vision
www.freedomvision.net
(800) 961-1334 or (650) 961-6541

Health Care Services
(304) 525-9184

HumanWare USA
www.humanware.com
(800) 722-3393 or (925) 680-7100

Innoventions
www.magnicam.com
(800) 854-6554 or (303) 797-6554

LS&S
www.lssgroup.com
(800) 468-4789 or (847) 498-9777

Optelec
www.lowvision.com
(800) 828-1056 or (978) 857-2500

OVAC
www.ovac.com
(800) 325-4488 or (760) 321-9220

Virtual Vision Technologies (VVT)
www.virtualvisiontech.com
(610) 622-0728

Vision Cue
www.visioncue.com
(510) 451-2582

Your Low Vision Store
www.yourlowvisionstore.com/index.shtml
(800) 310-3938

Recorded textbooks

Recording for the Blind and Dyslexic
www.rfbd.org
(866) 732-3585 or (609) 452-0606

Screen magnification programs

Ai Squared
www.aisquared.com
(800) 859-0270 or (802) 362-3612

Dolphin Computer Access
www.yourdolphin.com
(866) 797-5921 or (609) 803-2171

Freedom Scientific
www.freedomscientific.com
(800) 444-4443 or (727) 803-8000

Gregory Braun
www.gregorybraun.com
(800) 999-2734 or (719) 576-0123

JBliss Low Vision Systems
www.jbliss.com
(888) 452-5477 or (650) 327-5477

Specialized scanning systems

ABISee
www.abisee.com
(800) 681-5909 or (978) 201-9302

Bookbinder Group
(800) 535-9436 or (212) 369-5360

Dolphin Computer Access
www.yourdolphin.com
(866) 797-5921 or (609) 803-2171

Freedom Scientific
www.freedomscientific.com
(800) 444-4443 or (727) 803-8000

Guerilla Technologies
www.guerillatechnologies.com
(772) 283-0500

HumanWare USA
www.humanware.com
(800) 722-3393 or (925) 680-7100

JBliss Low Vision Systems
www.jbliss.com
(888) 452-5477 or (650) 327-5477

Kurzweil Educational Systems
www.kurzweiledu.com
(800) 894-5374 or (781) 276-0600

Premier Assistive Technology
www.premierathome.com
(517) 668-8188

Technologies for the Visually Impaired
www.tvi-web.com
(631) 724-4479

Scientific calculator (talking)

American Printing House for the Blind
www.aph.org
(800) 223-1839 or (502) 895-2405

Captek dba Science Products
(800) 888-7400 or (610) 296-2111

Independent Living Aids
www.independentliving.com
(800) 537-2118 or (516) 937-1848

LS&S
www.lssgroup.com
(800) 468-4789 or (847) 498-9777

MaxiAids
www.maxiaids.com
(800) 522-6294 or (631) 752-0689

Orbit Research
www. orbitresearch.com
(888) 606-7248

Sight Enhancement Systems
www.sightenhancement.com
(519) 883-8400

ViewPlus Technologies
www.viewplus.com
(541) 754-4002

9

Follow-up: Implementing the Recommendations

CHAPTER OVERVIEW

Writing the IEP Goals

Considerations for Teaching Assistive Technology

- When to Start Assistive Technology Instruction
- Taking a Proactive Approach to Teaching
- Employing Diagnostic Teaching

Troubleshooting Technology Difficulties

- Hardware and Software Problems
- Operator Errors

Training for Teachers

- Awareness of Assistive Technology
- Operational Knowledge
- Instructional Strategies
- Planning for Training
- Training Other Staff and Families

As important as a careful and thorough assessment is, it may have little meaning without thoughtful and persistent follow-up. Implementing the recommendations arising from an assistive technology assessment can have a dramatic and beneficial impact on a student's performance in school and in daily life. However, the implementation process requires continued participation from everyone involved in the student's educational program to ensure successful use of the recommended technology tools. The steps in this process include the following:

- The assistive technology assessment report is presented to the IEP team for discussion, comment, and explanation.
- The IEP team writes goals and objectives based on the assistive technology assessment findings to implement the recommendations.

- Questions concerning the need for the technology and other issues are discussed and resolved between the team and the school system.
- The school system acquires the recommended technologies, based on the agreed goals and objectives.
- The school system arranges for the appropriate staff to receive training in the use of these tools.
- The IEP team formulates a troubleshooting plan for responding to technology problems that may arise.
- The teacher of students with visual impairments and the other designated staff members begin teaching the student how to use the technology, making use of *diagnostic teaching methods*, which means that they consciously monitor the effectiveness of their instruction during lessons to make sure the student is making progress (this concept is discussed later in the chapter).
- When the student achieves an acceptable level of competence with the technology, he or she can begin using it to accomplish tasks independently
- The IEP team periodically reviews the student's needs and how well the technology is meeting those needs.
- The IEP team addresses the student's future assistive technology needs by designing a plan that will monitor developments in the assistive technology industry to ensure that the student maintains a full complement of strategies and devices that can support him or her throughout the entire educational journey.

WRITING THE IEP GOALS

The final report of the assistive technology assessment team should be presented to the IEP team as soon as possible after its completion. The IEP team may wish to call a meeting specifically to review the report and discuss how to implement the recommendations. Discussing and understanding the report and its recommendations fully may take some time; some recommendations in the report will be easily understood, while others will require further explanation and discussion with members of the assistive technology assessment team.

The assessment team can provide a valuable service by helping everyone involved understand what might constitute a realistic timeline for implementing the recommendations. Some recommendations will be able to be implemented almost immediately, such as providing the student with priority seating in the classroom, making adjustments to computer operating system display settings, and providing classroom handouts in the student's preferred font and point size. Others may take longer because they will require the school system to purchase or otherwise acquire various pieces of new technology and then provide opportunities for training staff on the use of these devices. Still others may not be implemented until the student has acquired certain prerequisite skills necessary to take advantage of the recommended technology. These factors should not be interpreted as indicating that recommendations do not need to be implemented in a timely manner or until all recommendations can be implemented. On the contrary, the IEP team should write goals and objectives that reflect a realistic and prioritized timeline for implementing the recommendations.

Writing the IEP goals requires careful consideration. Goals should state the task to be accomplished with a certain type of assistive technology, but should avoid using specific brand names of devices, even when the team knows which specific device the student will be using. Instead, specifying the features of a device or a program that the student will learn to operate gives instructors and the school system more flexibility in meeting the student's needs. For example, Bill Alonso, whose assistive technology assessment recommendations and report were included in Chapter 8 (Appendixes 8A and 8B), might have the following goals with regard to the recommendation that he learn to use a portable video magnification system (recommendation #8):

- Bill will demonstrate the ability to set up the video magnifier system and his laptop computer accurately and safely in less than two minutes.
- Bill will demonstrate the ability to disconnect the video magnifier system from the computer and safely store it in its traveling case in less than one minute.
- Bill will demonstrate the ability to execute the commands and procedures necessary to view a printed page in the "live camera" mode of the video magnifier system.
- Bill will demonstrate the ability to execute the commands and procedures necessary to view a printed page in the "scan and read" mode of the video magnifier system.
- Bill will demonstrate the ability to execute the commands and procedures necessary to view information displayed on the classroom whiteboard using the video magnifier system.

Some recommended technologies will include so many features that an extended timeline will need to be designated specifically for that device or program, or short-term objectives can be identified for certain features only. For example, if an accessible personal digital assistant (PDA) with a refreshable braille display is recommended for a young student, it is reasonable that the initial annual goals relating to this device might only focus on the student's learning to open and close text files and enter friends' telephone numbers in the address book of the device, but not on using its scientific calculator. A member of the assistive technology assessment team who is knowledgeable about the specific device can assist in constructing a realistic sequence of IEP goals to better meet the student's needs.

Some goals will need to specify the environments in which the technology is to be used. For example, again considering Bill Alonso, his goals for learning the appropriate use of a reader (recommendation #9 in Appendix 8B) might specify the following:

- Bill will need to learn strategies for using human readers in various settings. Bill will demonstrate the ability to courteously request that someone read him information displayed on the board in the classroom when his video magnification system is not available.
- Bill will demonstrate the ability to schedule a reader for an extended reading task outside of class.
- Bill will demonstrate the ability to organize materials that need to be read by a paid or volunteer reader in order to use his and the reader's time efficiently.

In many cases, the teacher of students with visual impairments or other teachers may want to work on specific objectives in a controlled setting—for example, during a pull-out lesson or in the resource room—before the student begins to use a particular technology in the general classroom, to ensure that the student has had some success with the device or equipment in realistic practice sessions before needing to use it without assistance.

The IEP goals and objectives should also be carefully written to indicate what level of skill the student should acquire before being expected to use a device independently in class. Often, the newness and excitement of interesting technology tools entices students to try to use them immediately and to show the technology and all the "cool" things it can do to teachers, family, and friends. (See the Technology Tip, "'Show and Tell' with New Technology.") Although this is a great incentive for a student to practice using a device, the team should realize that the student needs

instruction and practice before he or she attempts to use a new piece of technology in class. It is important for the student to be comfortable enough with a device to be able to maintain concentration on the subject matter being presented and not be distracted by trying to remember how to operate the equipment or software program. For example, another goal for Bill's use of the video magnifier might specify, "Bill will demonstrate the ability to alternate between near viewing and distance viewing using the video magnifier before using it in his classes."

IEP goals should identify the length, quantity, or size of the task for which a particular technology is appropriate. Some of the tools recommended for a student are best suited for shorter assignments, while others are more appropriate for longer tasks. Clearly defining the appropriate uses for each tool in the student's goals and objectives can focus instruction on which

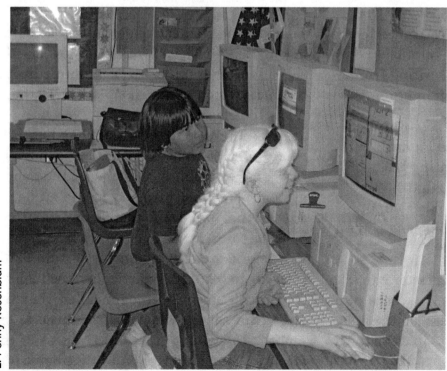

L. Penny Rosenblum

Before using any technology in class, a student needs to be comfortable enough to be able to concentrate on the subject matter being presented and not be distracted by trying to remember how to operate the equipment or software program.

TECHNOLOGY TIP

"SHOW-AND-TELL" WITH NEW TECHNOLOGY

When students are eager to show others their new technology devices, they should be encouraged to use the technology in a "show-and-tell" type activity in their class. A student can explain that he or she is learning about a device that has many functions and features, and that it will take some time before they are all mastered. Then the student can demonstrate one or two of the features that he or she is most comfortable executing.

An approach such as this might help everyone involved with the student—from classmates, classroom teachers, and administrators to the IEP team to family members—understand the need for appropriate training and skill acquisition before a device is used independently in the classroom. Too often students attempt to use technologies to work on assignments that have to be completed quickly before they have acquired the skills needed to do that task. This situation can be frustrating and embarrassing for the student and can possibly lead to a negative attitude about the technology that may result in the student's failure with it or unwillingness to use it. In most cases this kind of negative experience can be avoided by ensuring that the student has obtained a certain level of proficiency with a tool before relying on it to accomplish a specific task.

tools provide the greatest assistance to the student for different types of tasks. Two goals for Bill in the area of writing (recommendations #22 and #24) might state:

- Bill will demonstrate the ability to use bold-lined paper and a dark felt-tip pen to complete writing tasks of less than one page in length.
- Bill will use his accessible computer to complete writing tasks longer than one page in length.

A solid understanding of this factor can also help parents and classroom teachers support the student's awareness of the most appropriate tool to use for a given activity. Ultimately, the student will need to learn to

select the most effective devices for completing his or her schoolwork and develop the self-advocacy skills to communicate to teachers which adaptations are most helpful in the classroom.

It is likely that the recommended technology and instruction in its use may be new and unfamiliar to some of the school system personnel involved in the student's educational program. Instructors may not be able to estimate accurately how long it will take a student to master certain skills related to using a particular technology. Thus, it is strongly recommended that the IEP team set a review date of three to six months to evaluate the effectiveness of the interventions undertaken to that point and make appropriate plans to continue implementing the recommendations.

CONSIDERATIONS FOR TEACHING ASSISTIVE TECHNOLOGY

When to Start Assistive Technology Instruction

Taking a Proactive Approach to Teaching

- Intervening Early
- Knowing the General Education Curriculum
- Knowing about State Standards and Testing

Employing Diagnostic Teaching

- Progress Monitoring
- Periodic Reevaluation

Although IEP goals in the area of assistive technology give teachers a general guide to the skills to be taught, they do not usually identify the specific content, precise sequence, or exact strategies needed to be taught for each skill. Teachers will have some flexibility about how to teach the various technology skills and the particular order in which they should be taught. In most cases the responsibility for teaching assistive technology will fall to the teacher of students with visual impairments. However, he or she should investigate opportunities for the instruction of assistive technology to be provided by other trained personnel who may have more expertise in a particular technology. This applies particularly to students with additional disabilities who may be using multiple pieces of access technology not specifically designed

for students with vision loss. There are a number of general considerations that teachers should think about when designing instruction to implement the assistive technology recommendations.

WHEN TO START ASSISTIVE TECHNOLOGY INSTRUCTION

Many educators ask, "When should my student begin learning about assistive technology, and what should I teach first?" These are difficult questions to answer, because the answer always is: "It depends"—on the individual student, his or her specific needs, the tasks the student needs to accomplish at school and at home, and all the factors discussed throughout this book (particularly in Chapters 7 and 8). In general, students should start working on all the skills they need to use the technology that meets their needs as early as possible. Some technologies, such as the use of bold-lined paper, the braillewriter, optical devices, and many others can be taught to students in early elementary school. By upper elementary or middle school, most students will need to have mastered the basic operation of technologies, such as the use of a video magnifier, analog or digital recording, keyboarding, basic word processing, and basic functions with an accessible PDA, to name just a few. In high school, students *usually* refine their skills and learn more complex aspects of the technology, but some students may be working at that level in middle school. A comprehensive scope and sequence for teaching assistive technology to students who are blind or visually impaired is a subject that would require a separate book in itself.

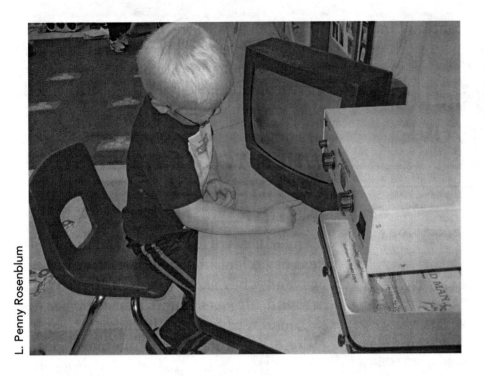

L. Penny Rosenblum

Students should start as early as possible to learn how to use the technology that meets their needs.

Although currently no research points to "best" ages to introduce assistive technology, a useful rule of thumb is to look at what children in the same age group as the student are doing. If their siblings, classmates, and friends are using technology, in all likelihood students who are blind or visually impaired will be ready to be exposed to computers and other technology in the same way as are typically sighted students. Today, very young children interact with computers and use technology for games and other activities. Students with visual impairments typically need more direct instruction, more hands-on experience, and more opportunities to practice than do students with unimpaired vision, so why wait?

Whenever possible, assistive technology skills being taught should be applied to tasks currently being assigned in the regular classroom. This will give the student opportunities to use the skills he or she has been practicing in an authentic context. Excellent communication between the classroom teacher and the teacher of students with visual impairments is critical to the success of this component of assistive technology instruction and use. The teacher of students with visual impairments will need to be fully aware of the classroom teacher's lesson plans so that, when feasible, the student can already have acquired the skills necessary to use the appropriate technology to complete the current activities assigned in the classroom.

TAKING A PROACTIVE APPROACH TO TEACHING

Intervening Early

Instruction in the use of assistive technology requires a two-pronged approach. The teacher of students with visual impairments needs to teach skills that can be learned in a relatively short period of time and used immediately to help the student perform his or her current schoolwork. At the same time, the teacher also needs to start teaching skills that may take longer to master and will be needed at a later time to use technology for more complex activities. The following example illustrates how this can be accomplished:

Savannah, a third-grade girl with low vision, has the following IEP goals among others relating to the use of technology to facilitate her writing skills:

- *Savannah will use bold-lined paper and a bold marker to complete writing tasks of less than one page in length.*
- *Savannah will demonstrate knowledge of the home row keys on the computer keyboard with 80% accuracy.*
- *Savannah will demonstrate the ability to open, save, and print documents using the word-processing program on her accessible computer.*

Marilyn, her teacher of students with visual impairments, decides to include instruction along three paths in her lesson plans. Part of each instructional period will be spent teaching Savannah to use low-tech writing devices, such as bold-lined paper with bold markers. Learning to use these tools should take a relatively short time.

Another part of the instructional period will be devoted to teaching beginning keyboarding skills. Al-though using a computer keyboard and word-processing software to produce written communication is an essential skill for Savannah to develop, it will take some time before she is ready to use a computer as an everyday writing tool.

A third portion of the instructional period will be spent on developing the skills necessary to use a video magnification system with distance viewing capabilities to view items on a chalkboard or whiteboard and then copy the information by writing or typing. Mastering the skills necessary to accomplish the last two tasks will take longer than mastering the skills for the first task, but Marilyn and Savannah can work on all of them simultaneously.

This multipronged strategy might be referred to as "proactive teaching." Savannah does not yet have a need to complete lengthy writing assignments in third grade, but her teacher of students with visual impairments knows that as she moves into higher grades, the low-tech writing tools that she is currently using will no longer be enough for her to keep up with her classmates. At that point, Savannah will need adequate keyboarding skills to use the computer and word-processing software to accomplish longer writing tasks.

There are two reasons why instruction for skills that will be needed in the future should begin at an early stage in the student's educational program. First, the necessary skills cannot be mastered in a short period of time. Keyboarding skills and the ability to use word-processing software, for example, require physical and cognitive skills that must be mastered over time, through repetition and practice, before a student can be expected to rely on them to complete complex tasks. Using the foregoing story, for example, there is a good chance that near the end of fourth grade and throughout the fifth grade, Savannah will need to use keyboarding and word-processing skills to complete some writing tasks. If the IEP team waits to introduce the use of assistive technology devices until Savannah needs to use that technology to complete her current educational assignments, she will be inefficient at using these tools and frustrated trying to keep up with school and homework. Many other skills also require time, practice, and feedback from an instructor before they are automatic and efficient. It is critical for the IEP team to be proactive and allow students to become proficient with assistive technology skills as early as possible so that they have mastered the skills by the time they need them.

The second reason why some instruction needs to be provided early is because certain sets of skills are cumulative. Some skills are fundamental and prerequisite, and others build on those initial skills. Therefore, mastering basic skills needs to be part of the student's program early on, because without them, the student will lack the foundation to develop the more advanced skills required later in secondary school. If instruction in keyboarding and word-processing skills, for example, is delayed until fifth grade, there will not be time for a student to learn all the other skills that will be necessary for middle school and beyond, such as notetaking, use of recorded and electronic materials, organization skills, and advocacy skills. If the teacher of students with visual impairments begins teaching all these skills well before the fourth or fifth grade, students will have ample time to master them before they will be required to use them in middle school and high school.

Knowing the General Education Curriculum

Another aspect of proactive teaching is becoming familiar with the general education curriculum in order to be able to anticipate a student's technology needs. For example, if the general education technology curriculum requires students to use a computer to search the Internet for resources and information to include in a report, students who are blind or visually impaired will need some prerequisite skills to participate in this part of the educational program. First, they will need to have a certain level of keyboarding skills to use a computer. These students will also need a basic knowledge of computer access technology and strategies. They most likely will need to know how to use screen-reading software or screen magnification software. And finally, the students will need to know enough about the access technology to use it effectively on the Internet. If the teacher of students with visual impairments knows when students will be expected to perform these tasks as part of the general curriculum, then the IEP team can plan the student's instructional program to ensure that the student will already have the prerequisite skills when they are needed.

Knowing about State Standards and Testing

Those involved with delivering assistive technology instruction also need to be proactive in relation to state standards and testing. Most states have specific standards for grade-level and other high-stakes tests, on which students have to demonstrate that they have mastered certain content in order to be promoted to the next higher grade. To demonstrate the competencies required for these exams, students who are blind or visually impaired may need to use certain types of assistive technology. A forward-thinking teacher of students with visual impairments will determine ahead of time the level of assistive technology knowledge necessary to complete the tasks required for the standards and begin instruction as soon as possible to prepare the student.

A good example of the need for advance planning around standardized exams is in the area of tactile graphics. In general, students are being required to work with more and more graphical information throughout their educational program. Students with low vision and students who are tactile learners can be at a definite disadvantage if they have not been taught to interpret graphs, charts, timelines, and other graphical information prior to testing on these concepts. Consequently, IEP goals specifying instruction in the use, creation, and interpretation of tactile graphics should be written beginning in preschool and throughout the student's educational career.

EMPLOYING DIAGNOSTIC TEACHING

The use of many assistive technology devices and software can be broken down into a series of skills that can be acquired in a step-by-step fashion. As mentioned earlier, teachers can make use of diagnostic teaching methods while instructing students to learn the use of assistive technology. Simply stated, diagnostic teaching involves carefully monitoring the effectiveness of instruction to make sure the student is making progress with the methods being used. If the student is not making adequate progress in learning skills and content, the teacher modifies his or her instruction to alter that outcome. This modification might mean changing teaching methods, the materials used, or the rate or intensity with which new material is presented. For example, if the teacher of students with visual impairments is teaching keyboarding skills

and the student is struggling to learn the correct fingering, the teacher can try a different teaching method (such as a computerized program or the color-coding system described in Chapter 4); perhaps a different size keyboard (a smaller keyboard on a laptop or a larger one that can connect to the laptop or computer) or a strategy of introducing fewer letters at a time or including more practice before introducing new letters will help.

The key to diagnostic teaching is for the teacher to constantly monitor how the student is doing, so that changes can be made to lesson plans as needed. The goal of effective instruction is not to rush the student through a program as quickly as possible, but to make sure the student learns the skills well. To ascertain the student's progress toward achieving goals, the teacher needs to collect specific data about the student's performance. This data can then be saved and shared with the student, parents, and the IEP team. For example, if the student is learning to keyboard, the teacher of students with visual impairments can keep a record of how many letters the student has learned, the student's accuracy level, and how many words per minute the student can type. This type of approach will allow the teacher to monitor the student's progress, diagnose any difficulties as they arise, and judge the student's progress on an objective basis. Careful attention to information about a student's performance is important, as this data can be used to make modifications in instruction to improve student outcomes.

Progress Monitoring

Progress monitoring during instruction and assessment is not only part of good teaching, it is also increasingly required by school systems and states as part of their accountability systems. Teachers are being held responsible for the progress that students make on the general curriculum, the state standards for learning, and the goals and objectives on a student's IEP. Accountability is a thorny issue in education. Although it appears to be a simple matter of demonstrating that education is "working" and that students are learning what they are supposed to learn, this seemingly simple concept leads to questions such as the following:

- What are students supposed to learn, and who decides?
- How do schools show that students are learning and what they have learned?
- How do we identify students who are not learning, and how do we help them?

In regard to assistive technology, teachers need to assess both how students are learning to use devices and what they are doing with them. That is, not only do teachers need to keep track of how students use various technology devices and software to see if students need additional instruction in how to use the technology, but also they need to keep track of the reading and writing skills that students are using with the technology to produce written papers, read assignments, and so forth.

As explained in "Monitoring Students' Assistive Technology Skills," there are a number of ways in which teachers can monitor students' progress in using different forms of assistive technology. Monitoring the end goal of technology use—the products that students produce using technology—involves looking at their class assignments. For example, when the teacher of students with visual impairments assesses how a student uses a computer equipped with screen-reading software to write a research paper, he or she also assesses the paper to make sure the student has formatted it correctly (using indented paragraphs and adding footnotes, headings, and page numbers) and used correct writing mechanics, such as capital letters and correct punctuation. The teacher of students with visual impairments and the classroom teacher need to work in close partnership to assess these elements. The teacher of students with visual impairments needs to know—and the classroom teacher should clearly communicate—the expectations for all the students in the class, so the teacher of students with visual impairments can teach and reinforce those skills. Teamwork among both teachers and the family is essential so that expectations remain high and instruction in essential skills is not accidentally omitted because each party assumed someone else had taught what the student needed!

Periodic Reevaluation

Assessment is an ongoing process, and students need to be reevaluated periodically concerning their assistive technology needs. Rather than specifying a set time period after which the student should be reevaluated, however, his or her IEP team needs to be alert to the variety of factors that might signal the need to reevaluate a student's assistive technology needs, including the following:

- **Change in vision or other medical condition:** If a student experiences a significant change in his or her visual functioning or other area of health or impairment, he or she may need to be reexamined. It is highly recommended that the IEP team should reassess the tools and methods used by the student to access print and electronic information and complete writing tasks, as well as the teachers' need to produce materials in alternate formats for the student.

- **Change in information the student must access:** The size of the print in the textbooks and other materials that students use generally

becomes smaller around the second or third grade. Some students with low vision may require different technology for reading when this happens. Or, a classroom teacher may begin to use presentation tools, such as a PowerPoint presentation projected on a screen, that make the information inaccessible to the student. These or

TECHNOLOGY TIP

MONITORING STUDENTS' ASSISTIVE TECHNOLOGY SKILLS

Many skills related to the use of assistive technology can be tracked through simple checklists, task analysis, and anecdotal records.

Checklists

Checklists for monitoring students' use of particular devices generally list the features of the devices in separate boxes. Teachers can check off the features that students are able to use independently or with assistance. Ready-made checklists are available from such sources as the web sites of the Texas School for the Blind and Visually Impaired and the California School for the Blind and from Special Education Technology—British Columbia (SET-BC; see the Resources section).

Task Analysis

A task analysis is a type of checklist that breaks down large tasks into small, manageable steps. Teachers can then check off which tasks—and how many steps of a task—students can do. Teachers can use ready-made forms or create their own. These forms can be used quantitatively in that the teacher can share with the IEP team how many steps the student is able do and how many still need to be mastered.

Anecdotal Records

Teachers can keep notes from each instructional session as a record of how a student does from day to day. Known as anecdotal records, this type of qualitative data can include information such as the student's motivation and frustration level, interest in the topic, questions the student asks that need follow-up, and other factors that led to the success of a lesson or that indicate changes might be needed.

similar changes might prompt a reevaluation to recommend better tools for the student to use to access information in the new or altered formats.

- **Change in the educational environment:** As students begin to work in a wider variety of environments, there may be a need to evaluate new or different tools for accessing the educational program. For example, a student may be moving from elementary to middle school and need more portable solutions as he or she begins to change classes within the school.
- **Availability of new technology:** As new technologies become available, some may have the potential to benefit to a student. The IEP team might schedule an assessment to evaluate the effectiveness of a new technology to meet a student's needs.

Any of these situations can trigger a reevaluation of a student's assistive technology needs. A scheduled periodic reevaluation may be recommended by the IEP team, usually every three years, but that should not deter the team from requesting a reevaluation if circumstances suggest the need for new or different tools.

In most cases where a reevaluation is indicated, a complete new assistive technology assessment may not be needed. The circumstances that initiate the reevaluation will also suggest the depth and detail needed. The team will need to assess how well the technology currently being used assists the student in accomplishing his or her educational tasks. In areas where these tools are working appropriately, there may be no need to reevaluate, but in areas in which the technology is not working out or

the student's needs have changed, a more extensive review may be necessary. If new technologies have become available, it may only be necessary to reevaluate the particular needs of the student that are addressed by those tools.

It is important for the team to keep in mind that students' needs change over time, as much as the students grow and mature physically and psychologically over the same period. It will always be necessary to evaluate students' progress in school, using assistive technology and other instructional materials, and to make changes to their programs as necessary. The effective technology solutions set up by the school for a student in a third-grade classroom may be completely inadequate for that same student as he or she enters middle school. They may need to be changed again as the student enters high school. No one expects that students would use the same textbooks for 12 years; so too, no one should expect that technology needs will remain the same from kindergarten through high school.

TROUBLESHOOTING TECHNOLOGY DIFFICULTIES

Hardware and Software Problems

Operator Errors

As teachers monitor a student's progress using assistive technology, there will be times when the student's progress in using a particular technology plateaus or even appears to regress. Such a situation can lead to a perplexing challenge for the instructor, the student, the parent, and the

IEP team, who may be wondering why the student is not more successful in using the technology and in learning to use it to perform appropriate tasks. The teacher will need to carefully observe the student's interactions with the technology to ascertain what difficulties the student might be having. These observations will help the teacher determine if the student's problems are a result of equipment malfunction or mistakes that the student is making in using the equipment—that is, operator error—or if other issues are hindering the student's progress (such as lack of motivation or difficulty with course content). But in cases where the student is eager to learn and practice with the device yet is still having difficulty with it, teachers should have a plan for systematic troubleshooting to uncover why the student is having problems.

HARDWARE AND SOFTWARE PROBLEMS

The first question to investigate is whether the technology is working properly, beginning with the most basic issues, such as whether all of the hardware is connected properly and plugged in. Will the device or the program perform its usual functions within the expected time frame? If not, the first step is for the teacher to try repeating the steps in the process the student was trying to perform—for example, printing out a document. If the teacher cannot reproduce the same error or achieve the desired result, the device should be powered down (or turned off) and restarted. If the problem is with a computer program that is not responding appropriately, the program should be closed and reopened or the computer system shut down completely and restarted.

If these simple interventions are not successful, then assistance will need to be solicited. Depending on the type of problem, one or all of the following sources might be helpful:

- The local school system assistive technology specialist
- The local educational agency (LEA) general technology specialist
- A state or regional assistive technology specialist
- Teachers of students with visual impairments in surrounding districts who use the same type of technology
- Visually impaired individuals in the school district or geographic area who use the same type of technology
- Assistive technology specialists providing services through state or private agencies
- Technical support services from the product's manufacturer
- State or national electronic mailing lists for professionals serving people who are blind or visually impaired
- Specialized electronic mailing lists dedicated to specific products
- Staff at state or local organizations or agencies that provide services to people who are visually impaired

In Chapter 6 the assessment team was encouraged to establish relationships with individuals, organizations, and vendors who might be helpful to the assessment team in locating technology that can be used for assessment purposes (see Sidebar 6.4). These resources will also be valuable assets when dealing with any type of technical problems.

Regardless of which resource is used to solicit assistance, the teacher should have the following information readily available before making the contact:

- Make and model number of all devices or hardware involved
- Name and version number of software or firmware for stand-alone devices (such as an accessible PDA)
- Operating system and software version for computer-related problems
- Detailed notes about the exact sequence of actions that occur just before the problem presents itself
- The exact wording of any error message that is presented, which can be copied and pasted into a word-processing file or e-mail message
- Information about any other unusual events that have been happening with the technology (for example, power surges in the building)

If at all possible, the teacher should have direct access to the inoperative technology when placing a call for technical assistance. When feasible, he or she should replicate the problem, shut down the system, and restart it. Once technical support has been reached and the teacher has provided a basic description of the problem and the technical information listed above, he or she should begin executing the steps that lead to the problem. Each action and the resulting response of the technology should be explained to the technical support person. This individual may ask the teacher to execute other actions along the way to help determine the cause of the problem. Most difficulties can be resolved through telephone technical support. In some situations, equipment may need to be returned for repair or software may need to be reinstalled on a device or computer, which may require having access to the CD, DVD, or floppy disk on which the source files of the software reside.

OPERATOR ERRORS

If it has been determined that the technology is functioning properly, the teacher will need to find out whether the student is making some kind of error in using the device. The teacher should have the student repeat the steps that led to the problem while monitoring these steps very carefully to ascertain if the student is making some type of mistake. If a document is failing to print, for example, the student should attempt to print it again, step by step, so the teacher can watch what he or she is doing to ensure that the steps are in the right order. Many technologies require the user to execute multiple steps in a certain order to complete tasks. It is easy for the user to forget one of the steps or to execute it inaccurately without realizing it. For this reason, it is strongly recommended that assistive technology instruction consist of a set of step-by-step directions whenever possible. If the teacher and student review such instructions one at a time, the cause of errors can usually be isolated and identified.

TRAINING FOR TEACHERS

Awareness of Assistive Technology

Operational Knowledge

Instructional Strategies

Planning for Training

Training Other Staff and Families

For many years, two major barriers to integrating technology into educational programs in this country were the lack of availability of equipment and the lack of funding to purchase it. Although these are still issues, particularly with very expensive equipment, one of the biggest concerns in education today is training for teachers in the use of technology (McDonald, 2005; NEA, 2008). Although university teacher preparation programs include coursework on assistive technology, many practicing teachers of all kinds have not had a great deal of instruction. Moreover, as technology changes so rapidly, teachers of students with visual impairments need to continually update their skills. Based on the definition of assistive technology services provided in the Individuals with Disabilities Education Act (IDEA; see Appendix A, "It's the Law"), it is critical that school systems work with teachers to ensure they have the skills to implement the recommendations of the assistive technology assessment in the student's IEP. Appropriate and adequate training is an essential element in the successful implementation of the assistive technology recommendations and the student's successful use of technology to access the educational curriculum.

Teachers of students with visual impairments have a number of ways to learn about assistive technology designed for students who are blind or visually impaired. Pursuing such learning opportunities can require some initiative, careful planning, and cooperation on the part of both the school system and the teacher, and perhaps some expense.

All teachers need to develop general computer and technology skills. Opportunities for this type of training are more readily available than specific training in assistive technology. Indeed, many school systems require teachers to be "computer literate," and some states require evidence of computer skill for teacher certification.

Many school systems and community colleges offer hands-on classes in basic computer applications such as word processing, e-mail, and Internet browsing that teachers can take advantage of. In addition, tutorials are available in books, online, and in a variety of electronic formats such as on CD or DVD. A basic knowledge of computers and technology, obtained from these types of training opportunities if necessary, will be of great assistance when the teacher begins to learn about specific assistive technology designed for students who are blind or visually impaired.

AWARENESS OF ASSISTIVE TECHNOLOGY

Knowledge about assistive technology can be divided into three levels: awareness, basic operational knowledge, and instructional strategies. General awareness about assistive technology can be acquired in a variety of ways. The Internet abounds with general descriptive information about the various types of assistive technology available. It is only necessary to enter the name of a category of assistive technology—such as "accessible PDA," "video magnifier," or "braille display"—into a search engine, and the results will offer some basic information about these types of technology. In addition, many organizations provide information about assistive technology. The Resources section of this book lists a number of organizations that teachers of students with visual impairments can contact for information and training, and "Resources for Learning about Assistive Technology" (Sidebar 9.1) provides more information on a variety of sources.

RESOURCES FOR LEARNING ABOUT ASSISTIVE TECHNOLOGY

There are a variety of resources available from organizations that focus on either visual impairment or assistive technology. They include books, web sites, conferences, and training opportunities. Information about the resources mentioned here can be found in the Resources section of this book.

Online and In Print

The assistive technology area of the American Foundation for the Blind's (AFB) web site (www.afb.org) provides helpful information about assistive technology designed for people who are blind or visually impaired. The information includes descriptions of different types of technology along with short videos, considerations for choosing a product, and evaluations of specific products. There is also an assistive technology database that provides specifications of individual products in each category of assistive technology and information about the manufacturer. (Please see the Resources section for a list of other useful web sites.)

In addition, *AccessWorld: Technology and People Who Are Blind or Visually Impaired*, a free online magazine (at www.afb.org/accessworld) published by AFB, specializes in technology specifically for people who are blind or visually impaired.

The AFB Career Connect program (www.afb.org/careerconnect) has developed a number of virtual worksites that offer general information about assistive technology and how it is used in various work settings. The site features videos that describe and demonstrate various types of assistive technology used by people who are blind or visually impaired. This site is not only an excellent source of information for teachers, but also a valuable tool that can be used with administrators, parents, students, employers, and other school system personnel.

Another resource for acquiring information about assistive technology is an AFB Press publication titled *AccessWorld: Guide to Assistive Technology Products*. This print and online publication covers all the major types of technology for people who are blind or visually impaired, with detailed information about current products.

Closing the Gap is a print and online subscription-based monthly magazine that offers information on a range of assistive technology.

Conferences

One of the best ways to learn about assistive technology is by attending conferences for professionals and for consumers who are blind or visually impaired. These conferences give teachers a great opportunity to network with other professionals who are using technology with their students. A big attraction of the conferences is the exhibit hall, where assistive technology vendors are available to demonstrate the latest advances in technology and attendees can try out various technologies and ask questions.

The organization that produces the periodical *Closing the Gap* also offers an annual assistive technology conference in Minnesota by the same name. Most of the sessions at the Closing the Gap conference are oriented toward education, although some are designed for service providers who work with adults. This conference is a well-established venue for learning about assistive technology for individuals with many types of disabilities, and includes sessions on vision-related technology, as well as technology used by individuals with multiple disabilities. It offers information at beginning, intermediate, and advanced levels, and various sessions provide hands-on training in specific pieces of technology.

The Association for Education and Rehabilitation of the Blind and Visually Impaired (AER), an organization of professionals in the blindness field, sponsors conferences that offer many opportunities to learn about assistive technology, in addition to numerous other topics. The Information and Technology Division of AER presents sessions that introduce various assistive technology devices and the latest developments in the field. Numerous opportunities for networking and visiting exhibitors are also available. AER has chapters throughout the United States and Canada, most of which have annual conferences at which technology presentations are often available, and most have vendors who exhibit the latest technology in the field.

The Council for Exceptional Children (CEC), a professional organization for special educators that holds an annual conference, has a division for Technology and Media that hosts sessions during the conference and publishes the informative *Journal of Special Education Technology*. Two major organizations representing consumers who are blind or visually impaired also offer conventions where educators can learn about technology. The American Council of the Blind (ACB) and the National Federation of the Blind (NFB) each holds a national annual convention that features exhibits by vendors who specialize in assistive technology for people who are blind or visually impaired.

An additional advantage of attending a consumer convention is the opportunity to see assistive technology being used by youths and adults. Many of the users are highly advanced and very knowledgeable about assistive technology and willing to share their knowledge and answer questions about the advantages and disadvantages of specific devices. At these conventions vendors often offer introductory, intermediate, and advanced training in the use of their products, which can be an excellent opportunity for teachers to improve their skills and gain additional training.

Two conferences run by technology organizations also offer training opportunities: the Technology and Persons with Disabilities Conference offered by California State University at Northridge (referred to as CSUN), and the Assistive Technology Industry Association Conference (ATIA). The CSUN conference, the first major conference on technology for people with disabilities, which began in October 1985, offers sessions on all areas of assistive technology, including numerous sessions on technology for people who are blind or

(continued on next page)

SIDEBAR 9.1 (CONTINUED)

visually impaired. The sessions cover general information as well as hands-on training with specific pieces of technology. The conference typically contains a very large exhibit area where attendees can see the latest assistive technology from around the world. The ATIA conference is organized and presented by manufacturers of assistive technology. Attendees will find numerous information sessions, along with additional opportunities for hands-on training. Many of the participating vendors sponsor two- or three-hour training sessions on their products.

OPERATIONAL KNOWLEDGE

A higher level of knowledge about assistive technology is understanding how to operate the technology. Individuals at this stage are learning which proverbial buttons to push to make the technology perform a desired operation or task. Familiarity with technology at this level is best achieved through face-to-face training in a hands-on setting where each learner can actually operate the hardware and software. This type of training may be more available in some areas than others, although it can be found at some of the national conferences discussed in Sidebar 9.1 and from an increasing number of organizations within the field of blindness and visual impairment.

Although most local school systems offer some hands-on training with general technology, few are able to offer the specialized training specific to children who are blind or visually impaired that is needed by teachers of students with visual impairments and other school system personnel. Most local educational agencies (LEAs) have state and local funding to provide professional development to their staff. If these LEAs cannot provide the specialized training needed by teachers of students with visual impairments it would seem reasonable for them to offer financial support to these teachers to acquire this training elsewhere. Some states have statewide training efforts to support special education teachers, including teachers of students with visual impairments. Funding should be provided to cover travel expenses and registration to attend conferences and hands-on training sessions when available.

It is reasonable for administrators to expect that teachers who receive financial assistance for training will then share the information with their colleagues and coworkers who also need the information. One option to explore is a cooperative effort among several school districts to obtain specific technology training for a teacher who then provides a workshop for other teachers from the cooperating districts. This "train-the-trainer" approach can be helpful, but its effectiveness can be limited because the teacher who received the training needs to have adequate time to assimilate and practice what was learned before attempting to train colleagues. Another cooperative effort that has been successful is pooling resources to hire a technology specialist to conduct training for teachers within a region, or even across state lines. (See the section on "Planning for Training" for more information on such efforts and how to set up a training program.)

In addition, online training opportunities can help teachers learn the skills they will need to operate the specialized assistive technology recommended for students who are blind or visually impaired. Some self-paced tutorials are accessible online and on CD (and a few still on cassette tape), which teachers can use to learn how to operate certain pieces of hardware and software. The Hadley School for the Blind provides free courses to professionals (as well as to parents and youths and adults who are blind). The Carroll Center for the Blind also provides online instruction on assistive technology specific to people who are blind. (See the Resources for more information.) In addition to the financial support needed to access these resources, districts will need to give teachers adequate release time to participate in online training activities and tutorials. However, because the training is not being delivered directly by a trained instructor, these options will most likely require additional time for staff to obtain the knowledge and master the skills needed to provide appropriate instruction to students.

There are also some online sites that provide other useful information for teachers, such as "cheat sheets" and lists of commands for various features of assistive technology devices. For example, the web site of Special Education Technology—British Columbia (SET-BC; see Resources) provides helpful information on using the Mountbatten Brailler, such as beginning lessons, lists of commands, and so forth. These resources can be helpful for teachers of students with visual impairments and others who might be learning how to use advanced features of the devices along with their students.

INSTRUCTIONAL STRATEGIES

The third level of training that teachers of students with visual impairments and other service providers need to achieve relates to instructional strategies that can be used to teach students how to effectively use assistive technology. There are not many formal opportunities for teachers to obtain training in this area, but one of the better ways to learn about instructional strategies is by networking with others who have taught assistive technology to students who are blind or visually impaired. Networking can take place at conferences and workshops, but in many cases it will need to occur through direct communications between service providers. One way to accomplish this is through the use of electronic mailing lists. There are dozens of active e-mail lists covering general and specific topics related to assistive technology. Some are sponsored by organizations in the field (see the Resources), and some can be found simply by searching the Internet for terms such as "e-mail list," "blind," and "assistive technology." Teachers should be encouraged to subscribe to these lists, ask questions, and participate in the discussions when appropriate. With technology permeating the education of students with visual impairments, many more books and articles may be written about instructional strategies for teaching assistive technology to them. In the meantime, teachers will have to be resourceful and creative in acquiring as much information as possible and developing their own instructional strategies that work with individual students.

Regardless of which training options are pursued, limits on the availability of technology training should not be allowed to delay the implementation of recommended assistive technology for the students and instruction in its use. Some assistive technology recommendations that require less expertise on the instructor's part can be implemented immediately or within a relatively short time. Instruction in other technologies can begin as soon as the teacher has mastered some of the basics of the assistive technology. If a comprehensive staff technology training plan has been implemented (as described in the next section), the teacher can begin by instructing the student in topics that the teacher has mastered. As the teacher learns about new features, they can be incorporated into the student's instructional program.

Although teachers of students with visual impairments need to be proficient in many areas of assistive technology knowledge and skills, especially for their younger students, they do not need to be technology experts, but rather they can learn some of the more advanced features of devices, equipment, and software along with their students. The teacher can serve as a role model for high school students and other students who have gained proficiency in several types of assistive technology devices by demonstrating how to use resources such as the "Help" feature, online or print manuals, or any tutorials that may be available that explain a device's advanced features. In fact, one of the most helpful strategies to employ is to teach students where to find the "Help" file, and encourage them to explore the menus and features of a device by themselves. This exposure will promote problem-solving strategies as students learn to figure out technology problems independently. Some students also learn from friends, and students who have some degree of comfort with technology can learn more about their devices and software by participating in mailing lists or online comment boards started by computer users who are blind or by manufacturers or users of specific products.

PLANNING FOR TRAINING

When teachers or school systems make arrangements to hire assistive technology specialists and organize their own training, the success of such an endeavor usually requires extensive planning to address the following items:

- **The technology training plan**: The first step is to determine the immediate and future needs for technology training among the staff members who are to participate in the training. If some individuals need general technology or computer training, this need should be addressed immediately as a prerequisite, before proceeding to the needs for assistive technology training. The planners will have to decide which training options (such as face-to-face workshops, CD or online tutorials, or private consultant) will be used to meet the assistive technology training needs of the staff. The specific needs and the training options may vary from teacher to teacher, but group training is usually a good option when possible. The technology training plan will need to focus on the long term. The array of technologies used by students who are blind or visually impaired cannot be learned in detail in just one or two sessions, but an overview of the general types of technology can be obtained. Some topics can be adequately covered in several two- to three-hour training sessions, while others will require more intense sessions of one to three days each. These training sessions will need to be scheduled on an ongoing basis to prepare teachers to meet the technology needs of their students. Not all of the training will need to be completed immediately, however. The teacher's training will need to progress over time, just as the student's training does, with basic skills learned first and more advanced skills added periodically.

- **The specific topic**: Training planners need to decide the level at which the training should be conducted, based on the prospective attendees' needs. If the training is to address general awareness of technology, the topic can be broader and can incorporate demonstrations of various technologies and their capabilities. If the training is to be at the operational or the instructional strategy level, one specific topic should be selected, limited to a specific piece of hardware or software or procedure.

- **Goals and objectives of the training**: The trainer will need to be made aware of the specific needs of the participants. Training sessions should be designed for beginning, intermediate, or advanced users. In addition, the objectives for the training will need to be clearly stated. In most cases, planners should select a limited number of features of a particular technology (about five to seven, depending on the length of the training session) and make sure that the trainer understands that the skills related to the use of these features are those the attendees should acquire during the

training. The planners of the training may wish to consult with other educators to determine appropriate objectives for a beginning, intermediate, or advanced training session.

- **Step-by-step instruction in writing**: An item that the planners should make sure to obtain from the trainer is a clear set of written, step-by-step instructions in an accessible format for each trainee. This material is extremely important because the trainees will need this information to refer to later as they practice and refine their skills using the technology.

- **Release time**: School administrators will need to allocate adequate release time for teachers to take full advantage of training opportunities. Some opportunities will be offered during work time. School systems that provide release time and financial support for teacher training will often find that dedicated teachers are willing to participate in some evening and weekend sessions, as well. The time required to participate in the training will vary greatly depending on the topic selected and the training option employed. Technology training at the operational level requires not only opportunities for hands-on instruction, but also practice activities after the training session to reinforce the new skills.

- **Appropriate space and equipment**: Planners of technology training will need to ensure that appropriate space and equipment will be available for the training. They should be aware that the assistive technology consultant providing the training will most likely need to meet with the school system's technology specialists to install software and configure hardware. These arrangements can be negotiated as part of the overall fees for the consultant or may be billed as a separate item depending on the complexity of the setup involved.

- **Availability of assistive technology and time to practice what is learned**: The assistive technology training plan will also need to ensure that staff have access to assistive technology devices after training to refine their skills with the new technologies. This access is essential for personnel receiving instruction at the operational level who seek to learn how to use devices and equipment, although it may not be mandatory for training at the awareness level.

Making sure that teachers of students with visual impairments are sufficiently knowledgeable about the assistive technology that their students need to use is an essential part of providing assistive technology services to students. In this way, teachers can provide appropriate training and support students in using the technology in the classroom. Acquiring this type of knowledge and training needs to be a joint responsibility shared by the teacher and the school system. Although teachers do not need to learn everything about all types of assistive technology all at once, it is a key area of their professional development.

TRAINING OTHER STAFF AND FAMILIES

For students to be successful in using assistive technology, other school system personnel and parents will also need to have some basic knowledge about the technology they are using, in addition to the teacher of students with visual impairments. Having parents and other service providers who work with the student "buy in" to the use of the technology is key to the successful implementation of the assessment team's recommendations. These individuals may not need to know all the operational features of devices or the strategies for using them, but they must be convinced of the technology's usefulness and its ability to assist the student in maximizing his or her educational and employment potential.

These individuals will need to have both general awareness and basic operational knowledge of the assistive technology being used by the student—although not to the same extent as the teacher of students with visual impairments. The necessary training can be provided in several ways. Some school system personnel, such as classroom teachers, assistive technology specialists, and paraeducators, may be able to take advantage of some of the same training opportunities that are available to the teacher of students with visual impairments. When this is not possible, the teacher of students with visual impairments may be able to provide the training. Such in-service training sessions can serve as good opportunities for the teacher to reinforce his or her own knowledge of assistive technology and to practice instructional techniques for teaching it to students. Training for parents and other family members has to be planned on a case-by-case basis, depending on the availability and interest of the individuals involved.

CONCLUSION

Although becoming familiar with the many types of assistive technology available may seem like a formidable challenge and matching a student's needs and circumstances with enabling solutions an even greater undertaking, there are few more important activities that educational professionals can undertake when working with students who are visually impaired. When teachers help their students learn how to use an accessible PDA or how to do an Internet search on a computer, they are doing so much more than helping them become comfortable with a new "techie" device—they are opening up the world for them. By taking on the critical process of showing students how to select the most effective way of accessing information and the universe around them and performing the tasks they need to do, they are in effect enabling those students to be active and successful citizens today. What greater contribution can someone make to another's life than to ensure that he or she has the tools to be an effective participant in school, in work, and in life? By accurately assessing students' assistive technology needs and thoughtfully implementing useful solutions, professionals are helping to lay the groundwork for their educational program and future as a whole. Congratulations for taking on this critically important assignment!

REFERENCES

McDonald, J. (2005). What school tech leaders say about professional development. Retrieved January 19, 2008, from www.eschoolnews.com

National Education Association (2008). Access, adequacy, and equity in education technology: Results of a survey of America's teachers and support professionals on technology in public schools and classrooms. Retrieved August 1, 2008, from www.nea.org/research/images/08gainsandgapsedtech.pdf

Thurlow, M., Quenemoen, R., Thompson, S., & Lehr, C. (2001). Principles and characteristics of inclusive assessment systems. *National Center on Educational Outcomes.* Retrieved January 3, 2007, from www.education.umn.edu/nceo/OnlinePubs/Synthesis40.html

It's the Law: Q&A about Assistive Technology and Special Education

This appendix provides answers to common questions about assistive technology and special education. Wherever possible the answers are taken from the controlling authority—the Individuals with Disabilities Education Act (IDEA) enacted into law by Congress and the regulations issued by the U. S. Department of Education that implement the statute and also have the force of law. At times reference is made to *Educating Blind and Visually Impaired Students*; *Policy Guidance* (henceforth, *Policy Guidance*), issued in June 2000, a statement of the Department of Education's interpretation of how IDEA applies to children and youths with visual impairments. Policy guidance documents interpret the regulations for implementing IDEA; they help state and local education agencies to meet the requirements of the law and therefore provide important information for families and educators, as well.

In general, the legal support for providing assistive technology devices and services to students in the schools is rooted in IDEA, the federal law that governs the provision of special education in the United States. The provision of assistive technology is also covered by other laws governing the civil rights of people with disabilities, such as the Americans with Disabilities Act and Section 504 of the Rehabilitation Act of 1973. Assistive technology devices and services are a required component of the free, appropriate public education (FAPE) guaranteed by IDEA. Specifically, assistive technology is included in the section of IDEA devoted to special factors that must be considered when developing the Individualized Education Program (IEP) for each student

Compiled by Mark Richert, Director; Barbara Jackson LeMoine, Policy Analyst; and Stacy Kelly, Policy Research Associate, American Foundation for the Blind Public Policy Center, Washington, D.C.; and Kay Alicyn Ferrell, Executive Director, National Center on Severe and Sensory Disabilities, University of Northern Colorado, Greeley.

(IDEA Sec. 614(d)(3)(B)(v)). Moreover, assistive technology is also included in the list of early intervention services that must be considered even for infants and toddlers with disabilities (IDEA Sec. 632(4)(E)(xiii)).

Q. What is assistive technology?

A. IDEA defines an assistive technology device as

> any item, piece of equipment, or product system, whether acquired commercially off the shelf, modified, or customized, that is used to increase, maintain, or improve functional capabilities of a child with a disability. (IDEA Sec. 602(1))

Neither the statute nor the regulations define assistive technology in more detail. The regulations state,

> The definition of assistive technology device does not list specific devices, nor would it be practical or possible to include an exhaustive list of assistive technology devices. Whether an augmentative communication device, playback devices, or other devices could be considered an assistive technology device for a child depends on whether the device is used to increase, maintain, or improve the functional capabilities of a child with a disability, and whether the child's individualized education program (IEP) team determines that the child needs the device in order to receive a free appropriate public education (FAPE).

This means that as new devices or other technologies are developed, they may be included as part of the IEP if they are determined by the IEP team to "increase, maintain, or improve" a child's abilities. The standard is whether the technology can or is likely to help the child access the curriculum.

Q. What are assistive technology services?

A. Assistive technology services are defined in the statute as

> any service that directly assists a child with a disability in the selection, acquisition, or use of an assistive technology device. (IDEA Sec. 602(2))

The term includes

- evaluation;
- acquiring a device for the child, either by purchase or lease;
- customizing the device to meet the child's needs;
- maintaining, repairing, or replacing the device;
- coordinating and using other therapies, interventions, or services with assistive technology devices, such as those associated with existing education and rehabilitation plans and programs;
- training or other assistance for the child, as well as the family, when appropriate;
- training for the educators, rehabilitation specialists, and employers working with the child.

Inclusion of assistive technology services within IDEA means that a child is entitled not just to the provision of various devices. It is insufficient to receive a device without training and follow up, as well. In discussing assistive technology services, the preamble to the regulations states that a service to support the use of Recordings for the Blind and Dyslexic [for example] on playback devices could be considered an assistive technology service if it assists a child with a disability in the selection, acquisition, or use of the device. If so, and if the child's IEP Team determines it is needed for the child to receive FAPE, the service would be provided. The definition of assistive technology service does not list specific services. (34 CFR Sec. 300.6)

Q. Would personal devices such as eyeglasses be considered assistive technology?

A. In the preamble to the regulations, the U.S. Department of Education explains:

> As a general matter, public agencies are not responsible for providing personal devices, such as eyeglasses or hearing aids that a child with a disability requires, regardless of whether the child is attending school. However, if it is not a surgically implanted device and a child's IEP Team determines that the child requires a personal device (e.g., eyeglasses) in order to receive FAPE, the public agency must ensure that the device is provided at no cost to the child's parents. (34 CFR Sec. 300.5)

As a general rule, eyeglasses are considered personal devices, because the child uses them out of school as well as during school hours. However, there may be cases where a student needs eyeglasses without which he or she would not be able to see the chalkboard, read the computer screen, or complete mathematics exercises. In such cases, the eyeglasses could be considered assistive technology and therefore provided at no cost

to the student's parents, whether or not the eyeglasses are also used outside the classroom. The IEP team is responsible for making this decision.

Q. Does IDEA cover assistive technology needed for use in settings other than the classroom?

A. Clarification of this issue is provided in the U.S. Department of Education's document, *Policy Guidance* (2000). This document informed local education agencies that decisions about assistive technology devices for students with vision loss should be made "on a case-by-case basis," and that

> consideration of the use of school-purchased assistive technology devices in a child's home or in other settings may be required. If the child's IEP team determines that the child needs to have access to a school-purchased device at home or in another setting in order to receive FAPE, a statement to this effect must be included in the child's IEP, the child's IEP must be implemented as written, and the device must be provided at no cost to the parents. (65 *Fed. Reg.* 36590)

The regulations (34 CFR Sec. 300.105(b)) further provide that such decisions are made by the child's IEP team on a case-by-case basis. The IEP team can determine that a child needs access to a school-purchased device outside of the classroom in order to receive a free, appropriate public education. If it is in the IEP, it must be provided at no cost to parents.

Q. What are the duties of an IEP team when considering assistive technology devices and services for children with vision loss?

A. IDEA requires that IEP teams consider all of the "academic, developmental, and functional needs of the child" (IDEA Sec. 614(d)(3)(A)(iv)), as well as specifically "consider whether the child needs assistive technology devices and services" (IDEA Sec. 614(d)(3)(B)(v)). The reference to assistive technology is included in a part of the statute called "special factors," the same section of the law that mandates consideration of instruction in braille. This means that every IEP team must at least discuss and determine whether or not assistive technology devices and services would help the child achieve a free, appropriate public education.

The Department of Education's *Policy Guidance* (2000) discusses the importance of assistive technology for students with vision loss and places it in the context of the IEP team's responsibility to address the student's ability to access information:

Issues related to accessing information frequently arise in the education of blind and visually impaired students. . . . Therefore, it is especially important that IEP teams for blind and visually impaired students give appropriate consideration to these students' needs for assistive technology and the full range of assistive technology devices and services that are available for them, and this consideration needs to occur as early as possible. . . . [A] blind or visually impaired student's ability to become proficient in the use of appropriate assistive technology could have a positive effect on the development of the student's overall self-confidence and self-esteem. Students taught the skills

necessary to address their disability-specific needs are more capable of participating meaningfully in the general curriculum offered to nondisabled students. (65 *Fed. Reg.* 36590)

The duties of the IEP team include providing access to information that results in a free, appropriate public education. If assistive technology devices and services contribute to that goal, then the IEP team should address them in the IEP.

Q. Are practitioners with special expertise about assistive technology devices and services part of a child's IEP team?

A. Given the legal requirements for the IEP team to consider assistive technology devices and services, a child with vision loss should receive an assistive technology evaluation as part of the development of the IEP. In many cases, the teacher of students with visual impairments will conduct this evaluation and will already be included on the IEP team. Other individuals can also be included on the IEP team, particularly if they have "knowledge or special expertise" about the child that can inform the discussion and development of the IEP (IDEA Sec. 614(d)(1)(B)(vi)).

Q. How do public agencies use assistive technology devices and services to ensure a free, appropriate public education?

A. The preamble to the regulations explains that each public agency is required to ensure that assistive technology devices (or assistive technology services, or both) are made available to a child with a disability if required as part of the child's special education, related services, or supplementary aids and services. This provision ties the definition to a child's educational needs, which public agencies must meet in order to ensure that a child with a disability receives a free appropriate public education. (34 CFR Sec. 300.105(a))

State and local education agencies ensure a free, appropriate public education by evaluating a child's need for assistive technology on a case-by-case basis, including those devices and services in the child's IEP, and providing them at no cost to parents. A free, appropriate public education is dependent on an individual child's ability to access information in the school environment.

Q. What collaborative responsibilities does the state education agency have in providing assistive technology devices and services to students with vision loss?

A. The state education agency is expected to work collaboratively with the state agency responsible for assistive technology programs (34 CFR Sec. 300.172(d)). The latter agency differs from state to state and is broadly interpreted as the agency funded by the Assistive Technology Act of 1998 to provide assistive technology services to individuals with disabilities. Provision of assistive technology is therefore not entirely the responsibility of the school district, and these other state resources should work together with the school district to make sure assistive technology is provided as needed.

Q. What is the responsibility of the school district or local education agency for assistive technology devices and services provided by public agencies other than educational agencies?

A. The school district or local education agency (LEA) is ultimately responsible for providing assistive technology devices and services. But other federal or state laws may require a device or service to be purchased by noneducation agencies. Such agencies cannot abrogate their responsibility even though the child is in school, and IDEA states that the financial responsibility of public noneducation agencies, including Medicaid and other public insurers obligated under federal or state law or assigned responsibility under state policy, always takes precedence over the financial responsibility of the LEA (IDEA Sec. 612(a)(12)(A)(i)). On the other hand, the LEA cannot simply wait for another agency to provide a service, particularly if there is a delay that jeopardizes the receipt of services listed in the child's IEP, thus preventing the provision of a free, appropriate public education. Although IDEA mandates that the chief executive officer of the state—such as the state superintendent of instruction or the commissioner of education—take responsibility for creating agreements among agencies to cover the costs of providing a free, appropriate public education, it also states that the LEA must provide the service in the interim (IDEA Sec. 612(a)(12)).

Q. When should assistive technology be considered for students with disabilities?

A. Assistive technology should be considered as early as possible, according to *Policy Guidance* (2000). Infancy is not too soon to consider assistive technology for students with vision loss. Assistive technology is included in the list of early intervention services that must be considered even for infants and toddlers with disabilities (IDEA Sec. 632(4)(E)(xiii)). For example, a variety of low- and high-tech tools can be used to facilitate early literacy experiences for infants and toddlers with vision loss.

Q. What funding sources can the state use to finance assistive technology devices and services?

A. States have considerable flexibility in funding. They are permitted to use funds "To support the use of technology, including technology with universal design principles and assistive technology devices, to maximize accessibility to the general education curriculum for children with disabilities" (34 CFR Sec. 300.704(b)(4)(iv)). The Department of Education's *Policy Guidance* also states, "In meeting the assistive technology needs of blind and visually impaired students, public agencies may use whatever State, local, Federal, and private sources of support are available in the State to finance required services" (34 CFR Sec. 300.103).

Q. What is the relationship between assistive technology and braille literacy?

A. Assistive technology devices and services are viewed as essential components of literacy for all students experiencing vision loss. As the U.S. Department of Education's *Policy Guidance* states:

> IEP teams must ensure that appropriate assistive technology is provided to facilitate necessary braille instruction. Likewise, for children with low

vision, instruction in the appropriate utilization of functional vision and in the effective use of low vision aids requires regular and intensive intervention from knowledgeable and appropriately trained personnel. (65 *Fed. Reg.* 36589)

The *Policy Guidance* document also acknowledges that braille readers may need assistive technology devices for writing and composition (65 *Fed. Reg.* 36589) and goes on to emphasize that decisions about assistive technology are individual determinations made by the IEP team according to the needs of the child. It should be remembered that the law requires the provision of instruction in braille and the use of braille unless the IEP team determines otherwise. In essence, this means that the law overwhelmingly presumes that braille is essential for literacy of students who are blind. However, the law does not contain a similar categorical requirement that assistive technology must be provided in the case of a child who is blind unless the IEP team goes out of its way to exclude it. Nevertheless, the strong presumption in favor of braille may be leveraged— that is, it can be used to obtain access to assistive technology devices and services that support instruction in and use of braille when developing and reviewing the IEP of a student who is blind student.

Q. How do IEP teams decide which assistive technologies will benefit blind and visually impaired children?

A. IEP teams consider multiple sources of information when composing an individual student's IEP, including

- the child's strengths;
- the parents' concerns;
- the most recent evaluation results;

- the academic, developmental, and functional needs of the child;
- consideration of special factors, such as braille and assistive technology. (IDEA Sec. 614(d)(3))

The team makes decisions about an individual child's IEP based on how the child will access the general education curriculum and ultimately how a free, appropriate public education will be achieved. Typically, they conduct an assistive technology assessment to evaluate how a student with vision loss accesses printed and electronic information as well as how he or she communicates through writing. Information is gathered about tasks the student has difficulty completing. Additional consideration is usually given to the effectiveness of assistive technology or other methods of modification the student may already be using to access information.

Q. What constitutes an assistive technology assessment for a student with vision loss?

A. The U.S. Department of Education's *Policy Guidance* refers to assessments that are unique to students with vision loss and connects them to assistive technology needs:

> An assessment of a child's vision status generally would include the nature and extent of the child's visual impairment and its effect, for example, on the child's ability to learn to read, write, do mathematical calculations, and *use computers and other assistive technology*, as well as the child's ability to be involved in and progress in the general curriculum. For children with low vision, this type

of assessment also generally should include an evaluation of the child's *ability to utilize low vision aids*, as well as a learning media assessment and a functional vision assessment. (65 *Fed. Reg.* 36587; emphasis added)

Q. What is the National Instructional Materials Accessibility Standard?

A. The National Instructional Materials Accessibility Standard (NIMAS) applies to print instructional materials published after August 18, 2006, and is defined as "the standard established by the Secretary to be used in the preparation of electronic files suitable and used solely for efficient conversion into specialized formats" (IDEA Sec. 674(e)(3)(B)). NIMAS creates a standardized electronic file format that publishers will use to allow their print materials to be converted to a variety of specialized formats that are accessible to students with print disabilities. Appendix C to Part 300 of the IDEA regulations explains, "The purpose of the NIMAS is to help increase the availability and timely delivery of print instructional materials in accessible formats to blind or other persons with print disabilities in elementary and secondary schools."

Q. What are a state's responsibilities under the National Instructional Materials Accessibility Standard?

A. A state is required to

- submit a plan that assures the Department of Education that the state has policies and procedures in place to adopt NIMAS (Sec. 612(a));
- provide materials to students with vision loss and other print disabilities in a timely manner, whether or not it coordinates with the National

Instructional Materials Access Center (NIMAC; Sec. 612(a)(23));

- contract with publishers to prepare and submit the NIMAS file (Sec. 612(a)(23)(C)(i));
- purchase materials from the publisher (Sec. 612(a)(23)(C)(ii));
- work collaboratively with the state agency responsible for assistive technology programs (Sec. 612 (a)(23)(D)).

Q. What is the National Instructional Materials Access Center and what are its duties?

A. The National Instructional Materials Access Center (NIMAC) was created by Sec. 674(e)(1) of IDEA 2004 at the American Printing House for the Blind. NIMAC's responsibilities are to

- receive and maintain a catalog of materials created in NIMAS format;
- provide accessible print instructional materials at no cost to students with disabilities in elementary and secondary schools;
- to develop, adopt and publish procedures to protect against copyright infringement. (IDEA Sec. 674(e)(2)(A)–(C))

Reference

Office of Special Education and Rehabilitative Services, U.S. Department of Education. (2000, June 8). *Educating Blind and Visually Impaired Students*; *Policy Guidance*; *Notice*. *Federal Register*, 65 (111) 36585-36594. www.ed.gov/legislation/FedRegister/other/2000-2/060800a.html.

B

Resources

The listings in this appendix represent a sampling of the extensive resources available on assistive technology. However, since assistive technology and related products are updated regularly, and web sites are subject to frequent change, this resources section constitutes simply a snapshot of what was available at the time it was compiled.

In addition to the listings included here, there are State Assistive Technology Act programs that work to improve the provision of assistive technology to individuals with disabilities of all ages through comprehensive statewide programs of technology-related assistance. These 56 state and territory programs are funded under the Assistive Technology Act of 1998. The programs support activities designed to maximize the ability of individuals with disabilities and their family members, guardians, and advocates to access and obtain assistive technology devices and services. A list of state programs and contact information can be found on the RESNA website at www.resna.org/projects.

NATIONAL ORGANIZATIONS

The national organizations listed here are, generally speaking, sources of information on assistive technology. Some also offer products, publications, services, consultation, or conferences. A separate list of organizations that provide information mainly through their web sites follows.

AbilityHub
c/o The Gilman Group, L.L.C.
P.O. Box 6356
Rutland, VT 05702-6356
(802) 775-1993 (phone)
(802) 773-1604 (fax)
info@abilityhub.com (e-mail)
http://abilityhub.com

Provides information on available adaptive equipment and alternative methods for accessing computers.

ABLEDATA

8630 Fenton Street, Suite 930
Silver Spring, MD 20910
(800) 227-0216 (phone)
(301) 608-8958 (fax)
(301) 608-8912 (TTY)
abledata@macrointernational.com (e-mail)
www.abledata.com

Provides information on assistive technology and rehabilitation equipment available from domestic and international sources to consumers, organizations, professionals, and caregivers within the United States.

AFB TECH

949 3rd Avenue, Suite 200
Huntington, WV 25701
(304) 523-8651 (phone)
AFBTECH@afb.net (e-mail)
www.afb.org

An office for the American Foundation for the Blind that develops information, through analysis, evaluation, and laboratory product testing, on a broad range of everyday and emerging devices. Evaluations are published in *AccessWorld: Technology and People with Visual Impairments*, as well as important related journals. Works with software developers, web site designers, and hardware manufacturers to help them better understand and address the needs of those who are blind or visually impaired. Both assistive technology products used by individuals who are blind or visually impaired and mainstream technology products are evaluated by AFB TECH staff. AFB TECH also operates CareerConnect, a web site and database of currently employed blind or visually impaired individuals who offer mentorship and support to blind or visually impaired people entering the workplace or pursuing an educational goal.

Information for parents, teachers, counselors, and employers is also provided, so they can better assist visually impaired people as they form and actualize their career plans.

Alliance for Technology Access (ATA)

1304 Southpoint Boulevard, Suite 240
Petaluma, CA 94954
(707) 778-3011 (phone)
(707) 765-2080 (fax)
(707) 778-3015 (TTY)
ATAinfo@ATAccess.org (e-mail)
www.ataccess.org

National network of community-based resource centers, product developers, vendors, service providers, and individuals that provides information and support services to children and adults with disabilities, and works to increase their use of technology.

American Foundation for the Blind

11 Penn Plaza, Suite 300
New York, NY 10001
(800) 232-5463 or (212) 502-7600 (phone)
afbinfo@afb.net (e-mail)
www.afb.org

Information clearinghouse that offers information about assistive technology on its web site as well as a searchable product database. AFB TECH, AFB's technology center in West Virginia, evaluates assistive technology and mainstream technology products used by individuals who are blind or visually impaired (see separate listing). Publishes a free online magazine, *Access World: Technology and People with Visual Impairments*. AFB's National Literacy Center develops teacher training curricula, provides up-to-date resources and workshops for professionals, and provides resources on braille, assistive technology, and low vision. The National Literacy

Center also publishes *Dots for Braille Literacy*, a free newsletter about new braille products, strategies for teaching, and resources for teachers, parents, family members, and anyone interested in braille literacy. AFB Press publishes a variety of materials including *AFB Directory of Services for Blind and Visually Impaired Persons in the United States and Canada*, available in print and in a searchable online version with sections on sources of assistive technology products and materials in alternate formats; "Technology Q&A," a regular column in AFB's *Journal of Visual Impairment & Blindness* designed to give readers practical information on assistive technology and how it is being used in education, on the job, and at home; and *AccessWorld Guide to Assistive Technology Products*, published by AFB Press and available in print and online, which provides descriptions of over 280 products for people who are blind or visually impaired and a resource list of product manufacturers and distributors. AFB Consulting is dedicated to working with manufacturers of mainstream technology and products to make them accessible to people who are blind or visually impaired.

American Printing House for the Blind

P.O. Box 6085
1839 Frankfort Avenue
Louisville, KY 40206-0085
(800) 223-1839 or (502) 895-2405 (phone)
(502) 899-2274 (fax)
info@aph.org (e-mail)
www.aph.org

Manufactures textbooks and other educational publications for students who are visually impaired and publications useful to adults, such as cookbooks and dictionaries in alternate formats. Also develops and manufactures hundreds of products, tools, and supplies that support students and adults who are visually impaired and increase their independence. Maintains the Louis database, which allows teachers, parents, and students to locate thousands of textbooks in braille, large print, recorded, and computer disc formats available from producers across the United States. Conducts ongoing research and product development activities in such areas as tactile graphics, braille reading readiness, and low vision. Hosts the National Instructional Materials Access Center (NIMAC), the central repository that contains source files from publishers that can be used to produce books in accessible formats for students with print disabilities.

Assistive Technology Industry Association (ATIA)

401 North Michigan Avenue
Chicago, IL 60611-4267
(877) 687-2842 or (312) 321-5172 (phone)
(312) 673-6659 (fax)
info@ATIA.org (e-mail)
www.atia.org

Membership organization of manufacturers, sellers, and providers of technology-based assistive devices and services. Holds a yearly conference on assistive technology.

California Transcribers and Educators of the Visually Handicapped

741 North Vermont Avenue
Los Angeles, CA 90029-3594
(323) 666-2211 (messages only)
www.ctevh.org

Membership organization of educators, transcribers, rehabilitation specialists, librarians, paraprofessionals, parents, and others who are interested in the needs of people who are blind and visually impaired. Holds annual conference and special workshops, and publishes a quarterly journal. Content experts, including experts in computer-assisted graphics and braille production, are available to respond to questions and offer assistance.

Carl and Ruth Shapiro Family National Center for Accessible Media (NCAM)
One Guest Street
Boston, MA 02135
(617) 300-3400 (phone)
(617) 300-1035 (fax)
(617) 300-2489 (TTY)
ncam@wgbh.org (e-mail)

Research and development facility dedicated to the issues of media and information technology for people with disabilities in their homes, schools, workplaces, and communities.

CAST (Center for Applied Special Technology)
40 Harvard Mills Square, Suite 3
Wakefield, MA 01880-3233
(781) 245-2212 (phone)
(781) 245-5212 (fax)
(781) 245-9320 (TTY)
cast@cast.org (e-mail)
www.cast.org
http://nimas.cast.org

Develops technology-based educational resources and strategies based on the principles of universal design for learning. CAST leads the NIMAS Development Center and the NIMAS Technical Assistance Center to further develop and support the implementation of the National Instructional Materials Accessibility Standard (NIMAS) to guide the development and distribution of digital instructional materials for students who are print disabled.

Center for Assistive Technology and Environmental Access (CATEA)
Georgia Institute of Technology
490 Tenth Street
Atlanta, GA 30332-0156
(404) 894-1414 (phone)
(800) 726-9119 (voice or TTY)
(404) 894-9320 (fax)
catea@coa.gatech.edu (e-mail)
www.catea.gatech.edu

Provides access to information on assistive technology devices and services, as well as other community resources for people with disabilities and the general public.

Center on Disabilities, California State University, Northridge (CSUN)
18111 Nordhoff Street, Bayramian Hall 110
Northridge, CA 91330-8340
(818) 677-2684 (phone)
(818) 677-4929 (fax)
conference@csun.edu (e-mail)
codss@csun.edu (e-mail)
www.csun.edu/cod

Holds CSUN, the annual International Conference on Assistive Technology and Persons with Disabilities, which provides an inclusive setting for researchers, practitioners, exhibitors, end users, speakers, and other participants to share knowledge and best practices in the field of assistive technology.

Closing the Gap
526 Main Street
P.O. Box 68
Henderson, MN 56044
(507) 248-3294 (phone)

(507) 248-3810 (fax)
www.closingthegap.com

Publishes a bimonthly newspaper that highlights hardware and software products appropriate for people with special needs. Holds an annual international conference.

Council for Exceptional Children (CEC)
1110 North Glebe Road, Suite 300
Arlington, VA 22201-5704
(800)224-6830 or (703) 620-3660 (phone)
(703) 264-9494 (fax)
(866) 915-5000 (TDD/TTY)
service@cec.sped.org (e-mail)
www.cec.sped.org
www.cecdvi.org (Division on Visual
   Impairments)
www.tamcec.org (Technology and Media
   Division)

Works to improve the educational success of individuals with disabilities and gifts and talents. CEC advocates for appropriate governmental policies, sets professional standards, provides professional development, advocates for individuals with exceptionalities, and helps professionals obtain conditions and resources necessary for effective professional practice. Holds an annual conference and publishes journals, newsletters, and books. Its 17 divisions include a Division on Visual Impairment, which publishes *D.V.I. Quarterly*, and the Technology and Media Division, which publishes the *Journal of Special Education Technology*.

Learning Independence through Computers (LINC)
1001 Eastern Avenue, 3rd Floor
Baltimore, Maryland 21202
(410) 659-5462 (phone)
(410) 659-5472 (fax)
www.linc.org/index.html

Computer resource center that provides opportunities for people with disabilities, their families, professionals, and members of the business community to explore adaptive technology, computer systems, software, and the Internet.

National Braille Association (NBA)
95 Allens Creek Road
Building 1, Suite 202
Rochester, NY 14618
(585) 427-8260 (phone)
(585) 427-0263 (fax)
nbaoffice@nationalbraille.org (e-mail)
www.nationalbraille.org

Membership organization for transcribers. Offers twice-yearly professional development conferences at various locations throughout the nation and offers assistance and resources regarding technical braille issues.

National Center for Technology Innovation (NCTI)
1000 Thomas Jefferson Street, NW
Washington, DC 20007-3835
(202) 403-5323 (phone)
(202) 403-5001 (fax)
(202) 333-3072 (TTY)
ncti@air.org (e-mail)
www.nationaltechcenter.org

Assists researchers, developers, and entrepreneurs in creating innovative learning tools for all students, with a special focus on students with disabilities. Funded by the Office of Special Education Programs (OSEP) at the U.S. Department of Education.

National Instructional Materials Access Center (NIMAC)
1839 Frankfort Avenue
Louisville, KY 40206-0085
(877) 526-4622 or (502) 899-2230 (phone)
nimac@aph.org (e-mail)
www.nimac.us

The federally funded national electronic file repository created under IDEA 2004 and established at the American Printing House for the Blind that makes National Instructional Materials Accessibility Standard (NIMAS) files available for the production of core print instructional materials in specialized formats for qualifying blind, visually impaired, or print-disabled students in elementary or secondary school.

National Library Service for the Blind and Physically Handicapped (NLS)
Library of Congress
1291 Taylor Street, NW
Washington, DC 20542
(800) 424-8567 or (202) 707-5100 (phone)
(202) 707-0712 (fax)
(202) 707-0744 (TDD/TTY)
nls@loc.gov (e-mail)
www.loc.gov/nls

National program to distribute free reading materials in braille, on recorded discs and cassettes, as Digital Talking Books, and in Web-Braille to blind and visually impaired persons who cannot use printed materials. Operates a reference section providing information on reading materials for disabled persons, offers braille transcription and proofreading courses, and maintains a music collection and music services for blind persons.

Recording for the Blind & Dyslexic
20 Roszel Road
Princeton, NJ 08540
(866) 732-3585 or (609) 452-0606 (phone)
custserv@rfbd.org (e-mail)
www.rfbd.org

Nonprofit volunteer organization serving people who cannot effectively read standard print because of visual impairment, dyslexia, or other physical disability. Lends audio or digital recorded textbooks and other educational materials at no charge. Recording is done in a network of studios across the country.

RESNA (Rehabilitation Engineering and Assistive Technology Society of North America)
1700 North Moore Street, Suite 1540
Arlington, VA 22209-1903
(703) 524-6686 (phone)
(703) 524-6630 (fax)
(703) 524-6639 (TTY)
www.resna.org

Membership organization of rehabilitation professionals, consumers, and students who are dedicated to promoting the exchange of ideas and information for the advancement of assistive technology. Holds an annual conference that brings together researchers, practitioners, policy specialists, manufacturers, educators, and consumers interested in the field.

WEB SITES

AccessIT: The National Center on Accessible Information Technology in Education
Box 357920
University of Washington
Seattle, WA 98195-7920
(206) 685-4181 (phone)
(206) 543-4779 (fax)
(866) 866-0162 (TTY)
accessit@u.washington.edu (e-mail)
www.washington.edu/accessit

A web site designed for educators, policymakers, librarians, technical support staff, and students and employees with disabilities and their advocates that promotes the use of electronic and information technology for students and employees with disabilities in educational institutions at all academic levels. Features a searchable database of questions and answers.

All Hotkeys
http://allhotkeys.com

Web site that collects and lists software keyboard shortcuts (hotkeys).

Apple, Inc.
One Infinite Loop
Cupertino, CA 95014
(408) 996-1010 (phone)
www.apple.com/accessibility/macosx/vision.
  html
www.apple.com/accessibility/resources/
  macosx.html

The accessibility section of the Apple web site offers information about the accessibility features of Macintosh computers. Within that section, a resources section offers a variety of accessibility solutions developed by third parties for the Macintosh operating system.

ASSIST with Windows (Accessible Step-by-Step Instructions for Speech Technology with Windows)
Iowa Department for the Blind
524 Fourth Street
Des Moines, IA 50309-2364
(515) 281-1357 (phone)
ASSIST@blind.state.ia.us (e-mail)

This project developed computer training materials written specifically for individuals who are blind, visually impaired, or deaf-blind. Although no longer developing new materials, the existing products are for sale,

including tutorials, keyboard guides and diagrams, and course packets. Some are available for free download. The training materials address all levels of users, from beginners to advanced users.

Assistive Technology Training Online Project (ATTO)
Center for Assistive Technology
School of Public Health and Health Professions
University of Buffalo
State University of New York
515 Kimball Tower
Buffalo, NY 14214
(716) 829-3141 (phone)
(716) 829-3217 (fax)
http://atto.buffalo.edu

Provides information on assistive technology applications that help students with disabilities learn in elementary classrooms.

Curtin University Centre for Accessible Technology
Building 204:216
Department of Electrical and Computer Engineering
Curtin University of Technology
Kent St Bentley
P.O. Box U1987
Perth 6845 WA
Australia
+61 8 9266 4540 (phone)
+61 8 9266 2584 (fax)
i.murray@curtin.edu.au (e-mail)
www.cucat.org

A multidisciplinary research group that develops both hardware and software solutions and methods of their application for people with print or vision disabilities, focusing on assistive technology and rehabilitation engineering solutions, with particular emphasis on e-Learning and educational requirements, techniques and curriculum development. The books section includes documentation on VoiceOver, the Macintosh screen readers, in accessible formats.

Family Center on Technology and Disability

Academy for Educational Development
1825 Connecticut Avenue, N.W.
Washington, DC 20009
202-884-8068 (Phone)
202-884-8441 (Fax)
fctd@aed.org (e-mail)
www.fctd.info

Supports organizations and programs that work with families of children and youth with disabilities. Offers a range of information and services on the subject of assistive technologies, including a searchable database of assistive technology resources.

Greg Kearney's Internet Services

Wyoming Medical Center
http://w3.wmcnet.org

This Internet page offers several applications and scripts especially for Macintosh computers, including braille software and VoiceOver-enabled software for the Apple Macintosh.

Microsoft Corporation

One Microsoft Way
Redmond, WA 98052-6399
(800) 642-7676; (800) 892-5234 (phone)
www.microsoft.com/enable/default.aspx
www.microsoft.com/enable/guides/vision.aspx

The accessibility section of Microsoft's web site devoted to accessibility of Microsoft programs (including the Windows operating system, Internet Explorer, Word, Microsoft Office, and Outlook). Includes tutorials and information about products compatible with Windows.

National Public Website on Assistive Technology

Center for Assistive Technology and Environmental Access
Georgia Institute of Technology
490 Tenth Street
Atlanta, GA 30332-0156
(800) 726-9119 or (404) 894-1414 (phone)
catea@coa.gatech.edu (e-mail)
http://assistivetech.net

Provides access to information on assistive technology devices and services, as well as other community resources for people with disabilities and the general public. The site is created and maintained through the collaboration of the Georgia Tech Center for Assistive Technology and Environmental Access (CATEA), National Institute on Disability and Rehabilitation Research (NIDRR), and the Rehabilitation Services Administration (RSA) of the U.S. Department of Education.

QIAT (Quality Indicators for Assistive Technology Services)

www.qiat.org

Nationwide grassroots group whose mission is to guide the development and delivery of quality assistive technology services by identifying, disseminating, and implementing a set of widely applicable quality indicators for assistive technology services in school settings.

Resources for Assistive Technology in Education

Joy Smiley Zabala
P.O. Box 3130
Lake Jackson, TX 77566

joy@joyzabala.com (e-mail)
http://sweb.uky.edu/~jszaba0/JoyZabala.html

Information about the SETT Framework, an organizational tool to help collaborative teams create Student-centered, Environmentally useful, and Tasks-focused Tool systems that foster the educational success of students with disabilities.

**Special Education Technology—
British Columbia (SET-BC)**
105-1750 West 75th Avenue
Vancouver, BC V6P 6G2
Canada
(604) 261-9450 (phone)
(604) 261-2256 (fax)
www.setbc.org

A program of the British Columbia Ministry of Education that assists school districts in educating students with physical disabilities, visual impairment, and autism through provision of assistive technology and training for students and educators. The Learning Centre section of the web site features a wide variety of resources for teachers on different kinds of assistive technology, including lesson plans, videos, and other information about teaching strategies and specific products.

**Texas School for the Blind and
Visually Impaired (TSBVI)**
1100 West 45th Street
Austin, TX 78756
(800) 872-5273 or (512) 454-8631 (phone)
(512) 206-9450 (fax)
(512) 206-9451 (TDD)
www.tsbvi.edu
www.tsbvi.edu/technology

The technology section of the TSBVI web site provides a wide variety of information on assistive technology, training, products, and technology assessment, including forms and checklists to evaluate students on specific products. The math section also contains information on adaptive tools and technology for mathematics and tactile graphics for mathematics.

**Web Accessibility Initiative (WAI) of
the World Wide Web Consortium (WC3)**
(617) 258-9741 (phone)
jbrewer@w3.org and w3t-pr@w3.org (e-mail)
www.w3.org/WAI

Works with organizations around the world to develop strategies, guidelines, and resources to help make the Web accessible to people with disabilities.

**Wisconsin Assistive Technology
Initiative (WATI)**
448 East High Street
Milton, WI 53563
(800) 991-5576 or (608) 758-6232, ext. 340 (phone)
(608) 868-6740 (fax)
info@wati.org (e-mail)
www.wati.org

Assists school districts and early intervention programs in providing assistive technology and with implementation of needed assistive technology devices and services. The web site offers a variety of information on assistive technology, including assessment guides, forms, and checklists. Sells manuals and other training materials on such topics as assessment, strategies for implementing assistive technology, assistive technology planning, autism, and transition.

TRAINING

**Assistive Technology Training Online
Project (ATTO)**
Center for Assistive Technology
School of Public Health and Health
Professions

University of Buffalo
State University of New York
515 Kimball Tower
Buffalo, NY 14214
(716) 829-3141 (phone)
(716) 829-3217 (fax)
http://atto.buffalo.edu

Provides step-by-step tutorials on how to use specific assistive technology products.

Carroll Center for the Blind

770 Centre Street
Newton, MA 02458
(800) 852-3131 or (617) 969-6200 (phone)
info@carroll.org (e-mail)
www.carroll.org
www.carrolltech.org

Offers online self-paced training through its distance learning web site, including instruction in the use of screen readers, screen magnification programs, scanners, braille translators and many of the applications that are part of the Microsoft Office suite and courses geared specifically for teachers of the visually impaired, rehabilitation teachers, and other professionals.

Hadley School for the Blind

700 Elm Street
Winnetka, IL 60093-2554 USA
(800) 323-4238 or (847) 446-8111 (phone)
(847) 446-0855 (fax)
info@hadley.edu (e-mail)
www.hadley-school.org

Offers classes free of charge to its blind and visually impaired students and their families and affordable tuition classes to blindness professionals in the mail or online. Includes courses on assistive technology and the Internet for students and professionals.

SOURCES OF ASSISTIVE TECHNOLOGY AND OTHER PRODUCTS

The companies listed in this section are manufacturers and developers of a wide variety of assistive technology products whose use is described in this book, as well as some distributors of products manufactured outside the United States. (Check manufacturers' web sites to locate additional local distributors.) Because technology changes so rapidly and it is impossible to enumerate all the products available, this list is just a sampling of what is available at the time of publication. An index to manufacturers by categories of products appears in the section that follows. For additional information and resources, visit the American Foundation for the Blind web site at www.afb.org/at.

ABISee, Inc.

52 Tanbark Road
Sudbury, MA 01776
(800) 681-5909 or (978) 201-9302 (phone)
(253) 595-3623 (fax)
info@abisee.com (e-mail)
www.abisee.com

Manufactures video magnifiers (Zoom Ex, Zoom Frog, Zoom Twix) and the Eye-Pal scanning machine.

Access Ingenuity

3635 Montgomery Drive
Santa Rosa, CA 95405
(877) 579-4380 or (707) 579-4380 (phone)
(707) 579-4273 (fax)
access@accessingenuity.com (e-mail)
www.accessingenuity.com

Offers a variety of assistive technologies from various manufacturers and an adjustable monitor arm stand for LCD monitors.

Ai Squared
130 Taconic Business Park Road
Manchester Center, VT 05255
(800) 859-0270 or (802) 362-3612 (phone)
(802) 362-1670 (fax)
sales@aisquared.com (e-mail)
www.aisquared.com

Manufactures screen magnification systems (ZoomText Magnifier, ZoomText Magnifier/Reader) and the ZoomText Large Print Keyboard. Also distributes a variety of video magnifiers.

American Printing House for the Blind (APH)
P.O. Box 6085
1839 Frankfort Avenue
Louisville, KY 40206-0085
(800) 223-1839 or (502) 895-2405 (phone)
(502) 899-2274 (fax)
info@aph.org (e-mail)
www.aph.org

Manufactures Digital Talking Book players (Book Wizard Producer, Book Wizard Reader); accessible personal digital assistants (Braille+ Mobile Manager); low vision devices (Primer Electronic Magnifier, RollBuster); a speech product (Money Talks); slates and styli; Math Flash drill and practice software; a variety of reading and writing supplies; tactile graphics materials; and tactile maps.

American Thermoform Corporation
1758 Bracket Street
La Verne, CA 91750
(800) 331-3676 or (909) 593-6711 (phone)
(909) 593-8001 (fax)
sales@americanthermoform.com (e-mail)
www.americanthermoform.com

Manufactures Thermoform duplicators and supplies; braille embossers and production equipment and a variety of braille and tactile graphics materials. Distributes a variety of products, including products from Index Braille in Sweden.

Ann Arbor Publishers Limited
P.O. Box 1
Belford
Northumberland
NE71 7JX
England
+44 01668 214460 (phone)
+44 01668 214484 (fax)
www.annarbor.co.uk

Supplies educational assessment materials for children with learning difficulties, as well as resources for professionals dealing with these problems, including tracking materials.

Another Eye
1046 Wood Duck Court
Maineville, OH 45039
(888) 274-1862 or (866) 778-7523 (phone)
info@anothereye.com (e-mail)
www.anothereye.com

Manufactures video magnifiers (AE1, AE3, AE3M, AE50, AE6).

Apple, Inc.
One Infinite Loop
Cupertino, CA 95014
(408) 996-1010 (phone)
www.apple.com/accessibility/voiceover

Manufactures the VoiceOver screen reader.

Ash Technologies
B5, M7 Business Park

Naas, Co. Kildaire
Ireland
+353 45 882212
info@ashtech.ie (e-mail)
www.ashtech.ie
U.S. distributor: Freedom Vision

Manufactures video magnifiers (Andromeda, Eclipse, Fusion, Liberty Scholar, Liberty Solo, OPTi Lite, OPTi Mouse, OPTi Verso, Quicklook Zoom, The Prisma, TVi Color).

Audio Visual Mart
603 Williams Boulevard.
Kenner, LA 70062
(504) 712-0400 (phone)
(504) 712-0032 (fax)
info@av-mart.com (e-mail)
www.av-mart.com

Distributes a variety of products, including products from F. H. Papenmeier in Germany and Index Braille in Sweden.

Baum Retec AG
Schloss Langenzell
D-69257 Wiesenbach
Germany
+49 6223 4909-0 (phone)
+49 6223 4909-7321 (fax)
info@baum.de (e-mail)
www.baum.de
U.S. distributor: HumanWare USA

Manufactures braille displays (VarioPro 64, VarioPro 80) and the ScannaR optical character recognition system.

Beyond Sight, Inc.
5650 South Windermere Street
Littleton, CO 80120
(303) 795-6455 (phone)
(303) 795-6425 (fax)

bsistore@beyondsight.com (e-mail)
www.beyondsight.com

Manufactures LapTalk (speech product). Also distributes a variety of products.

Bierley Associates
19500 Graystone Lane
San Jose, CA 95120
(800) 985-0535 or (408) 365-8012 (phone)
(408) 351-8300 (fax)
info@bierley.com (e-mail)
www.bierley.com

Manufactures video magnifiers (Big Reader, ColorMouse, ColorMouse-USB, MonoMouse, MonoMouse-USB).

BlinkSoft
2707 Meadow Place North
Renton, WA 98056
(425) 430-8800 (phone)
(425) 204-6072 (fax)
www.blinksoft.biz

Distributes a variety of products, including products from Index Braille in Sweden.

Brailler Depot
107 Trimble Avenue
Clifton, NJ 07011
(973) 272-7667 (phone)
info@braillerdepot.com (e-mail)
www.braillerdepot.com

Distributes a variety of products, including products from Index Braille in Sweden.

Brytech
600 Peter Morand Crescent, Suite 240
Ottawa, ON K1G 5Z3
Canada
(613) 731-5800 (phone)
(613) 731-5812 (fax)
inquiries@brytech.com (e-mail)
www.brytech.com

Manufactures speech products (Note Teller2, ColorTeller).

Canon U.S.A.
1 Canon Plaza
Lake Success, NY 11042
(703) 807-3158 (phone)
accessibility@cusa.canon.com (e-mail)
www.usa.canon.com/gmd/section508.html

Manufactures the Canon Voice Operation Kit.

Captek dba Science Products
1043 Lincoln Highway
Berwyn, PA 19312
(800) 888-7400 or (610) 296-2111 (phone)
lee@captek.net (e-mail)

Manufactures the Sharp A440 Talking Cash Register.

Christal Vision
6303 Southern Hills
San Antonio, TX 78244
(800) 299-0700 or (210) 666-0700 (phone)
(210) 662-7559 (fax)
ed@satx.rr.com (e-mail)
www.christal-vision.com

Distributes a variety of products, including products from Index Braille in Sweden and Low Vision International in Sweden.

Clarity
2222 Park Place, Suite 1-C
Minden, NV 89423
(800) 575-1456 or (775) 782-5611 (phone)
(775) 783-0966 (fax)
clarity@clarityUSA.com (e-mail)
www.clarityUSA.com

Manufactures video magnifiers (Clarity CarryMate, Clarity Deskmate, Clarity Flexmate, Clarity Junior, Clarity PCMate, Discovery II).

Dancing Dots
1754 Quarry Lane
Valley Forge, PA 19482
(610) 783-6692 (phone)
(610) 783-6732 (fax)
info@dancingdots.com (e-mail)
www.dancingdots.com

Manufactures braille translators (GOOD-FEEL Braille Music Translator, GOOD-FEEL Lite), the CakeTalking screen reader, and Sibelius Speaking (speech product) and other materials related to braille music.

David Mielke
http://mielke.cc/brltty/details.html

Developed the BRLTTY screen reader.

Design Science, Inc.
140 Pine Avenue, 4th Floor
Long Beach, CA 90802
(800) 827-0685 (phone)
info@dessci.com (e-mail)
www.dessci.com/en/company

Manufactures MathPlayer and MathType.

Dolphin Computer Access Inc.
231 Clarksville Road, Suite 3
Princeton Junction, NJ 08550
(866) 797-5921 or (609) 803-2171 (phone)
(609) 799-0475 (fax)
info@dolphinusa.com (e-mail)
www.yourdolphin.com

Manufactures the Cipher Braille Translator, EasyReader Digital Talking Book player, Cicero Text Reader, screen magnification systems (Lunar Screen Magnifier, LunarPlus Enhanced Screen Magnifier, Supernova Pro, Supernova Reader Magnifier Standard), and screen readers (Dolphin Pen, Hal Professional, Hal Standard).

Don Johnston, Inc.
26799 West Commerce Drive
Volo, IL 60073
(800) 999-4660 or (847) 740-0749 (phone)
(847) 740-7326 (fax)
info@donjohnston.com (e-mail)
www.donjohnston.com

Manufactures and distributes a variety of educational products for literacy and communication students with disabilities, including the Write:OutLoud talking word processor and writing software program.

Duxbury Systems, Inc.
270 Littleton Road, Unit 6
Westford, MA 01886-3523
(978) 692-3000 (phone)
(978) 692-7912 (fax)
info@duxsys.com (e-mail)
www.duxburysystems.com

Manufactures braille translators (Duxbury Braille Translator, MegaDots).

Easy Talk
2201 Limerick Drive
Tallahassee, FL 32309
(850) 906-9821 (phone)
sales@easytalkcomputers.com (e-mail)
www.easytalkcomputers.com

Distributes a variety of products, including products from Index Braille in Sweden and Human Information Management Service in Korea.

EnableMart
Sales Office
c/o MRN, Inc.
5353 South 960 East, Suite 200
Salt Lake City, UT. 84117
(888) 640-1999 or (360) 695-4155 (phone)
(888) 254-1712 (fax)
www.enablemart.com

Develops and distributes a variety of educational software and low vision devices.

Enabling Technologies Company
1601 Northeast Braille Place
Jensen Beach, FL 34957
(800) 777-3687 or (772) 225-3687 (phone)
(772) 225-3299 (fax)
info@brailler.com (e-mail)
www.brailler.com

Manufactures braille embossers (Braille BookMaker, Braille Express, Braille Place, ET, Gemini, Juliet Classic, Juliet Pro, Marathon Brailler, PED-30, Romeo Attache, Romeo Attache Pro, Romeo Braille 25, Romeo Pro 50, Thomas. TranSend LT). Also distributes a variety of products.

Enhanced Vision Systems
5882 Machine Drive
Huntington Beach, CA 92649
(888) 811-3161 or (714) 374-1829 (phone)
(714) 374-1821 (fax)
info@enhancedvision.com (e-mail)
www.enhancedvision.com

Manufactures video magnifiers (Acrobat, Amigo, Flipper, Flipper Panel, FlipperPort, Jordy, Max, Merlin, Nemo).

En-Vision America
1845 West Hovey Avenue
Normal, IL 61761
(800) 890-1180) or (309) 452-3088 (phone)
(309) 452-3643 (fax)
envision@envisionamerica.com (e-mail)
www.envisionamerica.com

Manufactures speech products (i.d. Mate II, ScripTalk)

Exceptional Teaching
5673 West Las Positas Boulevard, Suite 207

Pleasanton, CA 94588
(800) 549-6999 or (925) 598-6999 (phone)
(925) 598-0086 (fax)
info@exceptionalteaching.com (e-mail)
www.exceptionalteaching.com

Develops and distributes a variety of educational products for students with visual impairments and other special needs, including Wikki Stix and other supplies for making tactile graphics, tracking materials, and the SAL2 System, an interactive braille learning station that runs on the Talking Tactile Tablet (see Touch Graphics).

F. H. Papenmeier GmbH & Co. KG
Reha Division
P.O. Box 1620-58211
Schwerte, Germany
+49 02304-205-0 (phone)
+49 02304-205-205 (fax)
info@papenmeier.de (e-mail)
www.papenmeier.de
U.S. distributors: Audio Visual Mart,
Technologies for the Visually Impaired

Manufactures the Braillex EL 2D-80 braille display and braille personal digital assistants (Braillex EL Braille Assistant-20-cell, Braillex EL Braille Assistant-32-cell).

Fonix Speech, Inc.
387 South 520 West, Suite 110
Lindon, UT 84042
(801) 553-6600 (phone)
(801) 553-6707 (fax)
www.fonixspeech.com

Distributes speech synthesizers (DECtalk Access32, DECtalk Express, DECtalk PC2).

Franklin Electronic Publishers
One Franklin Plaza
Burlington, NJ 08016-4907

(800) 266-5626 (phone)
(609) 239-5948 (fax)
service@franklin.com (e-mail)

Manufactures a variety of talking electronic products, including accessible talking dictionaries.

Freedom Scientific
11800 31st Court North
St. Petersburg, FL 33716
(800) 444-4443 or (727) 803-8000 (phone)
(727) 803-8001 (fax)
info@FreedomScientific.com (e-mail)
www.freedomscientific.com

Manufactures braille displays (Focus 40 Braille Display, Focus 80 Braille Display, PAC Mate 20 Display, PAC Mate 40 Display), digital Talking Book player (FSReader), optical character recognition systems (OpenBook, SARA Scanning and Reading Appliance; Wynn Wizard scanning and reading software), personal digital assistants—braille (Braille Lite M20 and M40, PAC Mate Omni BX400, PAC Mate Omni BX420, PAC Mate Omni BX440), personal digital assistants—speech (PAC Mate QX400, PAC Mate Omni QX420, PAC Mate Omni QX440), screen magnification systems (MAGic Professional with speech, MAGic Professional without speech, MAGic Standard with speech, MAGic Standard without speech), screen readers (JAWS for Windows Professional, JAWS for Windows Standard), speech products (ScanTalker), and video magnifiers (ONYX, ONYX Deskset 17, ONYX PC Edition, Opal, TOPAZ Desktop Video Magnifiers).

Freedom Vision
615 Tami Way
Mountain View, CA 94041
(800) 961-1334 or (650) 961-6541 (phone)

(650) 968-4740 (fax)
info@freedomvision.net (e-mail)
www.freedomvision.net

Distributes a variety of products from Ash Technologies.

gh, LLC
1305 Cumberland Avenue
West Lafayette, IN 47906
(866) 693-3687 or (765) 775-3776 (phone)
(765) 775-2501 (fax)
sales@ghbraille.com (e-mail)
www.ghbraille.com

Manufactures the gh Player software for playing Digital Talking Books.

Gregory Braun
P.O. Box 237
Elm Grove, WI 53122-0237
(800) 999-2734 or (719) 576-0123 (phone)
support@gregorybraun.com (e-mail)
www.gregorybraun.com

Developed the Screen Loupe screen magnification system.

Guerilla Technologies
5029 SE Horseshoe Point Road
Stuart, FL 34997
(772) 283-0500 (phone)
sales@guerillatechnologies.com (e-mail)
www.guerillatechnologies.com

Manufactures optical character recognition systems (Extreme Reader ER1, Extreme Reader XR1, Extreme Reader XR10, MobilEyes).

GW Micro
725 Airport North Office Park
Fort Wayne, IN 46825
(260) 489-3671 (phone)
(260) 489-2608 (fax)

sales@gwmicro.com (e-mail)
www.gwmicro.com
Manufactures the Window-Eyes screen reader, Small-Talk Ultra, and the Portable SenseView video magnifier.

Distributes a variety of products, including products from Human Information Management Service in Korea and Index Braille in Sweden.

Handy Tech Elektronik GmbH
Brunnenstrasse 10
D-72160 Horb, Germany
+49 7451 5546-0 (phone)
+49 7451 5546-67 (fax)
info@handytech.de (e-mail)
www.handytech.com
U.S. distributor: Handy Tech North America

Manufactures braille displays (Bookworm, Braille Star 40, Braille Star 80, Braille Wave, Easy Braille, Modular Evolution) and the Braillino with Bluetooth personal digital assistant.

Handy Tech North America
1349 Pike Lake Drive
New Brighton, MN 55112
(651) 636-5184 (phone)
(866) 347-8249 (fax)
info@handytech.us (e-mail)
www.handytech.us/contact.html

Distributes products from Handy Tech Elektronik GmbH in Germany and Index Braille in Sweden.

Health Care Services, Inc.
342 Fourth Avenue
Huntington, WV 25701
(304) 525-9184 (phone)
fredSilver@aol.com (e-mail)

Distributes a variety of video magnifiers from Low Vision International in Sweden.

Henter Math, LLC
P.O. Box 40430
St. Petersburg, FL 33743-0430
(888) 533-6284 or (727) 347-1313 (phone)
info@hentermatch.com (e-mail)
www.hentermath.com

Manufactures educational products (Virtual Pencil Algebra and Virtual Pencil Arithmetic).

Human Information Management Service
High-Tech Venture Hall 5105
53-3 Eoeun-dong, Yuseong-gu
Daejeon, 305-348
Korea
U.S. distributors: GW Micro, Easy Talk

Manufactures braille displays (Sync Braille-20 Cell, Sync Braille-32 Cell) and personal digital assistants (Braille Sense and Voice Sense).

HumanWare Canada
445, rue du Parc Industriel
Longueuil, PQ 4H 3V7
Canada
(888) 723-7273 or (819) 471-4818 (phone)
(819) 471-4828 (fax)
ca.info@humanware.com (e-mail)
www.humanware.ca/en-canada/contact

Manufactures digital Talking Book players (Victor Reader ClassicX Plus, Victor Reader Stream, Victor Reader Wave, Victor Reader Soft).

HumanWare USA
175 Mason Circle
Concord, CA 94520
(800) 722-3393 or (925) 680-7100 (phone)

(925) 681-4630 (fax)
info@humanware.com (e-mail)
www.humanware.com

Manufactures braille displays (Braille Connect 12, BrailleConnect 32, Braille Connect 40, Brailliant 24, Brailliant 32, Brailliant 40, Brailliant 64, Brailliant 80), personal digital assistants-braille (Braille Note mPower BT 18, BrailleNote mPower BT 32, BrailleNote mPower QT 18, BrailleNote mPower QT 32, BrailleNote PK), personal digital assistants-speech (VoiceNote mPower BT, VoiceNote mPower QT), and video magnifiers myReader2, PocketViewer, SmartView Xtend). Also distributes a variety of products, including products from Quantum Technology in Australia and HumanWare Canada.

Independent Living Aids
200 Robbins Lane
Jericho, NY 11753
(800) 537-2118 or (516) 937-1848 (phone)
(516) 937-3906 (fax)
can-do@independentliving.com (e-mail)
www.independentliving.com

Distributes a variety of braille displays, braille embossers, digital Talking Book players, educational products, low vision products, tactile and braille materials, tactile maps, talking products, and video magnifiers.

Index Braille
Hantverksvagen 20, Box 155
S-954 23 Gammelstad, Sweden
+46 920 20 30 80
order@indexbraille.com (e-mail)
info@indexbraille.com (e-mail)
www.braille.se
U.S. distributors: American Thermoform, Audio Visual Mart, BlinkSoft, Brailler Depot, Christal Vision, Easy Talk, Handy Tech North America, NanoPac, Virtual Vision

Manufactures braille embossers (4 Wave Professional, Index 4×4, Index Basic D, Index Basic S, Index Everest-D), braille translators (iBraille, WinBraille), and optical character recognition systems (Optical Braille Recognition).

Innovative Rehabilitation Technology
13467 Colfax Highway
Grass Valley, CA 95945
(800) 322-4784 or (530) 274-2090 (phone)
(530) 274-2093 (fax)
info@irti.net (e-mail)
www.irti.net

Manufactures digital Talking Book players (Plextalk PTN1, Plextalk PTR2, eClipse Reader, eClipseWater, eClipseWater Professional, eClipseWriter Personal Edition, eClipseWriter Professional). Also distributes a variety of products.

Innoventions
9593 Corsair Drive
Conifer, CO 80433-9317
(800) 854-6554 or (303) 797-6554 (phone)
(303) 727-4940 (fax)
magnicam@magnicam.com (e-mail)
www.magnicam.com

Manufactures video magnifiers (Magni-Cam, Triad Color Magni-Cam Electronic Magnifier).

InSiPhil (US) LLC
650 Vaqueros Avenue, Suite F
Sunnyvale, CA 94085
(800) 804-8004 or (408) 616-8700 (phone)
(408) 616-8720 (fax)
info@insiphil.com (e-mail)
www.telesensory.com

Manufactures the Ovation optical character recognition system and video magnifiers (Aladdin Apex, Aladdin Classic, Aladdin Rainbow Elite, Aladdin Sunshine, Aladdin Ultra, Atlas 600, Atlas 610, Genie Pro, Olympia, Pico).

IntelliTools
1720 Corporate Circle
Petaluma, CA 94954
(800) 899-6687 or (707) 773-2000 (phone)
(707) 773-2001 (fax)
info@intellitools.com (e-mail)
www.intellitools.com

Produces classroom tools for students with learning and physical disabilities, including alternative keyboards (IntelliKeys) and overlays.

InTouch Graphics
P.O. Box 75762
St. Paul, MN 55175-0762
(612) 220-6657 (phone)
www.intouchgraphics.com

Creates customized tactile maps with both low vision and tactile features.

JBliss Low Vision Systems
P.O. 7382
Menlo Park, CA 94026
(888) 452-5477 or (650) 327-5477 (phone)
info@jbliss.com (e-mail)
www.jbliss.com

Manufactures optical character recognition systems (ezVIP, VIP) and the PnC Net screen magnification system. Also distributes a variety of screen readers and video magnifiers.

Kirk Reiser and Andy Berdan
www.linux-speakup.org

Developed the Speakup screen reader.

K-NFB Reading Technology
15 Walnut Street, Suite 200
Wellesley Hills, MA 02481
(877) 547-1500 (phone)
www.knfbreader.com

Manufactures the Kurzweil–National Federation of the Blind Reader optical character recognition system.

Kurzweil Educational Systems
14 Crosby Drive
Bedford, MA 01730-1402
(800) 894-5374 or (781) 276-0600 (phone)
(781) 276-0650 (fax)
info@kurzweiledu.com (e-mail)
www.kurzweiledu.com

Manufactures optical character recognition (specialized scanning) systems (Kurzweil 1000, Kurzweil 3000).

LevelStar
1500 Cherry Street, Suite D
Louisville, CO 80027
(800) 315-2305 or (303) 926-4334 (phone)
(303) 926-1787 (fax)
info@levelstar.com (e-mail)
www.levelstar.com

Manufactures the Icon accessible personal digital assistant.

Low Vision International
Verkstadsgatan 5
352 46 Växjö
Sweden
+46 470 727700 (phone)
+46 470 727725 (fax)
info@lvi.se (e-mail)
www.lvi.se
U.S. distributors: Health Care Services, Inc. (HCSI), Vision Cue, Virtual Vision Technologies (VVT), and Christal Vision

Manufactures video magnifiers (Explorer PC, MagniLink C Reader, MagniLink C Split, MagniLink P, MagniLink S Reader, MagniLink S Student Addition, MagniLink S Student Classic, MagniLink U Split, MagniLink U Student, MagniLink X Reader, MagniLink X Split, MagniLink Zip).

LS&S
P.O. Box 673
Northbrook, IL 60065
(800) 468-4789 or (847) 498-9777 (phone)
(847) 498-1482 (fax)
(866) 317-8533 (TDD/TTY)
info@LSSProducts.com (e-mail)
www.lssgroup.com

Distributes a variety of products, including products from Reinecker Reha-Technik in Germany.

MagniSight
3631 North Stone Avenue
Colorado Springs, CO 80907
(800) 753-4767 or (719) 578-8893 (phone)
(719) 578-9887 (fax)
sales@magnisight.com (e-mail)
www.magnisight.com

Manufactures video magnifiers (Explorer, Journey)

MaxiAids
42 Executive Boulevard
Farmingdale, NY 11735
(800) 522-6294 or (631) 752-0689 (phone)
(631) 752-0689 (fax)
(800) 281-3555 (Toll-Free TDD)
sales@maxiaids.com (e-mail)
www.maxiaids.com

Distributes a variety of products, including products from Variscite in Israel.

Metroplex Voice Computing
P. O. Box 121984
Arlington, Texas 76012
(817) 543-1103 (fax)

mathtalk@mathtalk.com (email)
www.mathtalk.com

Produces voiced mathematics products, including MathPad and MathTalk.

Michael Curran
developers@nvda-project.org (e-mail)
www.nvda-project.org

Developer and distributor of the NVDA (Nonvisual Desktop Access) screen reader.

Microsoft
www.microsoft.com/speech/speech2007/default.mspx

Manufactures the Microsoft Speech Engine speech synthesizer.

National Aeronautics and Space Administration (NASA)
http://prime.jsc.nasa.gov/mathtrax

Developed MathTrax, a free downloadable graphing tool for middle school and high school students.

Next Generation Technologies
20006 Cedar Valley Road, Suite 101
Lynnwood, WA 98036-6334
(425) 744-1100 (phone)
(425) 778-5547 (fax)
www.ngtvoice.com

Manufactures J-Say Pro. Also distributes a variety of educational products.

Ocutech
109 Conner Drive, Suite 2105
Chapel Hill, NC 27514
(800) 326-6460 or (919) 967-6460 (phone)
(919) 967-8146 (fax)
info@Ocutech.com (e-mail)
www.ocutech.com

Manufactures bioptic telescopes.

Optek Systems
P.O. Box 277
Rydalmere, NSW 0176
Australia
terryk@mpx.com.au (e-mail)
http://members.optusnet.com.au/~terryk
U.S. distributor: Opus Technologies

Manufactures the Toccata music braille translator and tactile graphics materials (Nomad Mentor software and Nomad pad). Also distributes a variety of products.

Optelec USA
3030 Enterprise Court, Suite C
Vista, CA 92081
(800) 828-1056 or (978) 857-2500 (phone)
(800) 368-4111 (fax)
optelec@optelec.com (e-mail)
www.optelec.com

Manufactures braille displays (Alva 544 Satellite Traveller, Alva 570 Satellite, Alva 584 Satellite Pro, Alva BC640, Braille Voyager 44), the EasyLink 12 personal digital assistant, and video magnifiers (Clear Note, ClearView+, Compact+, The Traveller).

Optron Assistive Technologies
P.O. Box 5454
Morton, IL 61550
(888) 567-8756 or (309) 694-2077 (phone)
info@optronusa.com (e-mail)
www.optronusa.com

Manufactures video magnifiers (i-Stick, Optron Mobile, Optron Observer, Optron Pro, Optron Vision).

Opus Technologies
13333 Thunderhead Street
San Diego, CA 92129-2329
(858) 538-9401 (phone)
opus@opustec.com (e-mail)
www.opustec.com

Distributes braille translators from Optek Systems, Toccata braille music translators, and other books and material regarding braille music.

Orbit Research
3422 Old Capitol Trail, Suite 585
Wilmington, DE 19808
(888) 606-7248 (phone)
(208) 279-4576 (fax)
info@orbitresearch.com (e-mail)
www. orbitresearch.com

Developed the Orion TI-36X talking scientific calculator.

OVAC
67-555 East Palm Canyon Drive
Unit C103
Cathedral City, CA 92234
(800) 325-4488 or (760) 321-9220 (phone)
(760) 321-9711 (fax)
info@ovac.com (e-mail)
www.ovac.com

Manufactures a variety of video magnifiers (Color-Eye, Flex-Eye, Golden-Eye, Pro Zoomer, ZACC-S, Zoom Flex, Zoom-Eye).

Perfect Solutions Software, Inc.
2685 Treanor Terrace
Wellington, FL 33414
(800) 726-7086 (phone)
(561) 790-0108 (fax)
perfect@gate.net (e-mail)
www.perfectsolutions.com

PC6 portable dedicated word processor.

Perkins Products/Howe Press
Perkins School for the Blind
175 North Beacon Street
Watertown, MA 02172-2790
(877) 473-7546 or (617) 972-7308 (phone)
(617) 926-2027 (fax)

perkinsproducts@Perkins.org (e-mail)
www.perkinsstore.org

Manufactures the Perkins Brailler, slates, and braille accessories. Also distributes a variety of educational products.

Portset Systems
Southampton SO32 1AX
United Kingdom
+44 01489 893 919 (phone)
Brook Street, Bishops Waltham
+44 01489 893 320 (fax)
admin@portset.co.uk (e-mail)
www.portset.co.uk
U.S. distributor: Technologies for the Visually Impaired

Manufactures the Portset Reader optical character recognition system.

Premier Assistive Technology
13102 Blaisdell Drive
DeWitt, MI 48820
(517) 668-8188 (phone)
(517) 668-2417 (fax)
info@readingmadeeasy.com (e-mail)
www.premierathome.com

Manufactures optical character recognition systems (Complete Reading System, Text Cloner Pro) and a variety of talking and educational products.

Quantum Technology
5 South Street
P.O. Box 390
Rydalmere NSW 2116
Australia
+61 2 8844 9888 (phone)
+61 2 9684 4717 (fax)
info@quantumtechnology.com.au (e-mail)
www.quantech.com.au/contact_us/contact.htm

Manufactures the Mountbatten Brailler (braille embosser) and Jot a Dot braille writing device.

RC Systems
1609 England Avenue
Everett, WA 98203
(425) 355-3800 (phone)
(425) 355-1098 (fax)
info@rcsys.com (e-mail)
www.rcsys.com

Manufactures speech synthesizers (Double Talk, DoubleTalk LT, DoubleTalk PC).

Recording for the Blind and Dyslexic
20 Roszel Road
Princeton, NJ 08540
(866) 732-3585 or (609) 452-0606 (phone)
(609) 520-7990 (fax)
custserv@rfbd.org (e-mail)
www.rfbd.org

Distributes digital Talking Book players (Professor, Telex Scholar).

Rehan Electronics
Industrial Estate, Courtown Road
Gorey, Co. Wexford
Ireland
+ 353 053 9422013 (phone)
+ 353 053 9420732 (fax)
sales@rehanelectronics.ie (e-mail)
www.rehanelectronics.ie
U.S. distributor: Your Low Vision Store

Manufactures the Looky video magnifier.

Renaissance Learning, Inc.
P.O. Box 8036
Wisconsin Rapids, Wisconsin 54495-8036
(800) 338-4204 or (715) 424-3636 (phone)
(715) 424-4242 (fax)

Manufactures Alpha Smart dedicated word processors (Neo and Dana).

Repro-Tronics
75 Carver Avenue
Westwood, NJ 07675
(800) 948-8453 or (201) 722-1880 (phone)
(201) 722-1881 (fax)
sales@repro-tronics.com (e-mail)
www.repro-tronics.com

Manufactures tactile graphics materials (Tactile Image Enhancer, Flexi-Paper Tactile Imaging Paper, Thermo Pen II).

RJ Cooper & Associates
27601 Forbes Road
Suite 39
Laguna Niguel, CA 92677
(800) 752-6673) or (949) 582-2572 (phone)
(949) 582-3169 (fax)
info@rjcooper.com (e-mail)
techsupport@rjcooper.com (e-mail)
www.rjcooper.com/index.html

Manufactures educational products (Biggy, Biggy-Light, Find the Buttons) and speech products (Speak to Me, Talk 'n Scan Calculator).

Robotron
15 Stamford Road
Oakleigh 3166
Australia
+61 3 9568 2568 (phone)
+61 3 9568 1377 (fax)
http://sensorytools.com
U.S. distributor: SensAbility

Manufactures the Braille Master braille translator and the Simon Reading Machine (optical character recognition system).

SensAbility
299-B Peterson Road
Libertyville, IL 60048

(888) 669-7323 (phone)
(847) 367-4003 (fax)

Distributes products from Robotron.

Serotek Corporation
1128 Harmon Place, Suite 300
Minneapolis, MN 55403
(866) 202-0520 (phone)
sales@freedombox.info (e-mail)
www.freedombox.info

Manufactures screen readers (System Access Stand-alone, System Access Stand-alone Mobile, System Access Surfboard); and speech products (FreedomBox Stand-alone).

Shop Low Vision
3030 Enterprise Court, Suite D
Vista, CA 92081-8358
(800) 826-4200 (phone)
(800) 368-4111 (fax)
www.shoplowvision.com

Offers a variety of independent living and low vision products.

Sight Enhancement Systems
60 Bathurst Drive, Unit #17
Waterloo, ON N2V 2A9
Canada
(519) 883-8400 (phone)
(519) 883-8405 (fax)
sales@sightenhancement.com (e-mail)
www.sightenhancement.com

Developers of video-based assistive technologies for people with vision loss. Manufactures the Sci Plus talking scientific calculators and the Wat-Cam video camera unit for distance viewing and close-up reading and writing tasks.

Society for the Blind
2750 24th Street
Sacramento, CA 95818

(916) 452-8271 (phone)
store@societyfortheblind.org (e-mail)
www.shopsftb.org/servlet/StoreFront

Distributes variety of braille writing materials and talking products.

Springer Design
3160 Crow Canyon Place, Suite 145
San Ramon, CA 94583
(925) 242-0310 (phone)
(925) 242-0357 (fax)
sales@bookcourier.com (e-mail)

Manufactures the BookCourier Digital Talking Book player.

Sun Microsystems
Accessibility Program Office
4150 Network Circle
Santa Clara, CA 95054 USA
(800) 786-0404 or (650) 960-1300 (phone)

Manufactures the Screen Reader and Magnifier screen readers.

TACK-TILES Braille Systems
P.O. Box 475
Plaistow, NH 03865
(800) 822-5845 (phone)
(603) 382-1748 (fax)
www.tack-tiles.com

Manufactures the Tack-tiles Braille System.

Technologies for the Visually Impaired
9 Nolan Court
Hauppauge, NY 11778
(631) 724-4479 (phone)
(631) 724-4479 (fax)
contact@tvi-web.com (e-mail)
www.tvi-web.com

Distributes a variety of products, including products from Index Braille in Sweden,

Papenmeier in Germany, and Portset Systems in the United Kingdom.

Touch Graphics

330 West 38th Street, Suite 1204
New York, NY 10018
(800) 884-2440 or (212) 375-6341 (phone)
(646) 452-4211 (fax)
info@touchgraphics.com (e-mail)
www.touchgraphics.com

Manufactures educational products and games based on the Talking Tactile Tablet and other computer products for visually impaired students and adults.

Variscite

P.O. Box 465
Nesher 36603
Israel
972-4-8200727 (phone)
info@variscite.com (e-mail)
U.S. distributor: MaxiAids

Manufactures the TADI Talking Organizer personal digital assistant (speech).

VideoEye Corporation

9465 West Emerald
Boise, ID 83704
(800) 416-0758 or (208) 323-9577 (phone)
(208) 658-1762 (fax)
sales@videoeye.com (e-mail)
www.videoeye.com/about.asp

Offers a variety of video magnifiers.

Videospec

Old Working, Surrey GU22 9ER
United Kingdom
+44 01483 722273 (phone)
30A High Street
+44 01483 728343 (fax)
www.videospec.co.uk
sales@videospec.co.uk

Manufactures the EEZEE Reader video magnifier.

VIEW International Foundation

230 Peach Tree Drive
West Monroe, LA 71291
(318) 396-1853 (phone)
ttsinfo@earthlink.net (e-mail)
www.viewinternational.org

Offers a collection of files for creating tactile diagrams.

ViewPlus Technologies

853 SW Airport Avenue
Corvallis, OR 97330
(541) 754-4002 (phone)
(541) 738-6505 (fax)
info@viewplus.com (e-mail)
www.viewplus.com

Manufactures braille embossers (Emprint SpotDot, Tiger embossers, ViewPlus Cub Embosser, ViewPlus Cub Jr Embosser, View Plus Max Embosser, ViewPlus Pro Embosser); and educational products (Audio Graphing Calculator, DotsPlus, Tiger Braille Math, IVEO speaking tactile diagram system).

Vision Technology

8501 Delport Drive
St. Louis, MO 63114
(800) 560-7226 or (314) 890-8300 (phone)
(314) 890-8383 (fax)
vti@vti1.com (e-mail)
www.visiontechnology.com

Manufactures video magnifiers (Premier, ProSeries, Select, SelectUltra, View, VTI InSight CCTV).

Xerox Corporation
Xerox Office Group Headquarters
P.O. Box 1000

MS 7060-583
Wilsonville, OR 97070
(800) 835-6100 (support)
(503) 682-2980 (fax)
www.office.xerox.com/software-
solutions/xerox-copier-assistant/enus.html

Manufactures the Xerox Copier Assistant
(speech product).

Your Low Vision Store
1794 East Main Street
Ventura, CA 93001
(800) 310-3938 (phone)
info@yourlowvisionstore.com (e-mail)
www.yourlowvisionstore.com/index.shtml

Distributes a variety of products, including
products from Rehan Electronics in Ireland.

ASSISTIVE TECHNOLOGY MANUFACTURERS BY CATEGORY

The general categories in this listing can be
used to find manufacturers and distributors
whose contact information appears in the
previous section that may sell a specific
type of technology being sought.

Braille Displays
Baum Retec AG
F. H. Papenmeier GmbH & Co. KG
Freedom Scientific
Handy Tech Elektronik GmbH
Human Information Management Service
HumanWare USA
Optelec USA

Braille Embossers
American Thermoform Corporation
Enabling Technologies Company
Index Braille

Nippon Telesoft
Quantum Technology
ViewPlus Technologies

Braille Translators
Dancing Dots
Dolphin Computer Access
Duxbury Systems, Inc.
Index Braille
Optek Systems
Robotron

CCTVs/Video Magnifiers
ABISee, Inc.
Another Eye
Ash Technologies
Bierley Associates
Clarity
Enhanced Vision Systems
Freedom Scientific
GW Micro
HumanWare USA
Innoventions
InSiPhil (US) LLC
Low Vision International
MagniSight
Optelec
Optron Assistive Technology
OVAC
Rehan Electronics
Reinecker-Reha-Technik
Sight Enhancement Systems
VideoEye Corporation
Videospec
Vision Technology, Inc.

Digital Talking Book Players
American Printing House for the Blind
Dolphin Computer Access
Freedom Scientific
gh
HumanWare Canada
Innovative Rehabilitation Technology
Recording for the Blind & Dyslexic
Springer Design

Educational Technology and Materials
American Printing House for the Blind
American Thermoform Corporation
Ann Arbor Publishers
Design Science
Don Johnston
EnableMart
Exceptional Teaching, Inc.
Franklin Electronic Publishers
Henter Math
IntelliTools
InTouch Graphics
Metroplex Voice Computing
National Aeronautics and Space
   Administration
Optek Systems
Orbit Research
Perfect Solutions Software
Perkins Products/Howe Press
Repro-Tronics
Premier Assistive Technology
Quantum Technology
Renaissance Learning
Repro-Tronics
RJ Cooper
Sight Enhancement Systems
Touch Graphics
View International
ViewPlus Technologies

Low Vision Devices
Ai Squared
American Printing House for the Blind
Independent Living Aids
LS&S
MaxiAids
Ocutech

Optical Character Recognition Systems and Reading Machines
Baum Retec AG
Freedom Scientific
Guerilla Technologies

Index Braille
InSiPhil (US) LLC
JBliss Imaging Systems
K-NFB Reading Technology, Inc.
Kurzweil Educational Systems
Portset Systems, Ltd.
Premier Assistive Technology
Robotron

Personal Digital Assistants
American Printing House for the Blind
F. H. Papenmeier GmbH & Co. KG
Freedom Scientific
Handy Tech Elektronik GmbH
Human Information Management Service
HumanWare USA
LevelStar
Optelec USA, Inc.
Variscite

Screen Magnification Systems
Ai Squared
Dolphin Computer Access
Freedom Scientific
Gregory Braun
JBliss Imaging Systems

Screen Readers
Apple
Accessibility Program Office of Sun
   Microsystems
Dancing Dots
David Mielke
Dolphin Computer Access
Freedom Scientific
GW Micro
Kirk Reiser and Andy Berdan
Michael Curran
Serotek

Speech Products
American Printing House for the Blind
Beyond Sight

Brytech
Canon USA
Captek dba Science Products
Dancing Dots
En-Vision America
Franklin Electronic Publishers
Freedom Scientific
GW Micro
Next Generation Technologies
Premier Assistive Technology
Serotek
Sight Enhancement
Xerox

Speech Synthesizers

Apple
Access Solutions
Eloquence
Fonix Speech, Inc.
Microsoft Speech Engine
RC Systems

SOURCES OF MATERIALS IN ALTERNATE FORMATS

The organizations listed in this section produce reading material for people who are blind or visually impaired in a variety of formats, including large print, braille, audio recording, and digital formats, as well as tactile graphics.

American Printing House for the Blind (APH)

1839 Frankfort Avenue
Louisville, KY 40206-0085
(800) 223-1839 or (502) 895-2405 (phone)
(502) 899-2274 (fax)
info@aph.org (e-mail)
www.aph.org

Maintains a repository of accessible materials for people who are blind or visually impaired. The Louis database on APH's web site allows teachers, parents, and students to locate thousands of textbooks in braille, large print, recorded, and computer disc formats available from producers across the United States. The Image Library Database may be accessed by teachers, transcribers, students, families, and paraprofessionals to find tactile graphics that can be enhanced for their needs. Administers the federal quota system to provide braille and other materials to students who are blind and houses the National Instructional Materials Access Center (NIMAC), the central repository that contains source files from publishers that can be used to produce books in accessible formats for students with print disabilities.

Audio Studio for the Reading Impaired (ASRI)

1403 Park Road
Anchorage, KY 40223
(502) 245-5422 (phone)
director@audio-studio.org (e-mail)
www.audio-studio.org

Produces recordings of printed material for anyone who is physically unable to read standard print or unable to hold a book.

Bookshare.org

480 California Avenue, Suite 201
Palo Alto, CA 94306
(650) 644-3400 (phone)
info@bookshare.org (e-mail)
www.bookshare.org

Online library of digital books for people with visual disabilities with a collection that includes fiction, nonfiction, reference material, textbooks, as well as newspapers and magazines. Members download books directly and read them with any available assistive hardware device or software application that supports digital text. Also provides an assistive software application for free.

Braille Co., Inc.
65-B Town Hall Square
Falmouth, MA 02540
(508) 540-0800 (phone)
braillinc@capecod.net (e-mail)
http://home.capecod.net/~braillinc

Specializes in transcription services for vocational and educational needs.

Braille Institute of America (BIA)
741 North Vermont Avenue
Los Angeles, CA 90029
(800) 272-4553 or (323) 663-1111, ext. 3112 (phone)
biainfo@brailleinstitute.org (e-mail)
www.brailleinstitute.org

Maintains a library with more than 60,000 books available in braille and on cassette, consisting of recreational and informational titles for adults and children. BIA's Universal Media Services also offers a variety of braille production services such as transcription into braille of electronic files, hard copy, or highly formatted or technical material; reproduction of multiple braille copies; and creation of tactile graphics.

Braille International
3290 Southeast Slater Street
Stuart, FL 34997
(888) 336-3142 or (772) 286-8366 (phone)
(772) 286-8909 (fax)
info@brailleintl.org (e-mail)
www.brailleintl.org

The William A. Thomas Braille Bookstore offers fiction and nonfiction braille books for children and adults. Also offers braille transcription and embossing services.

Braille Jymico
70 West Madison Street
Three First National Plaza, Suite 1400
Chicago, IL 60602
(312) 214-2380 (phone)
(312) 214-3110 (fax)
www.braillejymico.com

Produces illustrations, graphics, and spatial representations adapted to touch recognition for people who are blind.

Future Aids: The Braille Superstore
2190 Dolphin Crescent
Abbotsford, BC V2T 3T1
Canada
(800) 987-1231 or (604) 852-6341 (phone)
www.braillebookstore.com

Source of many braille books and devices, low vision devices, and speech software.

Horizons for the Blind
2 North Williams Street
Crystal Lake, Illinois 60014-4401
(800) 318-2000 or (815) 444-8800 (phone)
(815) 444-8830 (fax)
mail@horizons-blind.org (e-mail)
www.horizons-blind.org/index.php

Provides braille, large print, and audiocassette and CD instruction in crafts, gardening, food preparation, recreational reading, and the operation of household appliances as well as braille signage for public facilities.

Kenneth Jernigan Library for Blind Children
American Action Fund for Blind Children and Adults (AAF/BCA)
18440 Oxnard Street
Tarzana, CA 91356
(818) 343-2022 (phone)
twinvisionkjl@aol.com (e-mail)
www.actionfund.org/kjlibaps.htm

Has more than 40,000 braille and Twin Vision books, which are loaned free of charge to blind children, blind parents who have sighted children, schools, regional libraries for the blind, institutions serving the blind, and schools and libraries in many foreign countries.

Library Reproduction Service

14214 South Figueroa Street
Los Angeles, CA 90061-1034
(800) 255-5002 or (310) 354-2610 (phone)
(310) 354-2601 (fax)
lrsprint@aol.com (e-mail)
www.lrs-largeprint.com

Produces large-print textbooks, laboratory manuals, study guides, tests, and reference and general reading materials.

National Association for Visually Handicapped (NAVH)

22 West 21st Street 6th Floor
New York, NY 10010
(212) 255-2804 (phone)
(212) 727-2931 (fax)
navh@navh.org (e-mail)
www.navh.org

507 Polk Street, Suite 420
San Francisco, CA 94102
(415) 775-6284 (6284) (phone)
(415) 346-9593 (fax)
staffca@navh.org (e-mail)

Maintains a library with a large variety of large-print books in such categories as literature, language, mathematics, reading, science, social studies, spelling, and leisure reading.

National Braille Press

88 St. Stephen Street
Boston, MA 02115
(617) 266-6160 or (800) 548-7323 (phone)

(617) 437-0456 (fax)
orders@nbp.org (e-mail)
www.nbp.org

Offers a braille production service; produces braille textbooks and tests and tactile graphics. Sells a variety of print-braille books for young children and also offers the Children's Braille Book Club.

National Library Service for the Blind and Physically Handicapped (NLS)

Library of Congress
1291 Taylor Street, NW
Washington, DC 20542
(202) 707-5100 or (800) 424-8567 (phone)
nls@loc.gov (e-mail)
www.loc.gov/nls

Has a lending library of print/braille books, materials in braille, recorded discs and cassettes, Digital Talking Books, Web-Braille, and music for blind and visually impaired persons who cannot use printed materials. Distributes other braille books through state and regional libraries for the blind.

Readings for the Blind (RBMI)

29350 Southfield Road, Suite 130
Southfield, MI 48076-2060
(888) 766-1166 or (248) 557-7776 (phone)
rftb@sbcglobal.net (e-mail)
www.readingsfortheblind.org

Records books not available elsewhere for the visually impaired, learning disabled, and those physically unable to hold a book or turn a page. Recordings are available on cassette (2-track and 4-track) and CD.

Recording for the Blind & Dyslexic (RFB&D)

20 Roszel Road
Princeton, NJ 08540

(866) 732-3585 or (609) 452-0606 (phone)
custserv@rfbd.org (e-mail)
www.rfbd.org

Maintains an extensive collection of audio book titles in a broad variety of subjects, from literature and history to math and the sciences, at all academic levels, from kindergarten through post-graduate and professional. Also records books in major fields of study on request.

SCALARS Publishing

P.O. Box 382834
Germantown, TN 38183-2834
(901) 737-0001 (phone)
(901) 624-7995 (fax)
ScalarsPub@comcast.net (e-mail)
www.scalarspublishing.com/index.html

Publishes several books that teach the literary braille code and a print dictionary of words that contain braille contractions, *The Braille Enthusiast's Dictionary*.

Seedlings Braille Books for Children (SBBC)

14151 Farmington Road
Livonia, MI 48154-4522
(734) 427-8552 (phone)
(800) 777-8552

seedlink@aol.com (e-mail)
www.seedlings.org

Produces braille books at each level of development, from toddler board books to classic literature for older children. The Rose Project offers *World Book Encyclopedia* articles in braille, free of charge for blind students in grades 1-12.

T-Base Communications, Inc.

19 Main Street
Ottawa, ON K1S 1A9
Canada
(800) 563-0668 or (613) 236-0866 (phone)
(613) 236-0484 (fax)
info@tbase.com (e-mail)
www.tbase.com

Transcribes, publishes, and distributes documents into braille, large print, e-text, and audio formats.

TFB Publications

234 Lafayette Avenue
Cliffside Park, NJ 07010
(201) 313-8905 (phone)
tfb@panix.com (e-mail)

Offers braille transcription of materials submitted electronically. Also distributes braille books such as children's books, cook books, and sewing books.

Case Study: Semena

The case study of Semena Thomas is presented here because she is an elementary school student with no usable vision, in contrast to Bill Alonso, whose example was presented in Chapters 6–8 and is a high school student with usable vision. Thus, since Semena's primary learning medium is differ-

ent from Bill's, her assistive technology assessment would involve carrying out some different procedures, as represented on the forms completed for Semena on the following pages. The recommendations presented here for Semena also suggest some different technologies and incorporate different rationales.

Background Information for Assistive Technology Assessment

Student's Name: _Semena Thomas_   Birthdate: _1/22/1980_   Grade: _3_
Name of parent(s)/guardian(s): _Seth and Maryanne Thomas_
School: _Main Street Elementary School_
Teacher of students with visual impairments: _Samantha Higgins_
Referred by: _Samantha Higgins_
Reason for Referral: _Difficulty completing assignments_
_____

Initial or Ongoing Assessment (I) O
Additional Disabilities: Y /(N) Describe: _____
Current medication(s): _none_
Reported/observed visual side effects: _____
_____

Eye Report Summary (see Eye Report)
Dr.: _Sarah Johnson_   O.D.   Date of last examination: _2/15/06_
Eye condition: _retinopathy of prematurity_
Prognosis: _stable_

Visual Acuity

	Distance		Near	
	Without Correction	With Correction	Without Correction	With Correction
OD	NLP			
OS	NLP			
OU	NLP			

Field restriction(s): Y / N   Degrees: _____   Location: _____

Recommendations   Not applicable
Eyeglasses   ❑ Wear/Use Constantly   ❑ Wear/Use as Needed
Contact Lenses
   For distance?   Y / N   ❑ Wear/Use Constantly   ❑ Wear/Use as Needed
   For near?   Y / N   ❑ Wear/Use Constantly   ❑ Wear/Use as Needed
Low Vision Device(s) (specify): _____
Other: _____

Information from Learning Media Assessment
Primary learning channel: ❑ visual   ☑ tactile   ❑ auditory
Secondary learning channel: ❑ visual   ❑ tactile   ☑ auditory
Other: _____

(continued on next page)

Background Information *(continued)*

Other current accommodations and technology _(see Considerations Checklist)_ _____

_____

_____

Reading Preferences (if reported): Not applicable

Preferred visual format without device (specify): _____

    Point size: _____   Font: _____   Distance: _____

      Approximate reading rate: _____ wpm

Preferred visual format with device (specify): _____

    Point size: _____   Font: _____   Distance: _____

      Approximate reading rate: _____ wpm

Lighting preferences: _____

Braille: approximate reading rate: _____ wpm oral   _____ wpm silent

Experiences visual/physical fatigue after reading _____ minutes

Relevant information from functional low vision assessment: _Not applicable_ _____

_____

_____

Relevant information from medical, psychological, and academic evaluations: _No auditory_ _deficits or processing problems were reported in Semena's psychological evaluation._ _____

_____

Relevant information from teachers' observations and assessments: _Teachers report that_ _Semena needs additional time to complete lengthy writing assignments._ _____

_____

Additional comments: _____

_____

_____

ASSISTIVE TECHNOLOGY CONSIDERATIONS CHECKLIST

Student: _Semena Thomas_   School: _Main Street Elementary_

DIRECTIONS

1. Complete the student information section below to provide information on the student's needs, abilities, and difficulties as well as environments and barriers to success.
2. Please check (❑) the instructional or access areas in Column A that are appropriate for the student. Please leave blank any areas that are not relevant to the student. Specify all relevant tasks (for example, copying notes from board, responding to teacher questions, and so on) within each area in the space provided. Check the settings in which the task is required. GEC: General Education Classroom; SEC: Special Education Classroom; COM: Community; and HOM: Home.
3. In Column B, specify the standard classroom tools (low technology to high technology) used by the student to complete relevant tasks identified in Column A. Place a check (✔) in the boxes in Column B if the student is able to independently complete the tasks with standard classroom tools. For areas in which the student can complete the tasks independently, it will not be necessary to complete Columns C or D.
4. In Column C, specify the accommodations/modifications and assistive technology solutions that are currently being utilized. Place a check (✔) in the boxes in Column C if the student can adequately complete the tasks specified in Column A using the identified accommodations/modifications and assistive technology solutions.
5. Complete Column D if the student cannot adequately complete the task with accommodations/modifications and assistive technology solutions specified in Column C.

Student needs, abilities, and difficulties: _Semena is functioning at grade level in all academic areas but experiences difficulty in completing lengthy writing assignments in a form that her teachers can access._

Student environments:

☑ General Education Classroom (List all classes): _____

_____

❑ Special Education Classroom (List all classes): _____

_____

❑ Community (List all settings): _____

_____

❑ Home: _____

_____

Barriers to student performance and achievement: _Semena's writing assignments in braille cannot be immediately read by her classroom teachers. These assignments must be interlined by her teacher of visually impaired students and returned to the classroom teachers. This creates a delay in providing feedback about her work and progress._

(continued on next page)

Source: Reprinted with permission from the Georgia Project for Assistive Technology, Georgia Department of Education, Atlanta.

Assistive Technology Considerations Checklist *(continued)*

A. Instructional or Access Areas	B. Independent with Standard Classroom Tools	C. Completes Tasks with Accommodations/ Modifications and/or Assistive Technology Solutions Currently in Place		D. Additional Solutions/Services Needed, Including Assistive Technology
		Accommodations/ Modifications	Assistive Technology Solutions	
☑ Writing ☐ GEC ☐ SEC ☐ COM ☐ HOM		Semena uses a standard Perkins braillewriter to complete most written assignments		Accessible computer word processor for longer written assignments
☑ Spelling ☐ GEC ☐ SEC ☐ COM ☐ HOM				Talking dictionary
☑ Reading ☐ GEC ☐ SEC ☐ COM ☐ HOM	Yes, but needs additional opportunities for reading braille	Braille books and other materials		Accessible PDA with refreshable braille display
☐ Math ☐ GEC ☐ SEC ☐ COM ☐ HOM				
☐ Study/ Organizational Skills ☐ GEC ☐ SEC ☐ COM ☐ HOM				
☑ Listening ☐ GEC ☐ SEC ☐ COM ☐ HOM	Yes, but needs additional opportunities for reading braille			Introduce recorded and synthesized speech
☐ Oral Communication ☐ GEC ☐ SEC ☐ COM ☐ HOM				
☐ Aids to Daily Living ☐ GEC ☐ SEC ☐ COM ☐ HOM				

A. Instructional or Access Areas	B. Independent with Standard Classroom Tools	C. Completes Tasks with Accommodations/ Modifications and/or Assistive Technology Solutions Currently in Place		D. Additional Solutions/Services Needed, Including Assistive Technology
		Accommodations/ Modifications	Assistive Technology Solutions	
☐ Recreation and Leisure ☐ GEC ☐ SEC ☐ COM ☐ HOM				
☐ Prevocational/ Vocational ☐ GEC ☐ SEC ☐ COM ☐ HOM				
☐ Seating, Positioning, and Mobility ☐ GEC ☐ SEC ☐ COM ☐ HOM				
☐ Other (specify): ☐ GEC ☐ SEC ☐ COM ☐ HOM				

Consideration Outcomes:

☐ Student independently accomplishes tasks in all instructional areas using standard classroom tools. No assistive technology is required.

☐ Student accomplishes tasks in all instructional areas with accommodations and modifications. No assistive technology is required.

☐ Student accomplishes tasks in all instructional areas with currently available assistive technology. Assistive technology is required.

☑ Student does not accomplish tasks in all instructional access areas. Additional solutions including assistive technology may be required.

Specify any assistive technology services required by this student.
Requesting an assistive technology assessment to determine what assistive technology
might be of greatest benefit to Semena.

Consideration Checklist Completed by: Position: Date:

Samantha Higgins   _Teacher of Visually_   _5/23/08_
                                          Impaired Students

ASSISTIVE TECHNOLOGY ASSESSMENT CHECKLIST
FOR STUDENTS WITH VISUAL IMPAIRMENTS

Student's Name _Semena Thomas_   Person Completing Checklist _Samantha Higgins_

Student's Grade _3rd_   Position _Teacher of Visually Impaired Students_

Student's Date of Birth _1/22/1980_   Date(s) of assessment _9/3 & 9/10/2008_

This document is a summary of information collected during the above-named student's assistive technology evaluation. Information for this assessment was obtained from the student's learning media assessment, the clinical low vision evaluation, the functional low vision evaluation, and from observation and assessment of the student's use of specific devices, as outlined below.
The assessment covers three main areas:

- **Section I: Accessing Print**, which covers how the student uses visual, tactile, and/or auditory tools to access textbooks, workbooks, assigned novels, and other printed information generally used in the classroom, including information presented on chalkboards or whiteboards
- **Section II: Accessing Electronic Information**, which covers how the student uses visual, tactile, and/or auditory tools to obtain information from electronic means, such as computers, electronic dictionaries and similar devices, digital books, and electronic braille devices
- **Section III: Communication through Writing**, which includes manuscript (print) and cursive writing, braille writing, and the use of electronic writing tools

The assessment sections of this document are followed by a recommendations section. The notations made will become part of the final written report detailing the rationale for each recommendation submitted to the student's Individualized Education Program team.

Directions: Indicate in the space provided the date each section is completed. All items not assessed should be marked NA.

Source: Adapted with permission from the "Assistive Technology Vision Aids Assessment," from the Georgia Project for Assistive Technology, Georgia Department of Education, Atlanta.

* Sections that deal solely with visual access have been omitted from this version of the checklist since the student has no usable vision.

Section I: Accessing Print

B. Tactile Access and Braille   **Date completed** _9/3/2008_

When accessing graphical information the student is able to discriminate tactilely
- ☑ solid lines of various thickness.
- ☑ dashed lines.
- ☑ dotted lines.
- ☑ raised-line drawings of simple shapes.
- ☑ the boundary between two clearly defined textured fill patterns.
- ☐ the boundary between three clearly defined textured fill patterns.
- ☐ the boundary between four clearly defined textured fill patterns.

The student is able to identify tactile information most accurately when it is presented as a simple tactile graphic
- ☑ tooled onto braille paper.
- ☑ produced as a collage of varying textures.
- ☑ thermoformed onto plastic.
- ☑ embossed as dots and lines onto braille paper by a computer-controlled braille embosser.
- ☑ produced as raised lines and patterns on capsule paper.

The student is able to read materials in
- ☑ uncontracted braille.
- ☑ contracted braille.

☑ Results of formal or informal braille assessments conducted by the teacher of students with visual impairments are attached.
   Student's oral braille reading rate is _28_ words per minute (wpm).
   Student's silent braille reading rate is _35_ wpm.

When accessing print information with a refreshable braille display, the student is able to
- ☑ read instructional-level text.
- ☑ press correct key combination to issue forward and reverse navigation commands
  - ☑ with verbal prompt.
  - ☑ without verbal prompt.
- ☑ read _25_ wpm orally and _30_ wpm silently.

The student is willing to use these devices (the examiner may wish to list these separately)
- ☑ to complete assignments in the regular classroom.
- ☑ at home to complete school assignments.
- ☑ while working with the teacher of students with visual impairments.

Comments: _____

_____

_____

(continued on next page)

C. Auditory Access

1. Live Readers and Recorded Information   **Date completed** *9/3/2008*

When listening to instructional level information read aloud by the evaluator, the student is able to
- ☑ repeat words and simple phrases without having them repeated more than twice.
- ☑ paraphrase the information (a sentence or story).
- ☑ answer simple comprehension questions.

When listening to an analog or digital recording of a story, the student is able to
- ☑ repeat words and simple phrases without having them repeated more than twice.
- ☑ paraphrase the information (a sentence or story).
- ☑ accurately answer simple comprehension questions.

When using an analog or digital player-recorder, the student is able to
- ☑ insert and remove a tape or CD from the player-recorder.
- ☑ inactivate play, pause, stop, fast forward, and rewind functions (underline those demonstrated).
- ☐ understand and comprehend compressed or "fast" speech.
- ☑ manipulate variable speed and pitch controls.
- ☑ identify index tones, bookmarks, and page locators.

The student is able to
- ☐ listen to recorded speech and follow along with a print copy of the text.
- ☑ listen to recorded speech and follow along with a braille copy of the text.
- ☐ listen to synthesized speech and follow along with a print copy of the text.
- ☑ listen to synthesized speech and follow along with a braille copy of the text.

The student is able to read approximately
  40 words per minute (wpm) when listening and reading print or braille.

The student is willing to use these devices (the examiner may wish to list these separately)
- ☑ to complete assignments in the regular classroom.
- ☑ at home to complete school assignments.
- ☑ while working with the teacher of students with visual impairments.

Comments: _____
_____
_____

2. Specialized Scanning Systems for   **Date completed** *9/3/2008*
Accessing Print Information Auditorily

When accessing printed materials scanned into the computer with a specialized scanning system (such as Kurzweil 1000 and 3000, OpenBook, and WYNN), the student is able to
- ☐ adjust the rate and other speech parameters.
- ☐ navigate through the document when provided instruction by the evaluator.

❑ select items from the menus or tools from the toolbar when provided instruction by the evaluator.

When listening to text read by the program, the student is able to
- ☑ repeat words and simple phrases without having them repeated more than twice.
- ☑ paraphrase the information (sentence or story).
- ☑ accurately answer simple comprehension questions.

The student is willing to use these devices (the examiner may wish to list these separately)
- ☑ to complete assignments in the regular classroom.
- ☑ at home to complete school assignments.
- ☑ while working with the teacher of students with visual impairments.

When accessing printed materials using audio-assisted reading the student is able to read _____ words per minute (wpm).

Comments: _____
_____
_____

D. Reading Rates   Date completed _9/3/2008_

Optional; may be used to support use of various adaptations.

When accessing print information, the student is able to read
_____words per minute (wpm) orally when reading materials in 12-point type using prescribed spectacles or contact lenses.
_____wpm orally when reading materials in the optimum point size and font: _____-point print and _____font.
_____wpm orally when reading with a prescribed optical device.
_____wpm orally when reading with a video magnifier (CCTV).
_28_ wpm orally when reading braille.
_40_ wpm when using audio-assisted reading.

Comments: _____
_____
_____

E. Accessing Information Presented at a Distance

Date completed _9/3/2008_

When accessing information presented at a distance on a chalkboard or whiteboard or by an overhead or computer projector or TV/VCR/DVD, the student reported that he or she
- ❑ sits close enough to view the information, at a working distance of approximately _____ feet.

(continued on next page)

☐ uses a handheld or spectacle-mounted telescope.
☐ uses a video magnifier with distance-viewing capabilities.
☑ gets an accessible copy from the teacher.
☐ uses a peer notetaker.
☐ uses an electronic whiteboard connected to an accessible computer.
☑ has information read aloud by a peer or paraeducator and
  ☑ brailles information on a braillewriter.
  ☐ writes information on paper.
  ☐ inputs information into computer or accessible personal digital assistant.
  ☐ records information on tape recorder or digital recorder.
☐ other (specify): _____.

Are these options working adequately?

☑ Yes
☐ No

Explain briefly: <u>These options are working adequately for Semena at present, but they do not</u> <u>provide Semena the opportunity to develop independence in accessing this type of</u> <u>information in the future.</u>

The student is willing to use these devices and accommodations (the examiner may wish to list them individually)

☑ to complete assignments in the regular classroom.

Comments: _____
_____
_____

Section II: Accessing Electronic Information

A. Computer Access: Output Devices

1. Visual Access   **Date completed** <u>9/10/2008</u>

The student is able to view electronic information on a desktop computer or in the computer lab without additional adaptations and identify or read

☐ text   ☐ icon titles   ☐ menus   ☐ dialog boxes   ☐ other system items on a
  ☐ 17-inch monitor at approximately ___ inches.
  ☐ 19-inch monitor at approximately ___ inches.
  ☐ 21-inch monitor at approximately ___ inches.
  ☐ other (specify): _____

The student prefers viewing text in a word-processing program on the computer in
___-point type in   ☐ regular   ☐ bold print

- ❑ Arial
- ❑ APHont
- ❑ Tahoma
- ❑ Verdana
- ❑ other (specify): _____

displayed on a ___ -inch monitor at approximately ___ inches.

The student is able to view electronic information on a
___ -inch computer monitor with the use of
- ❑ screen magnification hardware at approximately ____ inches.
- ❑ an articulated flexible monitor stand at approximately ___ inches.

The student is able to view electronic information using the computer operating system's screen enhancements such as
- ❑ screen resolution (specify): _____.
- ❑ Windows Display Appearance Scheme (specify): _____.
- ❑ Windows Display Appearance Settings. *(Record specific settings selected on the Windows Display Properties Appearance Checklist appendix to this form.)*
- ❑ Microsoft Magnifier
    - ❑ magnification level: ____
    - ❑ other setting (specify): _____

    The student is able to use the Microsoft Magnifier to
    - ❑ identify screen elements.
    - ❑ read text in menus, dialog boxes, and text documents.
    - ❑ navigate around the screen.
    - ❑ locate the file names listed in the Open file dialog box.
    - ❑ select a requested file to open.

(If the school district uses Macintosh computers, complete the previous sections for the accessibility features provided in the computer's operating system.)

When using a dedicated screen magnification program, the student is able to
- ❑ read 12-point print enlarged to ___× magnification at a working distance of approximately 13 inches.
- ❑ locate and select menu items, buttons, and other screen elements with the mouse or other pointing device.
- ❑ locate and select menu items, buttons, and other screen elements using keyboard commands.
- ❑ navigate around the screen and maintain orientation.
- ❑ use an automatic reading feature at a speed setting of _____.

The student's color preference is _____ text on a _____ background.

- ☑ The student is unable to access the computer visually.

(continued on next page)

The student is willing to use these devices (the examiner may wish to list these separately)
- ☐ to complete assignments in the regular classroom.
- ☐ at home to complete school assignments.
- ☐ while working with the teacher of students with visual impairments.

Comments: _____
_____
_____

2. Tactile Access   **Date completed** 9/10/2008

When accessing electronic or computer-based information tactilely, the student is able to
- ☐ read braille text displayed on a dedicated braille display connected to a computer.
- ☑ read braille text displayed on an accessible PDA braille display connected to a computer.
- ☑ execute navigation commands with instruction.
- ☑ enter text through the braille keyboard, if available.

The student is willing to use these devices (the examiner may wish to list these separately)
- ☑ to complete assignments in the regular classroom.
- ☑ at home to complete school assignments.
- ☑ while working with the teacher of students with visual impairments.

Comments: _see report for details_ _____
_____
_____

3. Auditory Access   **Date completed** 9/10/2008

When accessing electronic information auditorily, the student is able to understand synthesized speech produced by

software synthesizers:
- ☑ Intellitalk
- ☐ TrueVoice
- ☐ OpenBook
- ☐ Other (specify): _____
- ☑ Write:Outloud
- ☐ DECTalk Access 32
- ☐ Microsoft Speech Engine
- ☑ Kurzweil
- ☐ Eloquence (JAWS)

hardware synthesizers:
- ☐ Type 'n Speak, Braille 'n Speak, Braille Lite
- ☐ Double Talk LT
- ☐ DECTalk Express
- ☑ Other (specify): _Braille Note mPower_

When accessing electronic information auditorily through synthesized speech and a screen reader the student is able to understand and identify
- ☑ sentences and lines.
- ☑ words.
- ☑ distinctive sounding letters (such as *a, f, h, o, s, w*) when spelled in words.
- ☐ similar sounding letters (*b, c, d, e, p, t, z*) when spelled in words.

☑ distinctive sounding letters (such as *a, f, h, o, s, w*) when spelled in isolation.
☐ similar sounding letters *(b, c, d, e, p, t, z)* when spelled in isolation.

When accessing electronic information auditorily through synthesized speech and a screen reader the student is able to execute navigation commands with instruction to
☑ read by characters.
☐ read by words.
☐ read by sentence and lines.
☑ move forward (to the next character, word, line).
☑ move backward (to the prior character, word, line).

☐ When accessing electronic information auditorily, the student was **not** able to grasp the concept of navigation.

The student is willing to use these devices (the examiner may wish to list these separately)
☑ to complete assignments in the regular classroom.
☑ at home to complete school assignments.
☑ while working with the teacher of students with visual impairments.

Comments: _____
_____
_____

B. Computer Access: Input Devices

1. Keyboard Use   **Date completed** 9/10/2008

☑ The student is able to use a standard keyboard without adaptation.

The student
☑ demonstrates keyboard awareness (has a general knowledge of the key locations).
☐ is able to search for keys and type individual letters.
☐ is able to locate and identify alphanumeric keys.
☐ is able to locate and identify function keys.
☐ is able to activate two keys simultaneously.
☐ is able to touch type while looking at his or her hands
    ☐ from dictation.
    ☐ from braille copy.
    ☐ from copy that is presented in the student's preferred font and point size and positioned on a flexible-arm copy holder.
☐ is able to touch type without looking at his or her hands
    ☐ from dictation.
    ☐ from braille copy.
    ☐ from copy that is presented in the student's preferred font and point size and positioned on a flexible-arm copy holder.
☐ does not demonstrate excessive miss-hits or key repeats.

(continued on next page)

    ❑ uses good mechanics when typing (posture, wrist elevation, etc.).

    ❑ types with ___ fingers of right hand and ___ fingers of left hand.

    ❑ is able to type approximately ___ words per minute (wpm)

        ❑ from dictation.

        ❑ from braille copy.

        ❑ from copy that is presented in the student's preferred font and point size and positioned on a flexible-arm copy holder.

❑ The student is able to utilize a standard computer keyboard with the following adaptations: *(Seek assistance from an occupational or physical therapist as needed.)*

    ❑ zoom caps   ❑ keyguard   ❑ tactile locator dots

    ❑ other (specify): _____

❑ The student is able to utilize a standard computer keyboard with the following keyboard utilities: *(Seek assistance from a assistive technology specialist, occupational therapist, or physical therapist to complete this section.)*

    ❑ sticky keys   ❑ repeat keys   ❑ slow keys

    ❑ mouse keys   ❑ toggle keys

❑ The student is **not** able to utilize a standard keyboard with or without adaptations. *(If checked, refer student for a computer access evaluation.)*

Comments: _____

_____

_____

C. Personal Digital Assistants (PDAs)   **Date completed** *9/10/2008*

The student is able to

❑ read the text displayed on a standard PDA.

❑ read the text displayed on a portable word processor with scalable fonts.

    Specify font _____ and point size _____.

☑ understand speech produced by a talking PDA, including

    ☑ sentences or lines.

    ☑ words.

    ☑ distinctive sounding letters (such as *a, f, h, o, s, w*).

    ❑ similar sounding letters (*b, c, d, e, p, t, z*).

☑ read the braille produced by a PDA with a refreshable braille display.

☑ execute navigation commands with instruction.

❑ execute navigation commands without instruction.

☑ enter text through the ☑ braille or ❑ QWERTY keyboard.

The student prefers using a/an
- ☐ portable word processor with scalable fonts.
- ☐ accessible PDA with speech output only.
- ☑ accessible PDA with refreshable braille display and speech output.

The student was able to answer simple comprehension questions about information presented on a/an
- ☐ portable word processor with scalable fonts.
- ☑ accessible PDA with speech output only.
- ☑ accessible PDA with refreshable braille display and speech output.

The student was able to read approximately
- _____ words per minute (wpm) when using a portable word processor with scalable fonts.
- _____ wpm when using an accessible PDA with speech output only.
- _____ wpm when using an accessible PDA with refreshable braille display and speech output.

The student is willing to use these devices (the examiner may wish to list these separately)
- ☑ to complete assignments in the regular classroom.
- ☑ at home to complete school assignments.
- ☑ while working with the teacher of students with visual impairments.

Comments: _____
_____
_____

D. Electronic Calculators and Dictionaries   Date completed 9/10/2008

The student is able to

- ☐ use a calculator with an enlarged display containing ___-inch numerals.
- ☐ accurately locate and press the keys on the calculator keypad.
- ☐ perform basic operations
    - ☐ with prompting.
    - ☐ without prompting.
- ☑ use a talking calculator and
    - ☑ demonstrate understanding of the synthesized speech by repeating
        - ☑ single digits spoken by the calculator.
        - ☑ whole numbers spoken by the calculator.
    - ☑ accurately locate and press the keys on the calculator keypad.
    - ☑ perform basic functions
        - ☑ with prompting.
        - ☐ without prompting.

(continued on next page)

When using a talking dictionary, the student is able to
- ☑ understand and identify distinctive sounding letters (such as *a, f, h, o, s, w*).
- ☐ understand and identify similar sounding letters (*b, c, d, e, p, t, z*).
- ☑ understand and identify individual words.
- ☑ understand definitions spoken as continuous speech.
- ☐ accurately locate and press the keys on the dictionary's keyboard.
- ☑ perform basic functions
    - ☑ with prompting.
    - ☐ without prompting.

The student is willing to use these devices (the examiner may wish to list these separately)
- ☑ to complete assignments in the regular classroom.
- ☑ at home to complete school assignments.
- ☑ while working with the teacher of students with visual impairments.

Comments: _____
_____
_____

Section III: Communicating Through Writing

A. Nonelectronic Tools for Producing Written Communication

2. Writing Tools for Students Using Tactile Access   Date completed *9/10/2008*

When using a manual braille-writing device, the student is able to use
- ☑ a standard Perkins Brailler to emboss characters, words, and sentences at the rate of
    20 words per minute (wpm) from dictation.
    8 wpm from copy.
- ☐ a manual brailler with extension keys to emboss characters, words, and sentences at the rate of
    ___ wpm from dictation.
    ___ wpm from copy.
- ☐ a unimanual brailler to emboss characters, words, and sentences at the rate of
    ___ wpm from dictation.
    ___ wpm from copy.
- ☐ a slate and stylus to emboss characters, words, and sentences at the rate of
    ___ wpm from dictation.
    ___ wpm from copy.

- ☐ The student is able to sign his or her name legibly in cursive using
    - ☐ a signature guide.
    - ☐ the edge of a card, ruler, or some other similar device.

The student is willing to use these devices (the examiner may wish to list these separately)
- ☑ to complete assignments in the regular classroom.
- ☑ at home to complete school assignments.
- ☑ while working with the teacher of students with visual impairments.

Comments: _____
_____
_____

B. Electronic Tools for Producing Written Communication

Date completed <u>9/10/2008</u>

When using a computer with a scanner and imaging software, the student is able to
  ❑ scan a worksheet or form.
  ❑ use the software text tool to insert text into the worksheet.

When using an accessible computer running a word-processing program, the student is able to enter characters, words, and sentences at the rate of
  ___ words per minute (wpm) from dictation.
  ___ wpm from copy.

When using the Mountbatten Brailler or another electronic braillewriter, the student is able to emboss characters, words, and sentences at the rate of
  ___ wpm from dictation.
  ___ wpm from copy.

When using an accessible PDA with a QWERTY keyboard, the student is able to enter characters, words, and sentences at the rate of
  ___ wpm from dictation.
  ___ wpm from copy.

When using an accessible PDA with a braille keyboard, the student is able to enter characters, words, and sentences at the rate of
  <u>18</u> wpm from dictation.
  <u>6</u> wpm from copy.

Comments: _____
_____
_____

Additional Assessment Information:
_____
_____
_____

ASSISTIVE TECHNOLOGY RECOMMENDATIONS FORM

Student Name: _Semena Thomas_

Date(s) of Assessment: _9/3 & 9/10, 2008_

Based on the results of the assistive technology assessment, the following recommendations are made regarding assistive technology to support this student's educational objectives.

Section I: Accessing Print

Students with visual impairments will use a combination of tools and strategies to access printed information. Some will be appropriate for short reading passages and others will be necessary for longer assignments.

A. Accessing Print Visually

Check all that apply.

❑ Student should use regular print materials with the following optical devices:

    ❑ prescribed eyeglasses or contact lenses

    ❑ prescribed handheld magnifier

        type: _____   _____ power   ❑ illuminated

    ❑ prescribed stand magnifier

        type: _____   _____ power   ❑ illuminated

    ❑ prescribed handheld telescope

        type: _____   _____ power

    ❑ prescribed spectacle-mounted telescope

        type: _____   _____ power

    ❑ other optical devices recommended in clinical low vision evaluation

        specify: _____

❑ Student should use materials written with felt-tip pen on regular blue-lined notebook paper.

❑ Student should use materials written with felt-tip pen on bold-lined paper.

❑ Student should use materials written with felt-tip pen on unlined paper.

❑ Student should use regular print materials enlarged on a photocopying machine.

    Specify: _____times at _____% enlargement

❑ Student should use large-print books.

❑ Student should use regular print materials scanned into a computer, edited, and printed in ___ point print in the _____ font.

- ❏ When possible, student should be provided with overhead lighting
    - ❏ from an incandescent bulb.
    - ❏ from a fluorescent bulb.
    - ❏ from a halogen bulb.
    - ❏ adjusted with a dimmer switch.
- ❏ When possible, student should be provided with window lighting adjusted with
    - ❏ blinds.
    - ❏ shades.
    - ❏ Other (specify): _____
- ❏ When possible, student should be provided with additional lighting from
    - ❏ desk lamp with a/an
        - ❏ incandescent bulb.
        - ❏ fluorescent bulb.
        - ❏ halogen bulb.
        - ❏ LED bulb.
    - ❏ floor lamp with a/an
        - ❏ incandescent bulb.
        - ❏ fluorescent bulb.
        - ❏ halogen bulb.
        - ❏ LED bulb.
- ❏ Student should use a book stand or reading stand. Specify type:
    - ❏ braille book stand
    - ❏ desktop model
    - ❏ portable model
    - ❏ floor model
- ❏ Student should use regular print materials with a video magnifier (CCTV). Specify type:
    - ❏ desktop model
    - ❏ flex-arm camera model
    - ❏ head-mounted display model
    - ❏ portable model
    - ❏ electronic pocket model
    - ❏ digital imaging model

(continued on next page)

Assistive Technology Recommendations Form *(continued)*

Specify essential features: _____
_____
_____

❑ Student should use regular print materials with the following type of scanner and imaging software:

   ❑ standard imaging program

   ❑ specialized scanning program

Additional comments or recommendations: _____
_____
_____

B. Accessing Print Tactilely

Check all that apply.

☑ Student should use materials in braille.

☑ Student should use an electronic refreshable braille display to access print and electronic information.

☑ Student should be provided opportunities to use tactile graphics created by various production techniques and in a variety of media, including real objects, models, collage, tooling and stenciling, thermoform, capsule paper and fuser, computer-generated, and commercially produced.

☑ Student should use tactile graphics to access maps, charts, and diagrams.

Additional comments or recommendations: _see written report for details_
_____
_____
_____

C. Accessing Print Auditorily

Check all that apply.

☑ Student should use a live reader for accessing certain materials.
   Specify: _see report_

☑ Student should use recorded materials for accessing some print information.
   Specify: _____

❑ Student should use a computer-assisted reading system such as Kurzweil 1000 or OpenBook.

Additional comments or recommendations: _____
_____
_____
_____

D. Accessing Information Presented at a Distance

Check all that apply.

- ☑ Student should be provided an accessible copy of information presented on chalkboards or whiteboards, overhead projectors, computer projection systems, and so forth.
- ☐ Student should use a handheld telescope for accessing chalkboards or whiteboards, overhead projectors, computer projection systems, and so forth.
- ☐ Student should use a video magnifier with distance viewing capabilities for accessing chalkboards or whiteboards, overhead projectors, computer projection systems, and so forth.
- ☐ Student should use a digital video camera connect to an appropriate size monitor for accessing chalkboards or whiteboards, overhead projectors, computer projection systems, and so forth.
- ☐ Student should use an electronic whiteboard connected to an accessible computer.
- ☑ Student should be provided audio-described videos when available.
- ☐ Student should be provided a separate ____-inch monitor for viewing DVDs, movies, and other video presentations.

Additional comments or recommendations: _____
_____
_____
_____

Section II: Accessing Electronic Information

A. Computer Access—Output Devices

1. Visual Access

Check all that apply.

- ☐ Student should use a standard computer monitor
  Optimal size: _____
- ☐ Student should use a standard computer monitor with the following hardware adaptations:
  - ☐ adjustable monitor arm
  - ☐ hardware screen magnifier
- ☐ Student should use a standard computer monitor with the following Windows or Macintosh Display Appearance Settings (list on separate page if needed):_____
  _____
- ☐ Student should use the following Accessibility options in the computer's operating system:
  - ☐ Macintosh   ☐ Windows Accessibility.
- ☐ Student should use the following screen magnification program provided in the computer's operating system:
  - ☐ Macintosh Zoom   ☐ Microsoft Magnifier.
- ☐ Student should use a dedicated screen magnification program.
  Specify essential features: _____

(continued on next page)

2. Tactile Access
- ❏ Student should use a refreshable braille display.
  Specify essential features: _____

3. Auditory Access
Check all that apply.

- ❏ Student should use a talking word processor to develop basic computer skills.
- ❏ Student should use the following screen-reading program provided in the computer's operating system:
  - ❏ Macintosh VoiceOver   ❏ Microsoft Narrator.
- ☑ Student should use a dedicated screen-reading program.

  Specify essential features: _support for refreshable braille display_____

  Additional comments or recommendations: _____
  _____
  _____

B. Computer Access—Input Devices

1. Keyboard Use
Check all that apply.

- ☑ Student should use a standard keyboard.
- ❏ Student should use a standard keyboard with
  - ❏ large-print labels, white text on black background.
  - ❏ large-print labels, black text on white background.
  - ❏ braille labels.
- ☑ Student should use a standard keyboard with locator dots to develop or improve keyboarding skills.
- ☑ Student should receive individual keyboarding instruction.
- ❏ Student should use a talking word processor for keyboarding instruction.
- ☑ Student should use a talking typing program for keyboarding practice and reinforcement of skills taught by instructor.
- ❏ Student should use a standard keyboard with Windows Accessibility or Macintosh Universal Access options:
- ❏ StickyKeys
- ❏ FilterKeys
- ❏ ToggleKeys
- ❏ Other (specify). _____
- ❏ Student should use a standard keyboard with hardware adaptations.
  Specify:_____
- ❏ Student should use an alternative keyboard.
  Specify:_____

2. Pointing Devices and Other Tools

Check all that apply.

- ❑ Student should use a standard pointing device like a mouse or trackball.
- ❑ Student should use an alternative pointing device.
  Specify:_____
- ❑ Student should use a voice recognition system to control the computer.
- ❑ Student should have access to a copyholder that allows printed materials to be positioned at a comfortable viewing distance.

Additional comments or recommendations: _____
_____
_____

C. Accessing Other Electronic Information

1. Specialized Scanning Systems
- ☑ Student should have access to a specialized scanning system.
  Specify essential features: *see report* _____

2. Accessible Personal Digital Assistant (PDA)
- ☑ Student should have access to a personal digital assistant with the following features:
  - ❑ scalable font display
  - ❑ screen magnification capability
  - ☑ synthesized speech output
  - ☑ refreshable braille display
  Specify essential features: _____

3. Other Electronic Tools
- ☑ Student should use a   ☑ basic   or   ❑ scientific talking calculator.
- ❑ Student should use a computer-based calculator program with
  - ❑ screen magnification software.
  - ❑ screen-reading software.
- ❑ Student should use a dictionary or thesaurus program on a computer with
  - ❑ screen magnification software.
  - ❑ screen-reading software.
- ☑ Student should use a portable talking dictionary.

Additional comments or recommendations: _____
_____
_____

(continued on next page)

Section III: Communicating Through Writing

Students who are blind or visually impaired will use a combination of tools and strategies to produce written communication. Some will be appropriate for short writing assignments and others will be necessary for longer assignments.

Check all that apply.

- ❑ Student should use pen or pencil and paper
  - ❑ for short writing assignments.
  - ❑ for most writing assignments.
- ❑ Student should use felt-tip pen or other bold marker.
- ❑ Student should use ❑ bold-lined ❑ raised-lined notebook paper.
- ❑ Student should use ❑ bold-lined ❑ raised-lined graph paper for math.
- ❑ Student should use crayons and a screen board for beginning handwriting.
- ❑ Student should use a whiteboard with erasable markers.
- ❑ Student should use a computer with a math writing and editing program.
- ❑ Student should use a computer with a scanner and imaging software to complete forms.
- ☑ Student should use an accessible computer with word-processing software.
- ❑ Student should use manual braillewriter.
- ❑ Student should use manual braillewriter with extension keys.
- ❑ Student should use a unimanual (one-handed) braillewriter.
- ❑ Student should use unimanual (one-handed) braillewriter with extension keys.
- ❑ Student should use slate and stylus.
- ❑ Student should use an electronic braillewriter.
  Specify: _____
- ☑ Student should use an adaptive analog or digital recorder for notetaking.
- ☑ Student should use an accessible PDA for notetaking and other short writing tasks.
- ❑ Student should use an accessible laptop or notebook computer for notetaking.

Additional comments or recommendations: _____

_____

_____

Section IV: Additional Hardware and Software

Student should be provided with access to the following hardware and software:

- ❑ Macintosh computer system with
  ____MB memory   ____ GB hard drive   ❑ CD/DVD drive
- ☑ Windows-compatible computer system with
  _2_ MB memory   _80_ GB hard drive   ☑ CD/DVD drive
- ☑ word processor   ☑ printer
- ☑ Internet access   ☑ flatbed scanner

other: _____

_____

_____

Equipment needed to produce materials for student in appropriate format:
- ☑ Macintosh or Windows-compatible computer system with
  _2Gb_ MB memory   _80_ GB hard drive   ☑ CD/DVD drive
  ☑ Internet access   ☑ flatbed scanner   ☑ OCR software
  ☑ word-processing software   ☑ braille translating software
  ☑ inkjet or laser printer   ☑ braille embosser or printer
  ☑ tactile graphics production equipment:
  Specify: _see report_ _____

Additional comments or recommendations: _____

_____

_____

The recommendations made here do not all have to be implemented immediately. These suggestions are designed for a two- to three-year plan in which the student masters certain skills and is provided access to additional technologies that can facilitate his or her educational program. During that time, new technologies are likely to become available that will enhance the student's ability to maximize his or her educational potential. The specific devices recommended may no longer be the most appropriate, but the assistance that they provide will continue to be a need for this student.

Samantha Higgins _____   _Teacher of students with visual impairments_
Assessment Completed by (signature)   Position

Beatrice Collins _____   _Assistive Technology Specialist_ _____
Assessment Completed by (signature)   Position

_____   _____
Assessment Completed by (signature)   Position

_____   _____
Assessment Completed by (signature)   Position

ASSISTIVE TECHNOLOGY ASSESSMENT REPORT AND RECOMMENDATIONS

Student's Name: _Semena Thomas_

Date(s) of assessment: _9/3, & 9/10/2008_

Semena is a third-grade student functioning on grade level in all academic areas. She has no usable vision. Semena uses braille as her primary learning medium and auditory information as her secondary medium. Many of Semena's educational objectives involve accessing printed information, accessing electronic information provided by the school's computers, and producing written communication that is accessible to both her and her teachers. An assistive technology assessment was requested and conducted to determine the tools that might assist Semena in accomplishing these educational objectives. To meet these objectives she will need a toolbox full of technology and the appropriate training to assist her in these tasks.

Some of the features of the devices and software recommended will be used by Semena and her service providers immediately and in the near future, while others will need to be learned over the next few years. Semena will need to master the basic functions of the technology in the next several years and then will need to develop competence and efficiency with their more advanced features in order to take advantage of her educational program in middle and high school. The variety and complexities of the recommended technology are such that Semena cannot be expected to be learning how to use them at the same time that she needs them to accomplish educational tasks. It is essential, therefore, that she be provided access to these tools in the next few years so that she has time to develop the required skills to use them proficiently.

Accessing Print Information
Semena uses braille as her primary method for accessing print information. She will need to continue to be provided with textbooks and other educational materials in braille. Continued improvement in her reading efficiency in braille will be essential for Semena to take full advantage of both her educational program and future employment opportunities. In order for Semena to improve her braille reading skills she will need additional opportunities to read materials in braille.

Currently Semena is provided braille in several ways: some textbooks are available in braille from the state Instructional Materials Center (IMC); textbooks not available from the IMC may have to be produced by and purchased from outside vendors; some textbooks are produced by Semena's teacher of visually impaired students, Samantha Higgins; almost all the supplemental educational materials used in her classes are produced in braille by Ms. Higgins; and a small number of books and magazines are available in braille from the National Library Service for the Blind and Physically Handicapped. These resources are not adequate to provide Semena with a free and appropriate public education as required by law. Semena's classmates have full access to all of their textbooks and any associated supplemental materials, while she does not. Furthermore, through the school's library and media center, Semena's classmates have access to hundreds or even thousands of volumes, while she only has access to a very small number of books and magazines in braille.

Several technologies can be recommended to assist Semena in accessing print information that she will need to meet her educational objectives.

1. Semena will need to use an accessible personal digital assistant (PDA) with a refreshable braille display. This device will serve as a major tool for accessing print information, accessing some electronic information, and producing written communication. It will also meet several of Semena's other educational needs, as discussed later in this report.

   a. An accessible PDA with a refreshable braille display can provide Semena with access to some of her textbooks. Textbooks, magazines, and a wide variety of other books are becoming available in electronic formats that can be downloaded into an accessible PDA and read with a refreshable braille display. This is the first feature of this device that Semena will need to learn to use. The teacher of visually impaired students will develop goals and objectives for Semena to acquire the skills necessary to use the other features of the accessible PDA during the next few years.

   b. This device can save the school system money by
      • reducing the number of books that will need to be produced and purchased in braille from outside vendors;
      • decreasing the number of books and materials that the TVI will need to produce in hard-copy braille.

2. Semena also needs access to the graphical information found in print materials. This type of information needs to be provided in the form of tactile graphics. Some tactile graphics are available in braille textbooks, but a great deal of the graphical information she will need is not. Some of these materials can be purchased from outside vendors, but many will need to be created by the teacher of visually impaired students. In order to produce and provide these tactile graphics, Ms. Higgins will need the following tools and materials:

   a. Tactile Graphics kit from the American Printing House for the Blind (APH)

   b. one of the following electronic fuser systems:
      • Pictures in a Flash (PIAF)—from HumanWare
      • Swell-Form Graphics Machine—from American Thermoform
      • Tactile Image Enhancer (TIE)—from Repro-Tronics

3. Semena will also need technology tools that will allow her to access print information auditorily. During the next few years, Semena will need to learn to use the tools and techniques to take full advantage of information in an auditory format.

(continued on next page)

    a. Semena will need to begin to receive instruction in the use of live readers, recorded speech, and synthesized speech.

    b. To begin this process she and Ms. Higgins will need access to a modified tape recorder such as the Handi-Cassette II available from APH on quota funds.

    c. As her auditory skills improve, Semena will need access to a Digital Talking Book player and Digital Talking Books. These tools will not replace her need for braille materials, but will supplement them as additional tools for accessing print information.

4. Semena will need to be provided with an accessible copy of information presented on chalk- or whiteboards, overhead projectors, and computer projection systems in the classroom. The teacher of visually impaired students will need to have access ahead of time to the information that is presented in class whenever possible so that she can provide it in braille for Semena. Semena can use some of the auditory skills she will develop, based on recommendation #3a, to make use of a reader. She can have someone read information to her and use one of the writing tools recommended later in this report to record the information for future reference.

5. Semena's classroom teacher and the school media specialist will need to search for videos with audio description when selecting videos to use in her class.

6. During middle school, Semena will need to learn to use a specialized scanning system (see recommendation #5 under Accessing Electronic Information).

7. Semena will need individualized instruction in the use of these technologies. In order for Semena to receive this instruction, her teacher of visually impaired students will need professional development opportunities to learn about these technologies and ample time to practice with them before beginning instruction.

Accessing Electronic Information

Semena will need to learn to use the school's computers to access electronic information. This will require her to develop skills in several areas:

1. Semena will need to learn to use the accessible PDA recommended in item #1 under Accessing Print Information as a tool for gaining tactile access to the school's computers. This is a long-term goal that should be completed by 7th or 8th grade.

2. Semena will need to receive instruction in the use of screen-reading software for the computer during the next few years. This will be facilitated by her development of keyboarding skills, as detailed in the following recommendations.

3. To develop the keyboarding skills necessary to access electronic information on the computer Semena will need the following tools:

    a. Standard keyboard with locator dots

    b. Screen-reading software

c. Word-processing software

d. Talking typing tutor software for drill and practice

4. Semena's teacher of visually impaired students will need to provide the keyboarding instruction. She should begin by teaching Semena to use the screen-reading software and a word processor. The synthesized speech provided by the screen-reading software will give Semena immediate feedback about the keys she presses, which in turn will enhance her ability to learn the keyboard. Using the word processor will give Semena an opportunity to print out her work to share with family and friends. It will also provide Ms. Higgins with a tool to track Semena's progress. Semena can use the talking typing tutor to practice letters and groups of letters that she has already learned when Ms. Higgins is not available.

5. During middle school, Semena will need to learn to use a specialized scanning system so that by the time she reaches high school she will be prepared to independently access both print and electronic information that is not available in alternate formats. Serena will use a computer with synthetic speech or her accessible PDA with refreshable braille to access the information that has been scanned.

6. Semena will need to have access to an accessible PDA to access electronic information. (See item #1 under Accessing Print Information.)

7. Semena will need access to a talking calculator later in her educational program. This is one of the additional features of the accessible PDA recommended in item #1 under Accessing Print Information.

8. Semena will need access to a full-featured talking dictionary such as the Franklin Speaking Language Master Special Edition. This is a tool that she can use now to check the spelling of words. As her needs and skills develop, she can learn to use some of the more advanced features of the device so that she will be proficient with them in middle and high school.

9. Semena will need individualized instruction in the use of these technologies. In order to receive this instruction, Semena's teacher of visually impaired students will need to have professional development opportunities to learn about these technologies and ample time to practice with them before beginning instruction.

Tools for Writing

1. Semena will need to learn to use an accessible computer with word-processing software for longer writing assignments.

2. Semena should continue to use a manual braillewriter as a personal writing tool for short writing assignments.

3. Semena will need to learn to use the slate and stylus as a portable writing tool.

4. As Semena moves into middle school, she will need to learn to use the features of a digital recorder for recording class lectures and notetaking. This can be

(continued on next page)

accomplished with the accessible PDA recommended in item #1 under Accessing Print Information.

5. As Semena moves into middle school, she will need to learn to use the word-processing features of the accessible PDA recommended in item #1 under Accessing Print Information as her primary tool for notetaking. She will need to begin learning the recording and notetaking features of this device so that she will be able to take notes independently when needed in middle school, high school, and beyond.

Additional Hardware and Software

1. Semena will need access to a Windows-based computer system with an adequate memory and hardware configuration to run the software noted in the previous recommendations.

2. To produce materials in braille and other alternate formats Semena's teacher of visually impaired students will need access to a Windows-based computer system with the following hardware and software:

   a. Adequate memory and storage capacity for all the software noted here
   b. Word-processing software; high-speed Internet and e-mail access; optical character recognition (OCR) software such as Omni Page Pro or Abbey Fine Reader; braille translation software such as Duxbury, MegaDots, Braille 2000, etc.; flatbed scanner; braille embosser

It is imperative that everyone involved in Semena's education be aware that these recommendations are designed to meet her current and future needs. Some items will need to be implemented as soon as possible, while others will need to be met during the next few years. Many of the technology tools that Semena will need to be successful in her educational pursuits cannot be learned in a short period of time. Therefore it will be necessary for Semena to begin learning the skills necessary to take advantage of these tools in the next several years. The goal will be for her to become competent in their use by the time she needs to rely on these tools to accomplish her educational objectives.

Semena's assistive technology needs will need to be addressed at each of her annual IEP reviews throughout her educational program. A partial or complete reevaluation will be required before she makes the transitions to middle school, to high school, and to college or work or any time that her program requires her to complete tasks that cannot be completed practically with the tools she is currently using.

Assessment Forms

Background Information for Assistive Technology Assessment

Student's Name: _____   Birthdate: _____   Grade: _____

Name of parent(s)/guardian(s): _____

School: _____

Teacher of students with visual impairments: _____

Referred by: _____   Reason for Referral: _____

_____

Initial or Ongoing Assessment: I / O

Additional Disabilities: Y / N Describe: _____

Current medication(s):_____

Reported/observed visual side effects: _____

_____

Eye Report Summary (see Eye Report)

Dr.: _____ O.D.   Date of last examination: _____

Eye condition: _____

Prognosis: _____

Visual Acuity

| | Distance | | Near | |
	Without Correction	With Correction	Without Correction	With Correction
OD	_____	_____	_____	_____
OS	_____	_____	_____	_____
OU	_____	_____	_____	_____

Field Restriction(s): Y / N   Degrees: _____   Location:_____

Recommendations

Eyeglasses   ❑ Wear/Use Constantly   ❑ Wear/Use as Needed

Contact Lenses

   For distance?   Y / N   ❑ Wear/Use Constantly   ❑ Wear/Use as Needed

   For near?   Y / N   ❑ Wear/Use Constantly   ❑ Wear/Use as Needed

Low Vision Device(s) (specify): _____

Other: _____

Information from Learning Media Assessment

Primary learning channel: ❑ visual   ❑ tactile   ❑ auditory

Secondary learning channel: ❑ visual   ❑ tactile   ❑ auditory

Other: _____

Other current accommodations and technology _____
_____
_____

Reading Preferences (if reported):
Preferred visual format without device (specify): _____
    Point size: _____   Font: _____   Distance: _____
      Approximate reading rate: _____ wpm
Preferred visual format with device (specify): _____
    Point size: _____   Font: _____   Distance: _____
      Approximate reading rate: _____ wpm
Lighting preferences: _____
Braille: approximate reading rate: _____ wpm oral   _____ wpm silent
Experiences visual/physical fatigue after reading _____ minutes

Relevant information from functional low vision assessment: _____
_____
_____

Relevant information from medical, psychological, and academic evaluations: _____
_____
_____

Relevant information from teachers' observations and assessments: _____
_____
_____

Additional comments: _____
_____
_____

ASSISTIVE TECHNOLOGY CONSIDERATIONS CHECKLIST

Student: _____   School: _____

DIRECTIONS

1. Complete the student information section below to provide information on the student's needs, abilities, and difficulties as well as environments and barriers to success.
2. Please check (❑) the instructional or access areas in Column A that are appropriate for the student. Please leave blank any areas that are not relevant to the student. Specify all relevant tasks (for example, copying notes from board, responding to teacher questions, and so on) within each area in the space provided. Check the settings in which the task is required. GEC: General Education Classroom; SEC: Special Education Classroom; COM: Community; and HOM: Home.
3. In Column B, specify the standard classroom tools (low technology to high technology) used by the student to complete relevant tasks identified in Column A. Place a check (❑) in the boxes in Column B if the student is able to independently complete the tasks with standard classroom tools. For areas in which the student can complete the tasks independently, it will not be necessary to complete Columns C or D.
4. In Column C, specify the accommodations/modifications and assistive technology solutions that are currently being utilized. Place a check (❑) in the boxes in Column C if the student can adequately complete the tasks specified in Column A using the identified accommodations/modifications and assistive technology solutions.
5. Complete Column D if the student cannot adequately complete the task with accommodations/modifications and assistive technology solutions specified in Column C.

Student needs, abilities, and difficulties: _____

_____

_____

Student environments:

❑ General Education Classroom (List all classes): _____

_____

❑ Special Education Classroom (List all classes): _____

_____

❑ Community (List all settings): _____

_____

❑ Home: _____

_____

Barriers to student performance and achievement: _____

_____

Source: Reprinted with permission from the Georgia Project for Assistive Technology, Georgia Department of Education, Atlanta.

A. Instructional or Access Areas	B. Independent with Standard Classroom Tools	C. Completes Tasks with Accommodations/ Modifications and/or Assistive Technology Solutions Currently in Place		D. Additional Solutions/Services Needed, Including Assistive Technology
		Accommodations/ Modifications	Assistive Technology Solutions	
❑ Writing ❑ GEC ❑ SEC ❑ COM ❑ HOM				
❑ Spelling ❑ GEC ❑ SEC ❑ COM ❑ HOM				
❑ Reading ❑ GEC ❑ SEC ❑ COM ❑ HOM				
❑ Math ❑ GEC ❑ SEC ❑ COM ❑ HOM				
❑ Study/ Organizational Skills ❑ GEC ❑ SEC ❑ COM ❑ HOM				
❑ Listening ❑ GEC ❑ SEC ❑ COM ❑ HOM				
❑ Oral Communication ❑ GEC ❑ SEC ❑ COM ❑ HOM				
❑ Aids to Daily Living ❑ GEC ❑ SEC ❑ COM ❑ HOM				

A. Instructional or Access Areas	B. Independent with Standard Classroom Tools	C. Completes Tasks with Accommodations/ Modifications and/or Assistive Technology Solutions Currently in Place		D. Additional Solutions/Services Needed, Including Assistive Technology
		Accommodations/ Modifications	Assistive Technology Solutions	
☐ Recreation and Leisure ☐ GEC ☐ SEC ☐ COM ☐ HOM				
☐ Prevocational/ Vocational ☐ GEC ☐ SEC ☐ COM ☐ HOM				
☐ Seating, Positioning, and Mobility ☐ GEC ☐ SEC ☐ COM ☐ HOM				
☐ Other (specify): ☐ GEC ☐ SEC ☐ COM ☐ HOM				

Consideration Outcomes:

☐ Student independently accomplishes tasks in all instructional areas using standard classroom tools. No assistive technology is required.

☐ Student accomplishes tasks in all instructional areas with accommodations and modifications. No assistive technology is required.

☐ Student accomplishes tasks in all instructional areas with currently available assistive technology. Assistive technology is required.

☐ Student does not accomplish tasks in all instructional access areas. Additional solutions including assistive technology may be required.

Specify any assistive technology services required by this student.

_____

_____

Consideration Checklist Completed by: Position: Date:

_____   _____   _____

ASSISTIVE TECHNOLOGY ASSESSMENT CHECKLIST
FOR STUDENTS WITH VISUAL IMPAIRMENTS

Student's Name _____   Person Completing Checklist _____

Student's Grade _____   Position _____

Student's Date of Birth _____   Date(s) of assessment _____

This document is a summary of information collected during the above-named student's assistive technology evaluation. Information for this assessment was obtained from the student's learning media assessment, the clinical low vision evaluation, the functional low vision evaluation, and from observation and assessment of the student's use of specific devices, as outlined below.
The assessment covers three main areas:

- **Section I: Accessing Print**, which covers how the student uses visual, tactile, and/or auditory tools to access textbooks, workbooks, assigned novels, and other printed information generally used in the classroom, including information presented on chalkboards or whiteboards
- **Section II: Accessing Electronic Information**, which covers how the student uses visual, tactile, and/or auditory tools to obtain information from electronic means, such as computers, electronic dictionaries and similar devices, digital books, and electronic braille devices
- **Section III: Communication through Writing**, which includes manuscript (print) and cursive writing, braille writing, and the use of electronic writing tools

The assessment sections of this document are followed by a recommendations section. The notations made will become part of the final written report detailing the rationale for each recommendation submitted to the student's Individualized Education Program team.

Directions: Indicate in the space provided the date each section is completed. All items not assessed should be marked NA.

Source: Adapted with permission from the "Assistive Technology Vision Aids Assessment," from the Georgia Project for Assistive Technology, Georgia Department of Education, Atlanta.

Section I: Accessing Print

A. Visual Access

1. Regular Print   Date completed _____

When accessing print information visually, the student is able to read passages on his or her independent reading level in regular print (12 point)

❑ without prescribed eyeglasses or contact lenses at a distance of

_____ inches, at approximately _____ words per minute (wpm).

❑ with prescribed eyeglasses or contact lenses at a distance of

_____ inches, at approximately _____ wpm.

❑ When reading this size print with or without prescribed eyeglasses or contact lenses the student experiences visual or physical fatigue after ____ minutes (as reported by student or teacher).

Comments: _____
_____
_____

From this point forward all items should be attempted with student's prescribed spectacles or contact lens in use.

2. Enlarged Print Produced on a Photocopier   Date completed _____

When accessing print information visually the student is able to read

❑ materials enlarged to ___% on

❑ 8 ½ × 11 inch paper   ❑ 8 ½ × 14 inch paper   ❑ 11 × 17 inch paper

at approximately _____ inches and at approximately _____ words per minute (wpm).

When reading this size print with or without prescribed eyeglasses or contact lenses the student experiences visual or physical fatigue after _____ minutes (as reported by student or teacher).

The student is willing to use materials enlarged by a photocopying machine on

❑ 8 ½ × 11 inch paper   ❑ 8 ½ × 14 inch paper   ❑ 11 × 17 inch paper

❑ to complete assignments in the regular classroom.

❑ at home to complete school assignments.

❑ while working with the teacher of students with visual impairments.

Comments: _____
_____
_____

3. Large Print   **Date completed** _____

The student is able to identify the following pictures of common objects:

_____ -inch high color photograph at a distance of approximately _____ inches.
❑ 3-inch high black-and-white line drawing at a distance of approximately ____ inches.
❑ 2-inch high black-and-white line drawing at a distance of approximately ____ inches.
❑ 1-inch high black-and-white line drawing at a distance of approximately ____ inches.

When accessing large print with prescribed eyeglasses or contact lenses (if appropriate) the student is able to read
❑ 72-point print at a distance of approximately _____ inches.
❑ 60-point print at a distance of approximately _____ inches.
❑ 48-point print at a distance of approximately _____ inches.
❑ 36-point print at a distance of approximately _____ inches.
❑ 30-point print at a distance of approximately _____ inches.
❑ 24-point print at a distance of approximately _____ inches.
❑ 18-point print at a distance of approximately _____ inches.
❑ 14-point print at a distance of approximately _____ inches.
❑ 12-point print at a distance of approximately _____ inches.

The student's preferred font is ❑ Arial ❑ APHont ❑ Tahoma ❑ Verdana
   ❑ Other (specify): _____

The student's preferred point size with prescribed eyeglasses or contact lenses is
   ❑ 14 ❑ 18 ❑ 24 ❑ 30 ❑ 36 ❑ 48 ❑ 60 ❑ 72

The student prefers text in
   ❑ regular style.
   ❑ bold style.

The student is able to read continuous text in preferred font and point size at approximately _____ words per minute.

When reading this size print with or without prescribed eyeglasses or contact lenses the student experiences visual or physical fatigue after ____ minutes (as reported by student or teacher).

The student is willing to use materials printed in the preferred font and point size on 8 ½ × 11 inch paper
   ____to complete assignments in the regular classroom.
   ____at home to complete school assignments.
   ____while working with the teacher of students with visual impairments.

Comments: _____
_____
_____

4. Nonoptical Devices   Date completed _____

When reading print information, the student prefers
- ❑ text written with a pen or pencil on standard lined notebook paper.
- ❑ text written with felt-tip pen on standard lined notebook paper.
- ❑ text written with felt-tip pen on bold-lined notebook paper.
- ❑ text written with felt-tip pen on unlined paper.
- ❑ other (specify): _____.

When reading handwritten information the student prefers
- ❑ manuscript (printed) writing.
- ❑ cursive writing.

When reading, the student
- ❑ prefers overhead lighting
    - ❑ from an incandescent bulb.
    - ❑ from a fluorescent bulb.
    - ❑ from a halogen bulb.
    - ❑ adjusted with a dimmer switch.
- ❑ prefers window lighting adjusted with
    - ❑ blinds.
    - ❑ shades.
    - ❑ other (specify): _____.
- ❑ experiences glare problems on
    - ❑ paper.
    - ❑ desktop.
    - ❑ computer or video magnifier monitor.
    - ❑ whiteboard.
    - ❑ chalkboard.
    - resulting from
        - ❑ overhead lighting.
        - ❑ window lighting (natural light, sunlight).
- ❑ prefers less lighting than currently available.
- ❑ prefers additional lighting from a
    - ❑ desk lamp with a/an
        - ❑ incandescent bulb.
        - ❑ fluorescent bulb.
        - ❑ halogen bulb.
        - ❑ LED bulb.

- ❑ floor lamp with a/an
    - ❑ incandescent bulb.
    - ❑ fluorescent bulb.
    - ❑ halogen bulb.
    - ❑ LED bulb.
- ❑ prefers the location of the lighting source to be
    - ❑ over the left shoulder.
    - ❑ over the right shoulder.
- ❑ prefers to have materials placed on a
    - ❑ desktop reading stand.
    - ❑ portable reading stand.
    - ❑ floor-standing reading stand.

The student is willing to use these devices and accommodations (the examiner may wish to list them individually)
- ❑ to complete assignments in the regular classroom.
- ❑ at home to complete school assignments.
- ❑ while working with the teacher of students with visual impairments.

Comments: _____

_____

_____

5. Optical Devices   Date completed _____

When accessing print materials with the use of a prescribed optical device, the student uses

❑ eyeglasses.

❑ contact lenses.

❑ handheld magnifier.

  type _____

  power _____

  ❑ illuminated   ❑ nonilluminated

❑ stand magnifier.

  type _____

  power _____

  ❑ illuminated   ❑ nonilluminated

❑ telescope.

  type _____

  power _____

- ❑ video magnifier (specify type):
  - ❑ desktop video magnifier.
  - ❑ flex-arm camera model.
  - ❑ portable model with handheld camera.
  - ❑ head-mounted display model.
  - ❑ electronic pocket magnifier.
  - ❑ digital imaging system.
  - ❑ other (specify): _____.

The student is able to read continuous text using the prescribed optical device at approximately

_____ words per minute without a reading stand.

_____ words per minute with a reading stand.

When reading regular-size print with the prescribed optical device the student experiences visual or physical fatigue after _____ minutes (as reported by student or teacher).

The student is willing to use these devices (the examiner may wish to list these separately)

- ❑ to complete assignments in the regular classroom.
- ❑ at home to complete school assignments.
- ❑ while working with the teacher of students with visual impairments.

Comments: _____

_____

_____

6. Video Magnifier (CCTV)   Date completed _____

Desktop Video Magnifier

When accessing print materials with the use of a desktop video magnifier (closed-circuit television or CCTV), the student is able to view a (insert a number to indicate the size)

___-inch-high graphic and ___-inch-high text on a ___-inch-monitor
at a working distance of approximately 10–13 inches.

___-inch-high graphic and ___-inch-high text on a ___-inch-monitor
at a working distance of approximately ___ inches.

The student's polarity preference when viewing text on a video magnifier is
- ❑ dark on light.
- ❑ light on dark.

The student's color preference is
_____ text on a _____ background.

The student is able to manipulate the controls of the video magnifier, with instructions from the examiner, to

- ❑ adjust the size of the image.
- ❑ focus the image if the unit does not have auto focus.

When using the video magnifier, the student is able to

- ❑ write a short sentence legibly on regular notebook paper while
  - ❑ looking at the screen or monitor.
  - ❑ looking at the paper.
- ❑ write a short sentence legibly on bold-lined paper while
  - ❑ looking at the screen or monitor.
  - ❑ looking at the paper.

When using the video magnifier, the student is able to read a 3- to 5-day-old sample sentence of his or her handwriting on

- ❑ blue-lined notebook paper.
- ❑ bold-lined writing paper.

The student is able to

- ❑ independently use an X-Y table for viewing materials with friction brake and margin stops are adjusted by examiner.

Comments: _____

_____

- ❑ independently adjust friction brake and margin stops after demonstration by examiner.

Comments: _____

_____

- ❑ independently manipulate the controls of the unit (knobs, buttons, switches, etc.).

Comments: _____

_____

The student is able to read approximately _____ words per minute (wpm) when the friction brake and margin stops are adjusted properly by the examiner.

When reading this size print with or without prescribed eyeglasses or contact lenses the student experiences visual or physical fatigue after _____ minutes (as reported by student or teacher).

The student is willing to use these devices (the examiner may wish to list these separately)

- ❑ to complete assignments in the regular classroom.
- ❑ at home to complete school assignments.
- ❑ while working with the teacher of students with visual impairments.

Comments: _____

_____

_____

Flex-Arm Camera Video Magnifier

When accessing print materials with the use of a flex-arm camera model video magnifier, the student is able to

- ❑ locate and operate the controls.
- ❑ use the device's X-Y table or manipulate the reading material without a table.
- ❑ rotate and adjust the camera for distance viewing.
- ❑ locate the distance target.
- ❑ identify the distance target.

The student is able to read approximately ___ wpm when the friction brake and margin stops are adjusted properly by the examiner.

When reading this size print with or without prescribed eyeglasses or contact lenses the student experiences visual or physical fatigue after ___ minutes (as reported by student or teacher).

The student is willing to use these devices (the examiner may wish to list these separately)

- ❑ to complete assignments in the regular classroom.
- ❑ at home to complete school assignments.
- ❑ while working with the teacher of students with visual impairments.

Comments: _____

_____

_____

Portable Video Magnifier with Handheld Camera

When accessing print materials through the use of a portable video magnifier with a handheld camera, the student is able to

- ❑ locate and operate the controls.
- ❑ maintain an angle of the camera with the text that is adequate for reading while moving the camera.

The student is able to read approximately ___ wpm when using this device.

When reading this size print with or without prescribed eyeglasses or contact lenses the student experiences visual or physical fatigue after ___ minutes (as reported by student or teacher).

The student is willing to use these devices (the examiner may wish to list these separately)

- ❑ to complete assignments in the regular classroom.
- ❑ at home to complete school assignments.
- ❑ while working with the teacher of students with visual impairments.

Comments: _____

_____

_____

Head-Mounted Video Magnifier

When accessing print materials through the use of a video magnifier with a head-mounted display, the student is able to

- ❑ locate and operate the controls.

❑ locate the distance target.
❑ identify the distance target.

Comments: _____
_____
_____

The student is willing to use these devices (the examiner may wish to list these separately)

❑ to complete assignments in the regular classroom.
❑ at home to complete school assignments.
❑ while working with the teacher of students with visual impairments.

Electronic Pocket Video Magnifier

When accessing print materials through the use of an electronic pocket video magnifier, the student is able to

❑ locate and operate the controls.
❑ maintain the camera at an adequate angle to the text for reading while moving the device.
❑ operate a model with the camera on the side of the unit.
❑ operate a model with the camera in the middle of the unit.

The student is able to read approximately _____ wpm when using this type of device.

When reading this size print with or without prescribed eyeglasses or contact lenses the student experiences visual or physical fatigue after _____ minutes (as reported by student or teacher).

The student is willing to use these devices (the examiner may wish to list these separately)
❑ to complete assignments in the regular classroom.
❑ at home to complete school assignments.
❑ while working with the teacher of students with visual impairments.

Comments: _____
_____
_____

Digital Imaging System

When accessing print materials through the use of a digital imaging system video magnifier, the student is able to

❑ locate and operate the controls.

The student is able to read approximately _____ wpm when using this type of device.

When reading this size print with or without prescribed eyeglasses or contact lenses the student experiences visual or physical fatigue after _____ minutes (as reported by student or teacher).

The student is willing to use these devices (the examiner may wish to list these separately)
❑ to complete assignments in the regular classroom.
❑ at home to complete school assignments.
❑ while working with the teacher of students with visual impairments.

Comments: _____
_____
_____

7. Scanning Systems for Accessing Print Information Visually   Date completed _____

When viewing print materials scanned into the computer using a standard imaging program (Microsoft Imaging, PaperPort, etc.), the student is able to

- ❑ operate the scanner.
- ❑ navigate the enlarged screen with the
  - ❑ keyboard.
  - ❑ mouse.

When viewing print materials scanned into the computer with a specialized scanning system (such as Kurzweil 1000 or 3000, OpenBook, or WYNN), the student is able to

- ❑ operate the scanner.
- ❑ adjust the magnification to the desired size using the
  - ❑ keyboard.
  - ❑ mouse.
- ❑ adjust the rate and other speech parameters.
- ❑ navigate the image horizontally and vertically using the
  - ❑ keyboard.
  - ❑ mouse.
- ❑ select items from the menus and tools from the toolbar with the
  - ❑ keyboard.
  - ❑ mouse.

The student is willing to use these devices (the examiner may wish to list these separately)

- ❑ to complete assignments in the regular classroom.
- ❑ at home to complete school assignments.
- ❑ while working with the teacher of students with visual impairments.

Comments: _____

_____

_____

8. Visual and Physical Fatigue   Date completed _____

The student experiences visual/physical fatigue after reading

- ❑ for ___ minutes **without** adaptations.
- ❑ for ___ minutes **with** adaptations.

Comments:
(*Please indicate fatigue factors for each visual access tool used by the student.*)

_____

_____

_____

B. Tactile Access and Braille   Date completed _____

When accessing graphical information the student is able to discriminate tactilely
- ❏ solid lines of various thickness.
- ❏ dashed lines.
- ❏ dotted lines.
- ❏ raised-line drawings of simple shapes.
- ❏ the boundary between two clearly defined textured fill patterns.
- ❏ the boundary between three clearly defined textured fill patterns.
- ❏ the boundary between four clearly defined textured fill patterns.

The student is able to identify tactile information most accurately when it is presented as a simple tactile graphic
- ❏ tooled onto braille paper.
- ❏ produced as a collage of varying textures.
- ❏ thermoformed onto plastic.
- ❏ embossed as dots and lines onto braille paper by a computer-controlled braille embosser.
- ❏ produced as raised lines and patterns on capsule paper.

The student is able to read materials in
- ❏ uncontracted braille.
- ❏ contracted braille.

❏ Results of formal or informal braille assessments conducted by the teacher of students with visual impairments are attached.
Student's oral braille reading rate is _____ words per minute (wpm).
Student's silent braille reading rate is _____ wpm.

When accessing print information with a refreshable braille display, the student is able to
- ❏ read instructional-level text.
- ❏ press correct key combination to issue forward and reverse navigation commands
  - ❏ with verbal prompt.
  - ❏ without verbal prompt.
- ❏ read ____ wpm orally and ____ wpm silently.

The student is willing to use these devices (the examiner may wish to list these separately)
- ❏ to complete assignments in the regular classroom.
- ❏ at home to complete school assignments.
- ❏ while working with the teacher of students with visual impairments.

Comments: _____
_____
_____

C. Auditory Access

1. Live Readers and Recorded Information   Date completed _____

When listening to instructional level information read aloud by the evaluator, the student is able to
- ❏ repeat words and simple phrases without having them repeated more than twice.
- ❏ paraphrase the information (a sentence or story).
- ❏ answer simple comprehension questions.

When listening to an analog or digital recording of a story, the student is able to
- ❏ repeat words and simple phrases without having them repeated more than twice.
- ❏ paraphrase the information (a sentence or story).
- ❏ accurately answer simple comprehension questions.

When using an analog or digital player-recorder, the student is able to
- ❏ insert and remove a tape or CD from the player-recorder.
- ❏ inactivate play, pause, stop, fast forward, and rewind functions (underline those demonstrated).
- ❏ understand and comprehend compressed or "fast" speech.
- ❏ manipulate variable speed and pitch controls.
- ❏ identify index tones, bookmarks, and page locators.

The student is able to
- ❏ listen to recorded speech and follow along with a print copy of the text.
- ❏ listen to recorded speech and follow along with a braille copy of the text.
- ❏ listen to synthesized speech and follow along with a print copy of the text.
- ❏ listen to synthesized speech and follow along with a braille copy of the text.

The student is able to read approximately
_____words per minute (wpm) when listening and reading print or braille.

The student is willing to use these devices (the examiner may wish to list these separately)
- ❏ to complete assignments in the regular classroom.
- ❏ at home to complete school assignments.
- ❏ while working with the teacher of students with visual impairments.

Comments: _____
_____
_____

2. Specialized Scanning Systems for   Date completed _____
Accessing Print Information Auditorily

When accessing print materials scanned into the computer with a specialized scanning system (such as Kurzweil 1000 and 3000, OpenBook, and WYNN), the student is able to
- ❏ adjust the rate and other speech parameters.
- ❏ navigate through the document when provided instruction by the evaluator.

- ❑ select items from the menus or tools from the toolbar when provided instruction by the evaluator.

When listening to text read by the program, the student is able to
- ❑ repeat words and simple phrases without having them repeated more than twice.
- ❑ paraphrase the information (sentence or story).
- ❑ accurately answer simple comprehension questions.

The student is willing to use these devices (the examiner may wish to list these separately)
- ❑ to complete assignments in the regular classroom.
- ❑ at home to complete school assignments.
- ❑ while working with the teacher of students with visual impairments.

When accessing printed materials using audio-assisted reading the student is able to read _____ words per minute (wpm).

Comments: _____
_____
_____

D. Reading Rates   Date completed _____

Optional; may be used to support use of various adaptations.

When accessing print information, the student is able to read
  _____ words per minute (wpm) orally when reading materials in 12-point type using prescribed spectacles or contact lenses.
  _____ wpm orally when reading materials in the optimum point size and font:
  ___-point print and _____ font.
  _____ wpm orally when reading with a prescribed optical device.
  _____ wpm orally when reading with a video magnifier (CCTV).
  _____ wpm orally when reading braille.
  _____ wpm when using audio-assisted reading.

Comments: _____
_____
_____

E. Accessing Information Presented at a Distance   Date completed _____

When accessing information presented at a distance on a chalkboard or whiteboard or by an overhead or computer projector or TV/VCR/DVD, the student reported that he or she
- ❑ sits close enough to view the information, at a working distance of approximately _____ feet.

- ❑ uses a handheld or spectacle-mounted telescope.
- ❑ uses a video magnifier with distance-viewing capabilities.
- ❑ gets an accessible copy from the teacher.
- ❑ uses a peer notetaker.
- ❑ uses an electronic whiteboard connected to an accessible computer.
- ❑ has information read aloud by a peer or paraeducator and
  - ❑ brailles information on a braillewriter.
  - ❑ writes information on paper.
  - ❑ inputs information into computer or accessible personal digital assistant.
  - ❑ records information on tape recorder or digital recorder.
- ❑ other (specify): _____.

Are these options working adequately?

- ❑ Yes
- ❑ No

Explain briefly:

_____

_____

_____

_____

The student is willing to use these devices and accommodations (the examiner may wish to list them individually)

- ❑ to complete assignments in the regular classroom.

Comments: _____

_____

_____

Section II: Accessing Electronic Information

A. Computer Access: Output Devices

1. Visual Access   Date completed _____

The student is able to view electronic information on a desktop computer or in the computer lab without additional adaptations and identify or read

❑ text ❑ icon titles ❑ menus ❑ dialog boxes ❑ other system items on a

- ❑ 17-inch monitor at approximately ___ inches.
- ❑ 19-inch monitor at approximately ___ inches.
- ❑ 21-inch monitor at approximately ___ inches.
- ❑ other (specify): _____

The student prefers viewing text in a word-processing program on the computer in ___-point type in ❑ regular ❑ bold print

❑ Arial
❑ APHont
❑ Tahoma
❑ Verdana
❑ other (specify): _____

displayed on a ___ -inch monitor at approximately ___ inches.

The student is able to view electronic information on a
___ -inch computer monitor with the use of
    ❑ screen magnification hardware at approximately ____ inches.
    ❑ an articulated flexible monitor stand at approximately ___ inches.

The student is able to view electronic information using the computer operating system's screen enhancements such as
    ❑ screen resolution (specify): _____
    ❑ Windows Display Appearance Scheme (specify): _____
    ❑ Windows Display Appearance Settings. *(Record specific settings selected on the Windows Display Appearance Checklist appendix to this form.)*

    ❑ Microsoft Magnifier
        ❑ magnification level: _____
        ❑ other setting (specify): _____
    The student is able to use the Microsoft Magnifier to
        ❑ identify screen elements.
        ❑ read text in menus, dialog boxes, and text documents.
        ❑ navigate around the screen.
        ❑ locate the file names listed in the Open file dialog box.
        ❑ select a requested file to open.

(If the school district uses Macintosh computers, complete the previous sections for the accessibility features provided in the computer's operating system.)

When using a dedicated screen magnification program, the student is able to
    ❑ read 12-point print enlarged to ___ magnification at a working distance of approximately 13 inches.
    ❑ locate and select menu items, buttons, and other screen elements with the mouse or other pointing device.
    ❑ locate and select menu items, buttons, and other screen elements using keyboard commands.
    ❑ navigate around the screen and maintain orientation.
    ❑ use an automatic reading feature at a speed setting of _____.

The student's color preference is _____ text on a _____ background.

❑ The student is unable to access the computer visually.

The student is willing to use these devices (the examiner may wish to list these separately)
- ❏ to complete assignments in the regular classroom.
- ❏ at home to complete school assignments.
- ❏ while working with the teacher of students with visual impairments.

Comments: _____
_____
_____

2. Tactile Access   Date completed _____

When accessing electronic or computer-based information tactilely, the student is able to
- ❏ read braille text displayed on a dedicated braille display connected to a computer.
- ❏ read braille text displayed on an accessible PDA braille display connected to a computer.
- ❏ execute navigation commands with instruction.
- ❏ enter text through the braille keyboard, if available.

The student is willing to use these devices (the examiner may wish to list these separately)
- ❏ to complete assignments in the regular classroom.
- ❏ at home to complete school assignments.
- ❏ while working with the teacher of students with visual impairments.

Comments: _____
_____
_____

3. Auditory Access   Date completed _____

When accessing electronic information auditorily, the student is able to understand synthesized speech produced by

software synthesizers:
- ❏ Intellitalk
- ❏ Write:Outloud
- ❏ Kurzweil
- ❏ TrueVoice
- ❏ DECTalk Access 32
- ❏ Eloquence (JAWS)
- ❏ OpenBook
- ❏ Microsoft Speech Engine
- ❏ Other (specify): _____

hardware synthesizers:
- ❏ Type 'n Speak, Braille 'n Speak, Braille Lite
- ❏ DECTalk Express
- ❏ Double Talk LT
- ❏ Other (specify): _____

When accessing electronic information auditorily through synthesized speech and a screen reader the student is able to understand and identify
- ❏ sentences and lines.
- ❏ words.
- ❏ distinctive sounding letters (such as *a, f, h, o, s, w*) when spelled in words.
- ❏ similar sounding letters (*b, c, d, e, p, t, z*) when spelled in words.

❑ distinctive sounding letters (such as *a, f, h, o, s, w*) when spelled in isolation.

❑ similar sounding letters *(b, c, d, e, p, t, z)* when spelled in isolation.

When accessing electronic information auditorily through synthesized speech and a screen reader the student is able to execute navigation commands with instruction to

❑ read by characters.

❑ read by words.

❑ read by sentence and lines.

❑ move forward (to the next character, word, line).

❑ move backward (to the prior character, word, line).

❑ When accessing electronic information auditorily, the student was **not** able to grasp the concept of navigation.

The student is willing to use these devices (the examiner may wish to list these separately)

❑ to complete assignments in the regular classroom.

❑ at home to complete school assignments.

❑ while working with the teacher of students with visual impairments.

Comments: _____

_____

_____

B. Computer Access: Input Devices

1. Keyboard Use   Date completed _____

❑ The student is able to use a standard keyboard without adaptation.

The student

❑ demonstrates keyboard awareness (has a general knowledge of the key locations).

❑ is able to search for keys and type individual letters.

❑ is able to locate and identify alphanumeric keys.

❑ is able to locate and identify function keys.

❑ is able to activate two keys simultaneously.

❑ is able to touch type while looking at his or her hands

  ❑ from dictation.

  ❑ from braille copy.

  ❑ from copy that is presented in the student's preferred font and point size and positioned on a flexible-arm copy holder.

❑ is able to touch type without looking at his or her hands

  ❑ from dictation.

  ❑ from braille copy.

  ❑ from copy that is presented in the student's preferred font and point size and positioned on a flexible-arm copy holder.

❑ does not demonstrate excessive miss-hits or key repeats.

- ❑ uses good mechanics when typing (posture, wrist elevation, etc.).
- ❑ types with ___ fingers of right hand and ___ fingers of left hand.
- ❑ is able to type approximately ___ words per minute (wpm)
  - ❑ from dictation.
  - ❑ from braille copy.
  - ❑ from copy that is presented in the student's preferred font and point size and positioned on a flexible-arm copy holder.

- ❑ The student is able to utilize a standard computer keyboard with the following adaptations: (*Seek assistance from an occupational or physical therapist as needed.*)
  - ❑ zoom caps   ❑ keyguard   ❑ tactile locator dots
  - ❑ other (specify): _____
- ❑ The student is able to utilize a standard computer keyboard with the following keyboard utilities: (*Seek assistance from an assistive technology specialist, occupational therapist, or physical therapist to complete this section.*)
  - ❑ sticky keys   ❑ repeat keys   ❑ slow keys
  - ❑ mouse keys   ❑ toggle keys

- ❑ The student is **not** able to utilize a standard keyboard with or without adaptations. (*If checked, refer student for a computer access evaluation.*)

Comments: _____

_____

_____

2. Pointing Device (Mouse)   **Date completed** _____

The student is able to visually locate the pointer on the screen when it is set to
- ❑ standard size
- ❑ standard large
- ❑ standard extra large

at approximately ___ inches on a ___-inch monitor.

The student is able to visually locate the pointer on the screen when it is set to
- ❑ black
- ❑ black large
- ❑ black extra large

at approximately ___ inches on a ___-inch monitor.

The student is able to visually locate the pointer on the screen set to
- ❑ inverted
- ❑ inverted large
- ❑ inverted extra large

at approximately ___ inches on a ___-inch monitor.
- ❑ other enlarged pointer (specify): _____

at approximately ___ inches on a ___-inch monitor.

The student is able to
- ❑ use the mouse to navigate the desktop and place the pointer on the desired screen element.
- ❑ maintain the mouse or pointer position while clicking or double-clicking.
- ❑ maintain eye contact with the mouse or pointer while navigating the desktop.

The student is able to select the following items with the mouse:
- ❑ pull-down menus
- ❑ toolbar buttons
- ❑ scroll bars
- ❑ tabs in multipage dialog boxes
- ❑ radio buttons
- ❑ edit fields
- ❑ edit combo box
- ❑ combo box
- ❑ edit spin box
- ❑ left-right slider
- ❑ checkbox
- ❑ other controls

❑ The student is able to perform most mouse functions using keyboard commands.

❑ The student is **not** able to physically use a standard mouse. (*If checked for a student with low vision using an enlarged pointer or screen magnification software, refer student for a computer access evaluation to determine a more accessible pointing device.*)

Comments: _____
_____
_____

C. Personal Digital Assistants (PDAs)   Date completed _____

The student is able to

❑ read the text displayed on a standard PDA.

❑ read the text displayed on a portable word processor with scalable fonts.
Specify font _____and point size _____.

❑ understand speech produced by a talking PDA, including
- ❑ sentences or lines.
- ❑ words.
- ❑ distinctive sounding letters (such as *a, f, h, o, s, w*).
- ❑ similar sounding letters (*b, c, d, e, p, t, z*).

❑ read the braille produced by a PDA with a refreshable braille display.

- ❑ execute navigation commands with instruction.

- ❑ execute navigation commands without instruction.

- ❑ enter text through the ❑ braille or ❑ QWERTY keyboard.

The student prefers using a/an
- ❑ portable word processor with scalable fonts.
- ❑ accessible PDA with speech output only.
- ❑ accessible PDA with refreshable braille display and speech output.

The student was able to answer simple comprehension questions about information presented on a/an
- ❑ portable word processor with scalable fonts.
- ❑ accessible PDA with speech output only.
- ❑ accessible PDA with refreshable braille display and speech output.

The student was able to read approximately
- ____ words per minute (wpm) when using a portable word processor with scalable fonts.
- ____ wpm when using an accessible PDA with speech output only.
- ____ wpm when using an accessible PDA with refreshable braille display and speech output.

The student is willing to use these devices (the examiner may wish to list these separately)
- ❑ to complete assignments in the regular classroom.
- ❑ at home to complete school assignments.
- ❑ while working with the teacher of students with visual impairments.

Comments: _____
_____
_____

D. Electronic Calculators and Dictionaries

Date completed _____

The student is able to

❑ use a calculator with an enlarged display containing ___-inch numerals.

❑ accurately locate and press the keys on the calculator keypad.

❑ perform basic operations
- ❑ with prompting.
- ❑ without prompting.

❑ use a talking calculator and
- ❑ demonstrate understanding of the synthesized speech by repeating
  - ❑ single digits spoken by the calculator.
  - ❑ whole numbers spoken by the calculator.
- ❑ accurately locate and press the keys on the calculator keypad.

- ❑ perform basic functions
    - ❑ with prompting.
    - ❑ without prompting. When using a talking dictionary, the student is able to
- ❑ understand and identify distinctive sounding letters (such as *a, f, h, o, s, w*).
- ❑ understand and identify similar sounding letters (*b, c, d, e, p, t, z*).
- ❑ understand and identify individual words.
- ❑ understand definitions spoken as continuous speech.
- ❑ accurately locate and press the keys on the dictionary's keyboard.
- ❑ perform basic functions
    - ❑ with prompting.
    - ❑ without prompting.

The student is willing to use these devices (the examiner may wish to list these separately)
- ❑ to complete assignments in the regular classroom.
- ❑ at home to complete school assignments.
- ❑ while working with the teacher of students with visual impairments.

Comments: _____

_____

_____

Section III: Communicating Through Writing

A. Nonelectronic Tools for Producing Written Communication

1. Writing Tools for Students Using Visual Access   Date completed _____

When using standard writing tools (pencil, pen, etc.), the student is able to

- ❑ write manuscript (print) legibly at the rate of
    - _____ words per minute (wpm) from dictation,
    - _____ wpm from copy, and
        - ❑ read his or her handwriting.
        - ❑ read a sample of his or her handwriting from 3 to 5 days earlier.

- ❑ write cursive legibly at the rate of
    - _____ wpm from dictation,
    - _____ wpm from copy, and
        - ❑ read his or her handwriting.
        - ❑ read a sample of his or her handwriting from 3 to 5 days earlier.

- ❑ space appropriately between letters and words.

- ❑ sign his or her name legibly in cursive using
    - ❑ a signature guide.
    - ❑ the edge of a card, ruler, or some other similar device.

❑ The student produces legible writing **laboriously** and **with great difficulty** when using standard writing tools.

Comments: _____
_____
_____

The student is able to produce legible **manuscript** (print) writing using

❑ bold-lined paper at the rate of
___wpm from dictation,
___wpm from copy, and:
   ❑ read his or her handwriting.
   ❑ read a sample of his or her handwriting from 3 to 5 days earlier.
❑ raised-lined paper at the rate of
___wpm from dictation,
___wpm from copy, and
   ❑ read his or her handwriting.
   ❑ read a sample of his or her handwriting from 3 to 5 days earlier.

❑ an erasable pen or   ❑ a thick, dark pencil such as a primary pencil at the rate of
___wpm from dictation,
___wpm from copy, and
   ❑ read his or her handwriting.
   ❑ read a sample of his or her handwriting from 3 to 5 days earlier.

❑ a felt-tip pen at the rate of
___wpm from dictation,
___wpm from copy, and
   ❑ read his or her handwriting.
   ❑ read a sample of his or her handwriting from 3 to 5 days earlier.

❑ a whiteboard and erasable marker at the rate of
___wpm from dictation,
___wpm from copy, and
   ❑ read his or her handwriting.
   ❑ read a sample of his or her handwriting from 3 to 5 days earlier.

❑ a video magnifier (specify writing tools and adaptations being used)
_____ at the rate of
___wpm from dictation,
___wpm from copy, and
   ❑ read his or her handwriting.
   ❑ read a sample of his or her handwriting from 3 to 5 days earlier.

___other (specify): _____

The student is able to produce legible **cursive** writing using

❏ bold-lined paper at the rate of
___wpm from dictation,
___wpm from copy, and
   ❏ read his or her handwriting.
   ❏ read a sample of his or her handwriting from 3 to 5 days earlier.

❏ raised-lined paper at the rate of
___wpm from dictation,
___wpm from copy, and:
   ❏ read his or her handwriting.
   ❏ read a sample of his or her handwriting from 3 to 5 days earlier.

❏ an erasable pen or   ❏ a thick, dark pencil such as a primary pencil at the rate of
___wpm from dictation,
___wpm from copy, and
   ❏ read his or her handwriting.
   ❏ read a sample of his or her handwriting from 3 to 5 days earlier.

❏ a felt-tip pen at the rate of
___wpm from dictation,
___wpm from copy, and
   ❏ read his or her handwriting.
   ❏ read a sample of his or her handwriting from 3 to 5 days earlier.

❏ a whiteboard and erasable marker at the rate of
___wpm from dictation,
___wpm from copy, and
   ❏ read his or her handwriting.
   ❏ read a sample of his or her handwriting from 3 to 5 days earlier.

❏ a video magnifier (specify writing tools and adaptations being used)
_____ at the rate of
___wpm from dictation,
___wpm from copy, and
   ❏ read his or her handwriting.
   ❏ read a sample of his or her handwriting from 3 to 5 days earlier.
❏ other (specify): _____

The student is willing to use these devices (the examiner may wish to list these separately)
   ❏ to complete assignments in the regular classroom.
   ❏ at home to complete school assignments.
   ❏ while working with the teacher of students with visual impairments.

Comments: _____
_____
_____

2. Writing Tools for Students Using Tactile Access   Date completed _____

When using a manual braille-writing device, the student is able to use

- ❑ a standard Perkins Brailler to emboss characters, words, and sentences at the rate of
  ___ words per minute (wpm) from dictation.
  ___ wpm from copy.

- ❑ a manual brailler with extension keys to emboss characters, words, and sentences at the rate of
  ___ wpm from dictation.
  ___ wpm from copy.

- ❑ a unimanual brailler to emboss characters, words, and sentences at the rate of
  ___ wpm from dictation.
  ___ wpm from copy.

- ❑ a slate and stylus to emboss characters, words, and sentences at the rate of
  ___ wpm from dictation.
  ___ wpm from copy.

- ❑ The student is able to sign his or her name legibly in cursive using
  - ❑ a signature guide.
  - ❑ the edge of a card, ruler, or some other similar device.

The student is willing to use these devices (the examiner may wish to list these separately)
- ❑ to complete assignments in the regular classroom.
- ❑ at home to complete school assignments.
- ❑ while working with the teacher of students with visual impairments.

Comments: _____
_____
_____

B. Electronic Tools for Producing Written Communication

Date completed _____

When using a computer with a scanner and imaging software, the student is able to
- ❑ scan a worksheet or form.
- ❑ use the software text tool to insert text into the worksheet.

When using an accessible computer running a word-processing program, the student is able to enter characters, words, and sentences at the rate of
___words per minute (wpm) from dictation.
___wpm from copy.

When using the Mountbatten Brailler or another electronic braillewriter, the student is able to emboss characters, words, and sentences at the rate of
___wpm from dictation.

___wpm from copy.

When using an accessible PDA with a QWERTY keyboard, the student is able to enter characters, words, and sentences at the rate of
  ___wpm from dictation.
  ___wpm from copy.

When using an accessible PDA with a braille keyboard, the student is able to enter characters, words, and sentences at the rate of
  ___wpm from dictation.
  ___wpm from copy.

Comments: _____
_____
_____

Additional Assessment Information:
_____
_____
_____

Appendix: Windows Display Properties Appearance Checklist

Items Adjusted
- ❏ 3D Objects
  - Color _____
- ❏ Active Title Bar
  - Size _____   Color _____
  - Font _____
    - ___Size _____Color ___Bold ___Italic
- ❏ Active Window Border
  - Size _____   Color _____
- ❏ Application Background
  - Color _____
- ❏ Caption Buttons
  - Size _____
- ❏ Desktop
  - Color _____
- ❏ Icons
  - Size _____
  - Font _____
    - ___Size ___Bold ___Italic
- ❏ Icon Spacing (Vertical)
  - Size _____
- ❏ Icon Spacing (Horizontal)
  - Size _____

❏ Inactive Title Bar

       Size _____   Color _____

       Font _____

           ____Size _____Color ____Bold ____Italic

❏ Inactive Window Border

       Size _____   Color _____

❏ Menu

       Size _____   Color _____

       Font _____

           ____Size _____Color ____Bold ____Italic

❏ Message Box

       Font _____

           ____Size _____Color ____Bold ____Italic

❏ Palette Title

       Size _____

       Font _____

      ____Size ____Bold ____Italic

❏ Scrollbar

       Size _____

❏ Selected Items

       Size _____   Color _____

       Font _____

           ____Size _____Color ____Bold ____Italic

❏ ToolTip

       Color _____

       Font _____

           ____Size _____Color ____Bold ____Italic

❏ Window

       Color _____

ASSISTIVE TECHNOLOGY RECOMMENDATIONS FORM

Student Name: _____

Date(s) of Assessment: _____

Based on the results of the assistive technology assessment, the following recommendations are made regarding assistive technology to support this student's educational objectives.

Section I: Accessing Print

Students with visual impairments will use a combination of tools and strategies to access printed information. Some will be appropriate for short reading passages and others will be necessary for longer assignments.

A. Accessing Print Visually

Check all that apply.

❑ Student should use regular print materials with the following optical devices:

  ❑ prescribed eyeglasses or contact lenses

  ❑ prescribed handheld magnifier

    type: _____   _____ power   ❑ illuminated

  ❑ prescribed stand magnifier

    type: _____   _____ power   ❑ illuminated

  ❑ prescribed handheld telescope

    type: _____   _____ power

  ❑ prescribed spectacle-mounted telescope

    type: _____   _____ power

  ❑ other optical devices recommended in clinical low vision evaluation

    specify: _____

❑ Student should use materials written with felt-tip pen on regular blue-lined notebook paper.

❑ Student should use materials written with felt-tip pen on bold-lined paper.

❑ Student should use materials written with felt-tip pen on unlined paper.

❑ Student should use regular print materials enlarged on a photocopying machine.

  Specify: _____times at _____% enlargement

❑ Student should use large-print books.

❑ Student should use regular print materials scanned into a computer, edited, and printed in ___ point print in the _____ font.

❑ When possible, student should be provided with overhead lighting

  ❑ from an incandescent bulb.

- ❑ from a fluorescent bulb.
- ❑ from a halogen bulb.
- ❑ adjusted with a dimmer switch.
- ❑ When possible, student should be provided with window lighting adjusted with
  - ❑ blinds.
  - ❑ shades.
  - ❑ other (specify): _____
- ❑ When possible, student should be provided with additional lighting from
  - ❑ desk lamp with a/an
    - ❑ incandescent bulb.
    - ❑ fluorescent bulb.
    - ❑ halogen bulb.
    - ❑ LED bulb.
  - ❑ floor lamp with a/an
    - ❑ incandescent bulb.
    - ❑ fluorescent bulb.
    - ❑ halogen bulb.
    - ❑ LED bulb.
- ❑ Student should use a book stand or reading stand (specify type):
  - ❑ braille book stand
  - ❑ desktop model
  - ❑ portable model
  - ❑ floor model
- ❑ Student should use regular print materials with a video magnifier (CCTV) (specify type):
  - ❑ desktop model
  - ❑ flex-arm camera model
  - ❑ head-mounted display model
  - ❑ portable model
  - ❑ electronic pocket model
  - ❑ digital imaging model

  Specify essential features: _____

  _____

  _____

  _____

❑ Student should use regular print materials with the following type of scanner and imaging software:

  ❑ standard imaging program
  ❑ specialized scanning program

Additional comments or recommendations: _____
_____
_____
_____

B. Accessing Print Tactilely

Check all that apply.

❑ Student should use materials in braille.

❑ Student should use an electronic refreshable braille display to access print and electronic information.

❑ Student should be provided opportunities to use tactile graphics created by various production techniques and in a variety of media, including real objects, models, collage, tooling and stenciling, thermoform, capsule paper and fuser, computer-generated, and commercially produced.

❑ Student should use tactile graphics to access maps, charts, and diagrams.

Additional comments or recommendations: _____
_____
_____
_____

C. Accessing Print Auditorily

Check all that apply.

❑ Student should use a live reader for accessing certain materials (specify):
_____

❑ Student should use recorded materials for accessing some print information (specify):
_____

❑ Student should use a computer-assisted reading system such as Kurzweil 1000 or OpenBook.

Additional comments or recommendations: _____
_____
_____
_____

D. Accessing Information Presented at a Distance

Check all that apply.

- ❑ Student should be provided an accessible copy of information presented on chalkboards or whiteboards, overhead projectors, computer projection systems, and so forth.
- ❑ Student should use a handheld telescope for accessing chalkboards or whiteboards overhead projectors, computer projection systems, and so forth.
- ❑ Student should use a video magnifier with distance viewing capabilities for accessing chalkboards or whiteboards, overhead projectors, computer projection systems, and so forth.
- ❑ Student should use a digital video camera connect to an appropriate size monitor for accessing chalkboards or whiteboards, overhead projectors, computer projection systems, and so forth.
- ❑ Student should use an electronic whiteboard connected to an accessible computer.
- ❑ Student should be provided audio-described videos when available.
- ❑ Student should be provided a separate _____-inch monitor for viewing DVDs, movies, and other video presentations.

Additional comments or recommendations: _____
_____
_____
_____

Section II: Accessing Electronic Information

A. Computer Access—Output Devices

1. Visual Access
Check all that apply.

- ❑ Student should use a standard computer monitor: Optimal size: _____
- ❑ Student should use a standard computer monitor with the following hardware adaptations:
  - ❑ adjustable monitor arm
  - ❑ hardware screen magnifier
- ❑ Student should use a standard computer monitor with the following Windows or Macintosh
- ❑ Display Appearance Settings (list on separate page if needed): _____
  _____
- ❑ Student should use the following Accessibility options in the computer's operating system:
  - ❑ Macintosh   ❑ Windows Accessibility
- ❑ Student should use the following screen magnification program provided in the computer's operating system:
  - ❑ Macintosh Zoom   ❑ Microsoft Magnifier
- ❑ Student should use a dedicated screen magnification program.
  Specify essential features: _____

2. Tactile Access

- ❏ Student should use a refreshable braille display.
  Specify essential features: _____

3. Auditory Access

Check all that apply.

- ❏ Student should use a talking word processor to develop basic computer skills.
- ❏ Student should use the following screen-reading program provided in the computer's operating system:
  - ❏ Macintosh VoiceOver   ❏ Microsoft Narrator
- ❏ Student should use a dedicated screen-reading program.

  Specify essential features: _____

  Additional comments or recommendations: _____
  _____
  _____

B. Computer Access—Input Devices

1. Keyboard Use

Check all that apply.

- ❏ Student should use a standard keyboard.
- ❏ Student should use a standard keyboard with
  - ❏ large-print labels, white text on black background.
  - ❏ large-print labels, black text on white background.
  - ❏ braille labels.
- ❏ Student should use a standard keyboard with locator dots to develop or improve keyboarding skills.
- ❏ Student should receive individual keyboarding instruction.
- ❏ Student should use a talking word processor for keyboarding instruction.
- ❏ Student should use a talking typing program for keyboarding practice and reinforcement of skills taught by instructor.
- ❏ Student should use a standard keyboard with Windows Accessibility or Macintosh Universal Access options:
- ❏ StickyKeys
- ❏ FilterKeys
- ❏ ToggleKeys
- ❏ Other (specify): _____
- ❏ Student should use a standard keyboard with hardware adaptations.
  Specify:_____
- ❏ Student should use an alternative keyboard.
  Specify:_____

2. Pointing Devices and Other Tools

Check all that apply.

- ❏ Student should use a standard pointing device like a mouse or trackball.
- ❏ Student should use an alternative pointing device.
  Specify:_____
- ❏ Student should use a voice recognition system to control the computer.
- ❏ Student should have access to a copyholder that allows printed materials to be positioned at a comfortable viewing distance.

  Additional comments or recommendations: _____
  _____
  _____

C. Accessing Other Electronic Information

1. Specialized Scanning Systems
- ❏ Student should have access to a specialized scanning system.
  Specify essential features: _____

2. Accessible Personal Digital Assistant (PDA)
- ❏ Student should have access to a personal digital assistant with the following features:
  - ❏ scalable font display
  - ❏ screen magnification capability
  - ❏ synthesized speech output
  - ❏ refreshable braille display

  Specify essential features: _____

3. Other Electronic Tools
- ❏ Student should use a ❏ basic or ❏ scientific talking calculator.
- ❏ Student should use a computer-based calculator program with
  - ❏ screen-magnification software.
  - ❏ screen-reading software.
- ❏ Student should use a dictionary or thesaurus program on a computer with
  - ❏ screen-magnification software.
  - ❏ screen-reading software.
- ❏ Student should use a portable talking dictionary.

  Additional comments or recommendations: _____
  _____
  _____

Section III: Communicating Through Writing

Students who are blind or visually impaired will use a combination of tools and strategies to produce written communication. Some will be appropriate for short writing assignments and others will be necessary for longer assignments.

Check all that apply.

- ❑ Student should use pen or pencil and paper
  - ❑ for short writing assignments.
  - ❑ for most writing assignments.
- ❑ Student should use felt-tip pen or other bold marker.
- ❑ Student should use ❑ bold-lined ❑ raised-lined notebook paper.
- ❑ Student should use ❑ bold-lined ❑ raised-lined graph paper for math.
- ❑ Student should use crayons and a screen board for beginning handwriting.
- ❑ Student should use a whiteboard with erasable markers.
- ❑ Student should use a computer with a math writing and editing program.
- ❑ Student should use a computer with a scanner and imaging software to complete forms.
- ❑ Student should use an accessible computer with word-processing software.
- ❑ Student should use manual braillewriter.
- ❑ Student should use manual braillewriter with extension keys.
- ❑ Student should use a unimanual (one-handed) braillewriter.
- ❑ Student should use unimanual (one-handed) braillewriter with extension keys.
- ❑ Student should use slate and stylus.
- ❑ Student should use an electronic braillewriter.
  Specify: _____
- ❑ Student should use an adaptive analog or digital recorder for notetaking.
- ❑ Student should use an accessible PDA for notetaking and other short writing tasks.
- ❑ Student should use an accessible laptop or notebook computer for notetaking.

Additional comments or recommendations: _____

_____

_____

Section IV: Additional Hardware and Software

Student should be provided with access to the following hardware and software:

- ❑ Macintosh computer system with
  ____MB memory   ____ GB hard drive   ❑ CD/DVD drive
- ❑ Windows-compatible computer system with
  ____MB memory   ____ GB hard drive   ❑ CD/DVD drive
- ❑ word processor   ❑ printer
- ❑ Internet access   ❑ flatbed scanner

  other: _____

_____

_____

Equipment needed to produce materials for student in appropriate format:

- ❑ Macintosh or Windows-compatible computer system with
  ___MB memory ___ GB hard drive ❑ CD/DVD drive
  - ❑ Internet access ❑ flatbed scanner ❑ OCR software
  - ❑ word-processing software ❑ braille translating software
  - ❑ inkjet or laser printer ❑ braille embosser or printer
  - ❑ tactile graphics production equipment:
    Specify:_____

Additional comments or recommendations: _____

_____

_____

The recommendations made here do not all have to be implemented immediately. These suggestions are designed for a two- to three-year plan in which the student masters certain skills and is provided access to additional technologies that can facilitate his or her educational program. During that time, new technologies are likely to become available that will enhance the student's ability to maximize his or her educational potential. The specific devices recommended may no longer be the most appropriate, but the assistance that they provide will continue to be a need for this student.

_____ _____
Assessment Completed by (signature) Position

_____ _____
Assessment Completed by (signature) Position

_____ _____
Assessment Completed by (signature) Position

_____ _____
Assessment Completed by (signature) Position

Index

About the Authors

Ike Presley, M.S., is National Project Manager at the American Foundation for the Blind (AFB) National Literacy Center in Atlanta, Georgia. He has worked in the field of blindness and visual impairment for over 30 years, starting as a teacher of visually impaired students and later as an assistive technology specialist for the Georgia Department of Education's Project for Assistive Technology, where he conducted assistive technology assessments of students with visual impairments throughout the state of Georgia and provided training to educators on the use of recommended technologies. He has also taught the use of assistive technology to visually impaired adults. In his work at AFB, Mr. Presley has developed and presented numerous professional development courses for service providers working with adults and youths who are blind or visually impaired. He has taught courses at Georgia State University on assistive technology for students who are blind or visually impaired and has given many national and international presentations on assistive technology and on literacy. He has also published articles and book chapters on assistive technology. Mr. Presley is a past chair of Division 5, Information and Technology, of the Association for Education and Rehabilitation of the Blind and Visually Impaired (AER).

Frances Mary D'Andrea, M.E., is a fellow of the National Center for Leadership in Visual Impairment, Salus University, Elkins Park, Pennsylvania, and a doctoral candidate at the University of Pittsburgh in special education with an emphasis in vision studies, where she also serves as instructor in the Vision Disabilities Program. Ms. D'Andrea started her career as a teacher of students with visual impairments and was formerly the director of the AFB National Literacy Center in Atlanta, Georgia. She is a coauthor of *Looking to Learn: Promoting Literacy for Students with Low Vision; The Braille Trail: An Activity Book* and *The Braille Trail Parent/Teacher Guide*; and *Instructional Strategies for Braille Literacy*, which won the 2000 C. Warren Bledsoe Award from AER as well as the 1998 Best New Professional/Scholarly Book in Nursing and Allied Health from the Association of American Publishers, Professional/Scholarly Publishing division. She was also consulting editor on *Braille Literacy: A Functional Approach*, by Diane Wormsley, and *Seeing Eye to Eye*, by Sandy Lewis and Carol Allman. Ms. D'Andrea was the editor of the *Dots for Braille Literacy* newsletter and has written articles and given numerous presentations on literacy for people who are blind or visually impaired. She serves as AFB's representative to the Braille Authority of North America (BANA); is a former chair of AER Division 16, Itinerant Teaching; is past president of the Georgia Chapter of AER; and is the recipient of the 2005 Holbrook-Humphries Literacy Award presented at the Getting in Touch with Literacy Conference.

CPSIA information can be obtained
at www.ICGtesting.com
Printed in the USA
FSOW02n1909200516
20687FS